To our Grandchildren
Alex, Ari, Christopher, Daniel, Kyle, Madelyn,
Maggie, Molly, Nicolas, Sarah, Todd, and Tracy

Cardiovascular
Physiology

The Mosby Physiology Monograph Series

Each book in this series presents normal physiology and selectively includes pathophysiology, with clinical examples highlighted in boxes/tables throughout. Chapters are summarized with key points; key words and concepts are listed; and each book contains a set of self-study questions. Two-color diagrams throughout the books illustrate basic concepts.

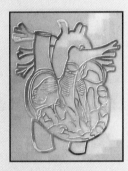

Berne and Levy:
Cardiovascular Physiology,
8th edition

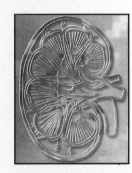

Koeppen and Stanton:
Renal Physiology,
3rd edition

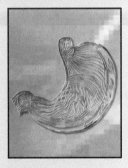

Johnson:
Gastrointestinal Physiology,
6th edition

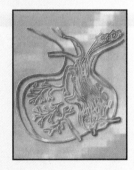

Porterfield:
Endocrine Physiology,
2nd edition

Coming Soon:
Blaustein: *Cellular Physiology*

A book designed to help medical students "bridge the divide between basic biochemistry, molecular and cell biology . . . and organ system physiology."

Cardiovascular Physiology

Eighth Edition

Robert M. Berne, MD, DSc (Hon)
Professor of Physiology, Emeritus
Department of Physiology
University of Virginia School of Medicine
Charlottesville, Virginia

Matthew N. Levy, MD
Senior Scientist
Rammelkamp Center
Professor Emeritus of Physiology and Biomedical Engineering
Case Western Reserve University
Cleveland, Ohio

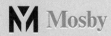 Mosby

A Harcourt Health Sciences Company

St. Louis   London   Philadelphia   Sydney   Toronto

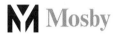

A Harcourt Health Sciences Company

Acquisitions Editor: William R. Schmitt
Project Manager: Carol Sullivan Weis
Production Editor: Rachel E. Dowell
Cover Art: Rokusek Design

EIGHTH EDITION
Copyright © 2001 by Mosby, Inc.

NOTICE
Medicine is an ever-changing field. Standard safety precautions must be followed, but as new research and clinical experience broaden our knowledge, changes in treatment and drug therapy may become necessary or appropriate. Readers are advised to check the most current product information provided by the manufacturer of each drug to be administered to verify the recommended dose, the method and duration of administration, and contraindications. It is the responsibility of the treating physician, relying on experience and knowledge of the patient, to determine dosages and the best treatment for each individual patient. Neither the publisher nor the editor assumes any liability for any injury and/or damage to persons or property arising from this publication.

Mosby, Inc.
A Harcourt Health Sciences Company
11830 Westline Industrial Drive
St. Louis, Missouri 63146

Printed in the United States of America

Library of Congress Cataloging-in-Publication Data

Berne, Robert M., 1918-
  Cardiovascular physiology / Robert M. Berne, Matthew N. Levy.—8th ed.
    p. ; cm.
  Includes bibliographical references and index.
  ISBN 0-323-01127-6 (alk. paper)
  1. Cardiovascular system—Physiology. I. Levy, Matthew N., 1922- II. Title.
  [DNLM: 1. Cardiovascular Physiology. WG 102 B525c 2000]
  QP101.B526 2000
  612.1—dc21   00-032430

01 02 03 04 05 CL/FF 9 8 7 6 5 4 3 2 1

Preface

This book is designed for medical students, graduate students, and cardiovascular fellows. Throughout the book we have incorporated the most recent information and have indicated which subjects are still controversial. Emphasis is placed on general concepts and control mechanisms with omission of extraneous isolated facts. To present a clear view of the various regulatory mechanisms, the component parts of the system are first discussed individually. Then, to show how the entire cardiovascular system operates in an intact subject, the last chapter describes how various individual components are coordinated. As examples we describe how the body responds to two important stresses—exercise and hemorrhage.

Normal physiology serves as a frame of reference that students of medicine must comprehend before they can understand the derangements caused by disease or toxic agents. Pathophysiology is considered very selectively in this text. Many examples of abnormal function are included to illustrate and clarify normal physiological processes. These clinical examples are scattered throughout the text and are emphasized by colored boxes.

The book has been updated and revised extensively. Some old figures have been deleted and some new figures have been added to facilitate comprehension of the textual material.

Carefully selected references appear at the end of each chapter. Review articles were preferred over scientific papers, and the scientific articles we included were chosen for their depth, clarity, timeliness, appropriateness, and bibliographies.

Throughout the book, *italics* are used to emphasize important facts and concepts, and **boldface type** is used for new terms and definitions. Each chapter includes a list of objectives at the beginning and a summary at the end to highlight key points. To help in review and to indicate clinical relevance of the material, case histories with multiple-choice questions are provided. Answers and a brief explanation appear at the end of the book.

We wish to thank our readers for their constructive comments in the past, and we hope that they will continue to provide the input necessary for us to improve future editions. We also wish to thank the numerous investigators and publishers who have granted us permission to use illustrations from their publications. In most cases these illustrations have been altered somewhat to increase their didactic utility. In some cases, unpublished data from our own investigations have been presented.

Robert M. Berne
Matthew N. Levy

Contents

Cardiovascular Physiology

CHAPTER 1

The Circuitry

Objectives

1. Indicate the compositions and functions of the blood vessels.

2. Indicate the relationship of vascular cross-sectional area to the velocity of blood flow in the various vascular segments.

3. Indicate the pressure changes and pathways of blood flow throughout the vasculature.

THE CIRCULATORY, ENDOCRINE, AND nervous systems constitute the principal coordinating and integrating systems of the body. Whereas the nervous system is primarily concerned with communications and the endocrine glands with regulation of certain body functions, the circulatory system serves to transport and distribute essential substances to the tissues and to remove by-products of metabolism. The circulatory system also shares in such homeostatic mechanisms as regulation of body temperature, humoral communication throughout the body, and adjustments of oxygen and nutrient supply in different physiological states.

The cardiovascular system that accomplishes these chores is made up of a pump, a series of distributing and collecting tubes, and an extensive system of thin vessels that permit rapid exchange between the tissues and the vascular channels. The primary purpose of this text is to discuss the function of the components of the vascular system and the control mechanisms (with their checks and balances) that are responsible for alteration of blood distribution necessary to meet the changing requirements of different tissues in response to a wide spectrum of physiological and pathological conditions.

Before considering the function of the parts of the circulatory system in detail, it is useful to consider it as a whole in a purely descriptive sense. The heart consists of two pumps in series: the right ventricle to propel blood through the lungs for exchange of oxygen and carbon dioxide **(the pulmonary circulation)** and the left ventricle to propel blood to all other tissues of the body **(the systemic circulation).** Unidi-

1

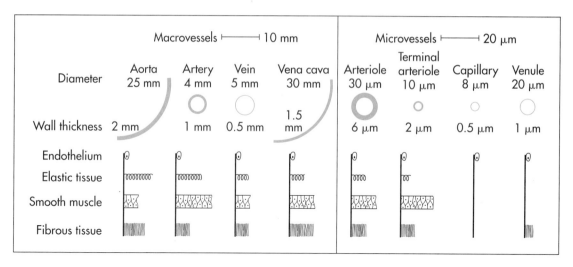

Figure 1-1 ▪ Internal diameter, wall thickness, and relative amounts of the principal components of the vessel walls of the various blood vessels that compose the circulatory system. Cross sections of the vessels are not drawn to scale because of the huge range from aorta and venae cavae to capillary. (Redrawn from Burton AC: *Physiol Rev* 34:619, 1954.)

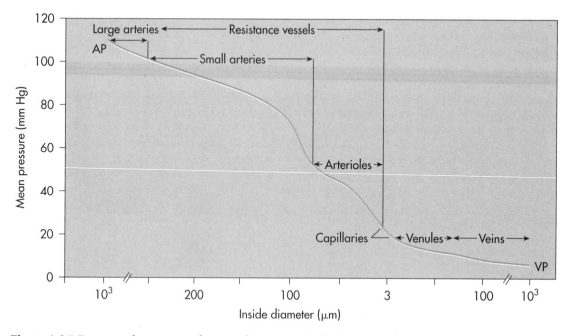

Figure 1-2 ▪ Pressure drop across the vascular system in the hamster cheek pouch. *AP,* Mean arterial pressure; *VP,* venous pressure. (Redrawn from Davis MJ, et al: *Am J Physiol* 250:H291, 1986.)

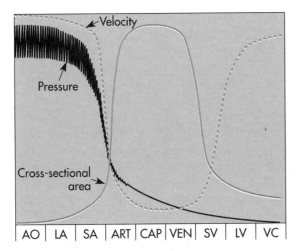

Figure 1-3 ▪ Phasic pressure, velocity of flow, and cross-sectional area of the systemic circulation. *The important features are the inverse relationship between velocity and cross-sectional area, the major pressure drop across the small arteries and arterioles, and the maximal cross-sectional area and minimal flow rate in the capillaries. AO,* Aorta; *LA,* large arteries; *SA,* small arteries; *ART,* arterioles; *CAP,* capillaries; *VEN,* venules; *SV,* small veins; *LV,* large veins; *VC,* venae cavae.

rectional flow through the heart is achieved by the appropriate arrangement of effective flap valves. Although the cardiac output is intermittent, continuous flow to the periphery occurs by distension of the aorta and its branches during ventricular contraction **(systole)** and elastic recoil of the walls of the large arteries with forward propulsion of the blood during ventricular relaxation **(diastole).** Blood moves rapidly through the aorta and its arterial branches. The branches become narrower and their walls become thinner and change histologically toward the periphery. From the aorta, a predominantly elastic structure, the peripheral arteries become more muscular until the muscular layer predominates at the arterioles (Figure 1-1).

In the large arteries, frictional resistance is relatively small, and pressures are only slightly less than in the aorta. However, the small arteries offer moderate resistance to blood flow, and this resistance reaches a maximal level in the arterioles, sometimes referred to as the stopcocks of the vascular system. Hence *the pressure drop is significant in the small arteries and is greatest in the arterioles* (Figure 1-2). Adjustment in the degree of contraction of the circular muscle of these small vessels permits regulation of tissue blood flow and aids in the control of arterial blood pressure.

In addition to a sharp reduction in pressure across the arterioles, there is also a change from pulsatile to steady flow as pressure continues to decline from the arterial to the venous end of the capillaries (Figure 1-3). *The **pulsatile arterial blood flow,** caused by the intermittency of cardiac ejection, is damped at the capillary level by the combination of distensibility of the large arteries and frictional resistance in the arterioles.*

BOX 1-1

In a patient with hyperthyroidism **(Graves disease),** the basal metabolism is elevated and is often associated with arteriolar vasodilation. This reduction in arteriolar resistance diminishes the dampening effect on the pulsatile arterial pressure and is manifest as pulsatile flow in the capillaries, as observed in the finger nail bed of patients with this ailment.

Many capillaries arise from each arteriole so that the *total cross-sectional area of the capillary bed is very large, despite the fact that the cross-sectional area of each capillary is less than that of each arteriole. As a result, blood flow velocity becomes quite slow in the capillaries (Figure 1-3), analogous to the decrease in velocity of flow seen at the wide regions of a*

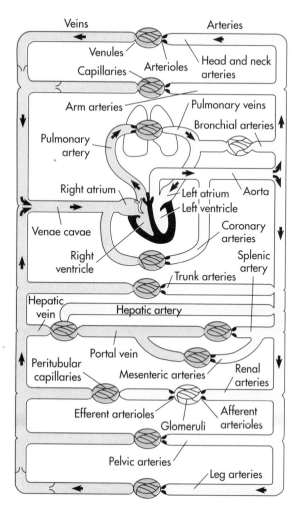

Veins
Arteries
Venules
Capillaries
Arterioles
Head and neck arteries
Arm arteries
Pulmonary veins
Bronchial arteries
Pulmonary artery
Right atrium
Left atrium
Aorta
Left ventricle
Venae cavae
Coronary arteries
Right ventricle
Splenic artery
Trunk arteries
Hepatic vein
Hepatic artery
Peritubular capillaries
Portal vein
Mesenteric arteries
Renal arteries
Efferent arterioles
Afferent arterioles
Glomeruli
Pelvic arteries
Leg arteries

Figure 1-4 ▪ Schematic diagram of the parallel and series arrangement of the vessels composing the circulatory system. The capillary beds are represented by thin lines connecting the arteries (on the right) with the veins (on the left). The crescent-shaped thickenings proximal to the capillary beds represent the arterioles (resistance vessels). (Redrawn from Green HD: In Glasser O, editor: *Medical physics*, vol 1, Chicago, 1944, Mosby–Year Book.)

river. Because the capillaries consist of short tubes whose walls are only one cell thick and because flow velocity is low, conditions in the capillaries are ideal for the exchange of diffusible substances between blood and tissue.

On its return to the heart from the capillaries, blood passes through venules and then through veins of increasing size with a progressive decrease in pressure until the blood reaches the right atrium (Figure 1-2). As the heart is approached, the number of veins decreases, the thickness and composition of the vein walls change (Figure 1-1), the total cross-sectional area of the venous channels diminishes, and the velocity of blood flow increases (Figure 1-3). Note that the velocity of blood flow and the cross-sectional area at each level of the vasculature are essentially mirror images of each other (Figure 1-3).

Data from a 20-kg dog* (Table 1-1) indicate that between the aorta and the capillaries the number of vessels increases about 3 billion-fold, and the total cross-sectional area increases about 500-fold. The volume of blood in the systemic vascular system is greatest in the veins and venules (67%). It is only 5% of the total blood volume in the capillaries and 11% in the aorta, arteries, and arterioles. In contrast, blood volume in the pulmonary vascular bed is about equally divided among the arterial, capillary, and venous vessels. The cross-sectional area of the venae cavae is larger than that of the aorta. Therefore, the velocity of flow is slower in the venae cavae than that in the aorta (Figure 1-3).

Blood entering the right ventricle via the right atrium is pumped through the pulmonary arterial system at a mean pressure about one seventh that in the systemic arteries. The blood then passes through the lung capillaries, where carbon dioxide is released and oxygen taken up. The oxygen-rich blood returns via the four pul-

---

*Similar relationships exist in humans.

TABLE 1-1

Vascular dimensions in a 20-kg dog

Vessels	No.	Total cross-sectional area (cm²)	Total blood volume (%)
Systemic			
Aorta	1	2.8 ⎫	
Arteries	40 to 110,000	40 ⎬	11
Arterioles	2.8×10^6	55 ⎭	
Capillaries	2.7×10^9	1357	5
Venules	1×10^7	785 ⎫	
Veins	660,000 to 110	631 ⎬	67
Venae cavae	2	3.1 ⎭	
Pulmonary			
Arteries and arterioles	1-1.5×10^6	137	3
Capillaries	2.7×10^9	1357	4
Venules and veins	2×10^6 to 4	210	5
Heart			
Atria	2		5
Ventricles	2		

Data from Milnor WR: *Hemodynamics,* Baltimore, 1982, Williams & Wilkins.

monary veins to the left atrium and ventricle to complete the cycle. Thus, in the normal intact circulation, the total volume of blood is constant, and an increase in the volume of blood in one area must be accompanied by a decrease in another. However, the distribution of the circulating blood to the different regions of the body is determined by the output of the left ventricle and by the contractile state of the arterioles (resistance vessels) of these regions. The circulatory system is composed of conduits arranged in series and in parallel (Figure 1-4).

SUMMARY

- The greatest resistance to blood flow, and hence the greatest pressure drop, in the arterial system occurs at the level of the small arteries and the arterioles.
- Pulsatile pressure is progressively damped by the elasticity of the arteriolar walls and the functional resistance of the arterioles, so that capillary blood flow is essentially nonpulsatile.

- Velocity of blood flow is inversely related to the cross-sectional area at any point along the vascular system.
- Most of the blood in the systemic vascular bed is located in the venous side of the circulation.

■ CASE 1

After a knife wound to the groin, a man develops a large arteriovenous (AV) shunt between the iliac artery and vein. Which of the following is not characteristic of his systemic circulation?

a. Blood flow in the capillaries of the finger nail bed is pulsatile.

b. The circulation time (antecubital vein to tongue) is increased.

c. The arterial pulse pressure (systolic minus diastolic pressure) is increased.

d. Greatest velocity of blood flow prevails in the aorta.

e. Pressure in the right atrium is less than in the inferior vena cava.

CHAPTER 2

Electrical Activity of the Heart

Objectives

1. Characterize the types of cardiac action potentials.

2. Define the ionic basis of cardiac action potentials.

3. Explain the temporal changes in cardiac excitability.

4. Explain the basis of automaticity.

5. Describe the spread of automaticity.

6. Explain the basis of reentry.

7. Describe the components of the electrocardiogram.

8. Explain various cardiac rhythm disturbances.

THE EXPERIMENTS ON "ANIMAL ELEC-
tricity" conducted by Galvani and Volta two
centuries ago led to the discovery that electrical
phenomena were involved in the spontaneous
contractions of the heart. In 1855 Kölliker and
Müller observed that when they placed the nerve
of an innervated skeletal muscle preparation in
contact with the surface of a frog's heart, the
muscle twitched with each cardiac contraction.

The electrical events that normally take place
in the heart initiate its contraction. Disorders in
electrical activity can induce serious and sometimes lethal rhythm disturbances.

■ CARDIAC ACTION POTENTIALS CONSIST OF SEVERAL PHASES

The electrical behavior of single cardiac muscle
cells has been investigated by inserting micro-
electrodes into the interior of the cell. The potential changes recorded from a typical ventricular muscle fiber are illustrated in Figure 2-1, *A*.
When two electrodes are placed in an electrolyte solution near a strip of quiescent cardiac
muscle, no potential difference (point *a*) is mea-
surable between the two electrodes. At point *b,*
one of the electrodes, a microelectrode, was inserted into the interior of a cardiac muscle fiber.
Immediately the galvanometer recorded a potential difference (V_m) across the cell membrane; the potential of the interior of the cell
was about 90 mV lower than that of the
surrounding medium. Such electronegativity of
the interior of the resting cell is also characteristic of skeletal and smooth muscles, nerves, and
indeed most cells within the body.

At point *c* the ventricular cell was excited by
an electrical stimulator. Very rapidly the cell
membrane became depolarized; actually, the

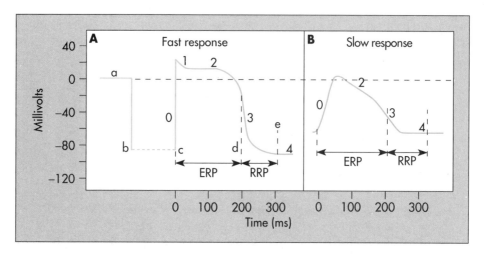

Figure 2-1 ▪ **Changes in transmembrane potential recorded from a fast-response** (A) **and slow-response** (B) **cardiac fiber in isolated cardiac tissue immersed in an electrolyte solution. A, At time** *a* **the microelectrode was in the solution surrounding the cardiac fiber. At time** *b* **the microelectrode entered the fiber. At time** *c* **an action potential was initiated in the impaled fiber. Time** *c* **to** *d* **represents the effective refractory period** *(ERP);* **time** *d* **to** *e* **represents the relative refractory period** *(RRP).* **B, An action potential recorded from a slow-response cardiac fiber. Note that compared with the fast-response fiber, the resting potential of the slow fiber is less negative, the upstroke (phase** *0)* **of the action potential is less steep, the amplitude of the action potential is smaller, phase** *1* **is absent, and the RRP extends well into phase** *4,* **after the fiber has fully repolarized.**

potential difference was reversed (positive overshoot), such that the potential of the interior of the cell exceeded that of the exterior by about 20 mV. The rapid upstroke of the **action potential** is designated phase 0. Immediately after the upstroke, there was a brief period of partial repolarization (phase 1), followed by a **plateau** (phase 2) that persisted for about 0.1 to 0.2 s. The potential then became progressively more negative (phase 3), until the resting state of polarization was again attained (at point *e*). **Repolarization** (phase 3) is a much slower process than is **depolarization** (phase 0). The interval from the end of repolarization until the beginning of the next action potential is designated phase 4.

The relationships between the electrical events and the actual mechanical contraction are shown in Figure 2-2. Rapid depolarization (phase 0) precedes force development, completion of repolarization coincides approximately with peak force, and the duration of contraction parallels the duration of the action potential.

Principal Types of Cardiac Action Potentials Are the Slow and Fast Types

Two main types of action potentials are observed in the heart, as shown in Figure 2-1. One type, the **fast response,** occurs in the ordinary atrial and ventricular myocytes and in the specialized conducting fibers **(Purkinje fibers).** The other type of action potential, the **slow response,** is found in the **sinoatrial (SA) node,** the natural pacemaker region of the heart, and in the **atrioventricular (AV) node,** the special-

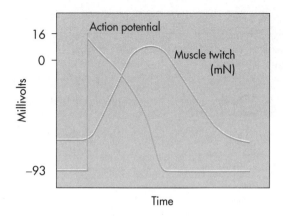

Figure 2-2 ■ **Time relationships between the mechanical force developed by a thin strip of ventricular muscle and the changes in transmembrane potential.** (Redrawn from Kavaler F, Fisher VJ, Stuckey JH: *Bull NY Acad Med* 41:592, 1965.)

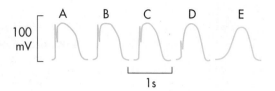

Figure 2-3 ■ **Effect of tetrodotoxin on the action potential recorded in a calf Purkinje fiber perfused with a solution containing epinephrine and 10.8 mM K^+. The concentration of tetrodotoxin was 0 M in A, 3×10^{-8} M in B, 3×10^{-7} M in C, and 3×10^{-6} M in D and E; E was recorded later than** D. (Redrawn from Carmeliet E, Vereecke J: *Pflugers Arch* 313:300, 1969.)

ized tissue that conducts the cardiac impulse from atria to ventricles.

As shown in Figure 2-1, not only is the **resting membrane potential** (phase 4) of the fast response considerably more negative than that of the slow response, but also the slope of the upstroke (phase 0), the amplitude of the action potential, and the extent of the overshoot of the fast response are greater than those of the slow response. The amplitude of the action potential and the steepness of the upstroke are important determinants of propagation velocity, as explained below. Hence in slow response fibers, conduction velocity is much slower than in fast response fibers. Slow conduction increases the likelihood of certain rhythm disturbances.

Ionic Basis of the Resting Potential

The various phases of the cardiac action potential are associated with changes in the **permeability** of the cell membrane, mainly to sodium, potassium, and calcium ions. Changes in cell membrane permeability alter the rate of ion pas-

BOX 2-1

Fast responses may change to slow responses under certain pathological conditions. For example, in patients with coronary artery disease, when a region of cardiac muscle is deprived of its normal blood supply, the K^+ concentration in the interstitial fluid that surrounds the affected muscle cells rises because K^+ is lost from the inadequately perfused (**ischemic**) cells. The action potentials in some of these cells may then be converted from fast to slow responses. An experimental conversion from a fast to a slow response by the addition of **tetrodotoxin,** which blocks fast Na^+ channels in the cardiac cell membranes, is illustrated in Figure 2-3.

sage across the membrane. *The permeability of the membrane to a given ion defines the net quantity of the ion that will diffuse across each unit area of the membrane per unit concentration difference across the membrane.* Changes

TABLE 2-1

**Intracellular and extracellular ion concentrations and equilibrium potentials
in cardiac muscle cells**

Ion	Extracellular concentrations (mM)	Intracellular concentrations (mM)*	Equilibrium potential (mV)
Na^+	145	10	70
K^+	4	135	−94
Ca^{++}	2	0.1	132

Modified from Ten Eick RE, Baumgarten CM, Singer DH: *Prog Cardiovasc Dis* 24:157, 1981.
*The intracellular concentrations are estimates of the free concentrations in the cytoplasm.

in permeability are accomplished by the opening and closing of **ion channels** that are specific for the individual ions.

Just as with all other cells in the body, the concentration of potassium ions inside a cardiac muscle cell, $[K^+]_i$, greatly exceeds the concentration outside the cell, $[K^+]_o$, as shown in Figure 2-4. The reverse concentration gradient exists for Na ions and for free Ca ions (not bound to protein). Estimates of the extracellular and intracellular concentrations of Na^+, K^+, and Ca^{++}, and of the equilibrium potentials (defined below) for these ions, are compiled in Table 2-1.

The resting cell membrane is relatively permeable to K^+, but much less so to Na^+ and Ca^{++}. Hence K^+ tends to diffuse from the inside to the outside of the cell, in the direction of the concentration gradient, as shown on the right side of the cell in Figure 2-4.

Any flux of K^+ that occurs during phase 4 takes place through certain specific **K^+ channels.** Several types of K^+ channels exist in cardiac cell membranes. Some of these channels are controlled (i.e., opened and closed) by the transmembrane potential, whereas others are controlled by some chemical signal (e.g., a neurotransmitter). The specific K^+ channel through which K^+ passes during phase 4 is a voltage-regulated channel that conducts the K^+ current, called i_{K1}, which is an in-

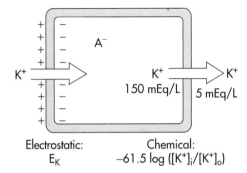

Figure 2-4 ▪ The balance of chemical and electrostatic forces acting on a resting cardiac cell membrane, based on a 30:1 ratio of the intracellular to extracellular K^+ concentrations and the existence of a nondiffusible anion (A^-) inside but not outside the cell.

wardly rectifying K^+ current, as explained below (Figure 2-5). Many of the anions (labeled A^-) inside the cell, such as the proteins, are not free to diffuse out with the K^+ (see Figure 2-4). Therefore, as the K^+ diffuses out of the cell and leaves the A^- behind, the deficiency of cations causes the interior of the cell to become electronegative.

Therefore two opposing forces are involved in the movement of K^+ across the cell membrane. A chemical force, based on the concentration gradient, results in the net outward diffusion of K^+. The counterforce is an electrostatic

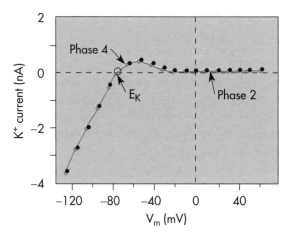

Figure 2-5 ■ **The K$^+$ currents recorded from a rabbit ventricular myocyte when the potential was changed from a holding potential of −80 mV to various test potentials. Positive values along the vertical axis represent outward currents; negative values represent inward currents. The V$_m$ coordinate of the point of intersection *(open circle)* of the curve with the X axis is the reversal potential; it denotes the Nernst equilibrium potential *(E$_K$)* at which the chemical and electrostatic forces are equal.** (Redrawn from Giles WR, Imaizumi Y: *J Physiol [Lond]* 405:123, 1988.)

one; the positively charged K ions are attracted to the interior of the cell by the negative potential that exists there, as shown on the left side of the cell in Figure 2-4. If the system came into equilibrium, the chemical and electrostatic forces would be equal.

This equilibrium is expressed by the **Nernst equation** for potassium:

$$E_K = -61.5 \log ([K^+]_i/[K^+]_o) \qquad (1)$$

The right-hand term represents chemical potential difference at the body temperature of 37° C. The left-hand term, E$_K$, represents the electrostatic potential difference that would exist across the cell membrane if K$^+$ were the only diffusible ion. E$_K$ is called the **potassium equilibrium potential.**

An experimental disturbance in the equilibrium between electrostatic and chemical forces imposed by **voltage clamping** would cause K$^+$ to move through the K$^+$ channels. If the transmembrane potential (V$_m$) were clamped at a level negative to E$_K$, the electrostatic forces would exceed the diffusional forces, and K$^+$ would be attracted into the cell (i.e., the K$^+$ current would be **inward**). Conversely, if V$_m$ were clamped at a level positive to E$_K$, the diffusional forces would exceed the electrostatic forces, and K$^+$ would leave the cell (i.e., the K$^+$ current would be **outward**).

When the measured concentrations of [K$^+$]$_i$ and [K$^+$]$_o$ for mammalian myocardial cells are substituted into the Nernst equation, the calculated value of E$_K$ equals about −94 mV (Table 2-1). This value is close to, but slightly more negative than, the resting potential actually measured in myocardial cells. Therefore the electrostatic force is slightly weaker than the chemical (diffusional) force, and K$^+$ tends to leave the resting cell.

The balance of forces acting on the Na ions is entirely different from that acting on the K ions in resting cardiac cells. The intracellular Na$^+$ concentration, [Na$^+$]$_i$, is much lower than the extracellular Na$^+$ concentration, [Na$^+$]$_o$. At 37° C, the **sodium equilibrium potential,** E$_{Na}$, expressed by the Nernst equation is:

$$-61.5 \log ([Na^+]_i/ [Na^+]_o) \qquad (2)$$

For cardiac cells, E$_{Na}$ is about 70 mV (Table 2-1). Therefore at equilibrium a transmembrane potential of about +70 mV would be necessary to counterbalance the chemical potential for Na$^+$. However, the actual polarization of the resting cell membrane is just the opposite. The resting membrane potential of myocardial fibers is about −90 mV (see Figure 2-1, *A*). Hence both chemical and electrostatic forces act to pull extracellular Na$^+$ into the cell. The influx of Na$^+$ through the cell membrane is small, however, because the permeability of the resting membrane to Na^+ is very low. Nevertheless, it is mainly this small inward current of positively charged Na ions that causes the potential on the inside of the resting cell membrane to be slightly less negative than the value predicted by the Nernst equation for K^+.

The steady inward leak of Na^+ would gradually depolarize the resting cell membrane were it not for the metabolic pump that continuously extrudes Na^+ from the cell interior and pumps in K^+. The metabolic pump involves the enzyme **Na^+, K^+-ATPase,** which is located in the cell membrane itself. Because the pump must move Na^+ against both a chemical and an electrostatic gradient, operation of the pump requires the expenditure of metabolic energy. Increases in $[Na^+]_i$ or in $[K^+]_o$ accelerate the activity of the pump. The quantity of Na^+ extruded by the pump exceeds the quantity of K^+ transferred into the cell by a $3:2$ ratio. Therefore the pump itself tends to create a potential difference across the cell membrane, and thus it is termed an **electrogenic pump.** If the pump is partially inhibited, as by **digitalis,** the resting membrane potential becomes less negative than normal.

The dependence of the transmembrane potential, V_m, on the intracellular and extracellular concentrations of K^+ and Na^+ and on the conductances (g_K and g_{Na}) of these ions is described by the **chord conductance equation:**

$$V_m = \frac{g_K}{g_K + g_{Na}} E_K + \frac{g_{Na}}{g_K + g_{Na}} E_{Na} \quad (3)$$

For a given ion (X), the conductance (g_x) is defined as the ratio of the current (i_x) carried by that ion to the difference between the V_m and the Nernst equilibrium potential (E_x) for that ion; that is,

$$g_x = \frac{i_x}{V_m - E_x} \quad (4)$$

The chord conductance equation reveals that the relative, not the absolute, conductances to

Na^+ and K^+ determine the resting potential. In the resting cardiac cell, g_K is about 100 times greater than g_{Na}. Therefore the chord conductance equation reduces essentially to the Nernst equation for K^+.

When the ratio $[K^+]_i/[K^+]_o$ is decreased experimentally by raising $[K^+]_o$, the measured value of V_m (Figure 2-6) approximates that predicted by the Nernst equation for K^+. For extracellular K^+ concentrations of about 5 mM and above, the measured values correspond closely with the predicted values. The measured levels of V_m are slightly less negative than those predicted by the Nernst equation because of the small but finite value of g_{Na}. For values of $[K^+]_o$ below about 5 mM, the effect of the Na^+ gradient on the transmembrane potential becomes more important, as predicted by equation 3. This increase in the relative importance of g_{Na} accounts for the greater deviation of the measured V_m from that predicted by the Nernst equation for K^+ at very low levels of $[K^+]_o$ (Figure 2-6).

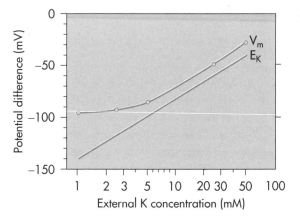

Figure 2-6 ■ **The transmembrane potential** (V_m) **of a cardiac muscle fiber varies inversely with the potassium concentration of the external medium** *(curved line).* **The straight line represents the change in transmembrane potential predicted by the Nernst equation for E_K.** (Redrawn from Page E: *Circulation* 26:582, 1962.)

The Fast Response Depends Mainly on Voltage-Dependent Sodium Channels

Genesis of the Upstroke Any process that abruptly changes the resting membrane potential to a critical value (called the **threshold**) will induce a propagated action potential. The characteristics of fast-response action potentials are shown in Figure 2-1, *A*. The rapid depolarization (phase 0) is related almost exclusively to the inrush of Na^+ by virtue of a sudden increase in g_{Na}. The **amplitude** of the action potential (the magnitude of the potential change during phase 0) varies linearly with the logarithm of $[Na^+]_o$, as shown in Figure 2-7. When $[Na^+]_o$ is reduced from its normal value of about 140 mM to about 20 mM, the cell is no longer excitable.

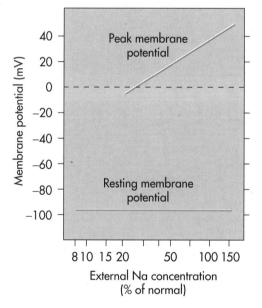

Figure 2-7 ■ The concentration of sodium in the external medium is a critical determinant of the amplitude of the action potential in cardiac muscle *(upper line)* but has relatively little influence on the resting potential *(lower line)*. (Redrawn from Weidmann S: *Elektrophysiologie der Herzmuskelfaser,* Bern, 1956, Verlag Hans Huber.)

The physical and chemical forces responsible for these transmembrane movements of Na^+ are explained in Figure 2-8. Panel *A* in this figure represents the resting state (phase 4) of a cardiac myocyte. The balance of chemical and electrostatic forces are such that the resting membrane potential is −90 mV. When the resting membrane potential, V_m, is suddenly changed to the threshold level of about −65 mV (panel B), the properties of the cell membrane change dramatically. The conductance of the cell membrane to Na^+ increases rapidly. Hence Na^+ begins to enter the cell, and the transmembrane potential becomes less negative (panel *B*). Specific **voltage-dependent Na^+ channels** (often called **fast Na^+ channels**) exist in the cell membrane. These channels can be blocked specifically by the puffer fish toxin **tetrodotoxin.**

When a suprathreshold stimulus is delivered to resting atrial or ventricular myocytes, the Na^+ current increases very rapidly. The upstroke of the action potential requires only 1 or 2 ms (see Figure 2-1, *A*). The processes that initiate the fast Na^+ current are referred to as **activation** of that current. Almost immediately after such activation, the reverse process takes place; that is, the fast Na^+ current rapidly diminishes. This opposing process is referred to as **inactivation.** The kinetics of inactivation are exponential. The inactivation of the Na^+ current proceeds rapidly at first, but the process gradually diminishes. Hence the inactivation process may persist for about 100 to 200 ms. Thus the **recovery from inactivation** may be an important determinant of the ability of a myocyte to be reexcited at a specific time after a previous excitation. This phenomenon is discussed below with regard to the refractoriness of a cardiac cell.

The movement of Na^+ through the fast Na^+ channels suggests that the Na^+ flux is controlled by two types of "gates" in each channel. One of

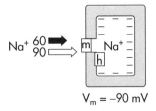

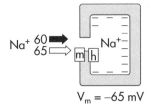

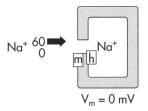

$V_m = -90$ mV

$V_m = -65$ mV

$V_m = 0$ mV

A, During phase 4, the chemical (60 mV) and electrostatic (90 mV) forces favor influx of Na$^+$ from the extracellular space. Influx is negligible, however, because the activation **(m)** gates are closed.

B, If V_m is brought to about −65 V, the **m** gates begin to swing open, and Na$^+$ begins to enter the cell. This reduces the negative charge inside the cell. The change in V_m also initiates the closure of inactivation **(h)** gates, which operate more slowly than the **m** gates.

C, The rapid influx of Na$^+$ rapidly decreases the negativity of V_m. As V_m approaches 0, the electrostatic force attracting Na$^+$ into the cell is neutralized. Na$^+$ continues to enter the cell, however, because of the substantial concentration gradient, and V_m begins to become positive.

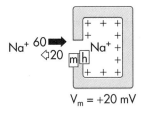

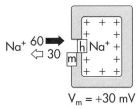

$V_m = +20$ mV

$V_m = +30$ mV

D, When V_m is positive by about 20 mV, Na$^+$ continues to enter the cell, because the diffusional forces (60 mV) exceed the opposing electrostatic forces (20 mV). The influx of Na$^+$ is slow, however, because the net driving force is small, and many of the inactivation gates have already closed.

E, When V_m reaches about 30 mV, the **h** gates have now all closed, and Na$^+$ influx ceases. The **h** gates remain closed until the first half of repolarization, and thus the cell is absolutely refractory during this entire period. During the second half of repolarization, the **m** and **h** gates approach the state represented by panel A, and thus the cell is relatively refractory.

Figure 2-8 ■ **The gating of a sodium channel in a cardiac cell membrane during phase 4 (A) and during various stages of the action potential upstroke (B to E). The positions of the m and h gates in the fast Na$^+$ channels are shown at the various levels of V_m. The electrostatic forces are represented by the white arrows and the chemical (diffusional) forces by the black arrows.**

these gates, the **m gate,** tends to open the channel as V_m becomes less negative than the threshold potential and is therefore called an **activation gate.** The other, the **h gate,** tends to close the channel as V_m becomes less negative and hence is called an **inactivation gate.** The m and h designations were originally employed

by Hodgkin and Huxley several decades ago in their mathematical model of ion conduction in nerve fibers.

A much more detailed and modern concept of the voltage-dependent Na$^+$ channel is shown in Figure 2-9. The individual cylinders (numbered 1 to 6) represent transmembrane α he-

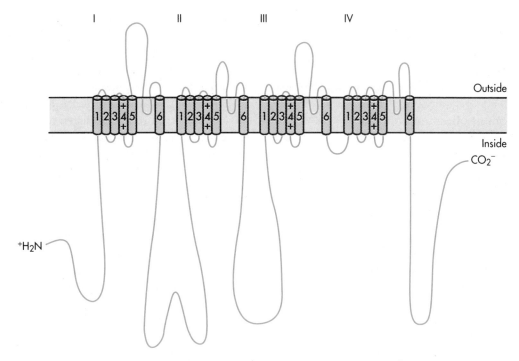

Figure 2-9 ■ **A two-dimensional model of the voltage-dependent Na⁺ channel protein.**

lices. The S4 helices (marked with plus signs) serve as voltage sensors, and their movements are responsible for activating the channel. The intracellular loop that connects domains III and IV functions as the inactivation gate. After depolarization, this loop swings into the mouth of the channel to block ion conduction. The extracellular portions of the loops that connect helices 5 and 6 in each domain participate in the determination of ion selectivity.

With the cell at rest, V_m is about -90 mV. At this level, the m gates are closed and the h gates are wide open, as shown in Figure 2-8, *A*. The concentration of Na⁺ is much greater outside than inside the cell, and the interior of the cell is electrically negative with respect to the exterior. Hence both chemical and electrostatic forces are oriented to draw Na⁺ into the cell.

The electrostatic force in Figure 2-8, *A* is a potential difference of 90 mV, and it is represented by the white arrow. The chemical force, based on the difference in Na⁺ concentration between the outside and inside of the cell, is represented by the black arrow. For a Na⁺ concentration difference of about 130 mM, a potential difference of 60 mV (inside more positive than the outside) is necessary to counterbalance the chemical, or diffusional, force, according to the Nernst equation for Na⁺ (equation 2). Therefore we may represent the net chemical force favoring the inward movement of Na⁺ in Figure 2-8 *(black arrows)* as equivalent to a potential of 60 mV. With the cell at rest the total electrochemical force favoring the inward movement of Na⁺ is 150 mV (panel *A*). The m gates are closed, however, and the conductance of the resting cell membrane to Na⁺ is very low.

Hence virtually no Na^+ moves into the cell; that is, the **inward Na^+ current** is negligible.

Any process that makes V_m less negative tends to open the m gates and thereby activates the fast Na^+ channels. The activation of the fast channels is therefore called a **voltage-dependent phenomenon.** The precise potential at which the m gates swing open is called the **threshold potential.** As V_m becomes less negative, the m gates open and Na^+ enters the cell (Figure 2-8, *B*) by virtue of the chemical and electrostatic forces. The entry of positively charged Na^+ into the interior of the cell neutralizes some of the negative charges inside the cell and thereby diminishes further the transmembrane potential, V_m (Figure 2-8, *B*).

The rapid opening of the m gates in the fast Na^+ channels is responsible for the large and abrupt increase in Na^+ conductance, g_{Na}, coincident with phase 0 of the action potential (see Figure 2-15). The rapid influx of Na^+ accounts for the steep upstroke of V_m during phase 0. The maximal rate of change of V_m varies from 100 to 200 V/s in myocardial cells and from 500 to 1000 V/s in Purkinje fibers. Although the quantity of Na^+ that enters the cell during one action potential alters V_m by over 100 mV, that quantity of Na^+ is too small to change the intracellular Na^+ concentration measurably. The chemical force remains virtually constant, and only the electrostatic force changes throughout the action potential. Hence the lengths of the black arrows in Figure 2-8 remain constant at 60 mV, whereas the white arrows change in magnitude and direction.

As Na^+ rushes into the cardiac cell during phase 0, the negative charges inside the cell are neutralized, and V_m becomes less negative. When V_m becomes zero (Figure 2-8, *C*), an electrostatic force no longer pulls Na^+ into the cell. As long as the fast Na^+ channels are open, however, Na^+ continues to enter the cell because of the large concentration gradient. This

continuation of the inward Na^+ current causes the inside of the cell to become positively charged (Figure 2-8, *D*). This reversal of the membrane polarity is the so-called **overshoot** of the cardiac action potential. Such a reversal of the electrostatic gradient tends to repel the entry of Na^+ (Figure 2-8, *D*). However, as long as the inwardly directed chemical forces exceed these outwardly directed electrostatic forces, the net flux of Na^+ will still be inward, although the rate of influx will be diminished.

The inward Na^+ current finally ceases when the h (inactivation) gates close (Figure 2-8, *E*). The opening of the m gates occurs very rapidly (in about 0.1 to 0.2 ms), whereas the closure of the h gates is slower, requiring 100 ms or more. Inactivation of the fast Na^+ channels is finally terminated when the h gates close. The h gates then remain closed until the cell has partially repolarized during phase 3 (at about time *d* in Figure 2-1, *A*). From time *c* to time *d,* the cell is in its **effective refractory period** and will not respond to excitation. This mechanism prevents a sustained, tetanic contraction of cardiac muscle. Such a sustained contraction precludes the normal intermittent pumping action of the heart. An ample period of myocardial relaxation, to permit the cardiac ventricles to fill with venous blood during each cardiac cycle, is just as essential to the normal pumping action of the heart as is a strong cardiac contraction.

About midway through phase 3 (time *d* in Figure 2-1, *A*), the m and h gates in some of the fast Na^+ channels resume the states shown in Figure 2-8, *A.* Such channels are said to have **recovered from inactivation.** The cell can begin to respond again to excitation (Figure 2-10). Application of a suprathreshold stimulus to a region of normal myocardium during phase 3 evokes an action potential. As the stimulus is delivered progressively later during the course of phase 3, the slopes of the action potential upstrokes and the amplitudes of the evoked action potentials progressively increase. Throughout the remainder of phase 3, the cell completes its recovery from inactivation. By time *e* in Figure 2-1, *A,* the h gates have reopened and the m gates have reclosed in the remaining fast Na^+ channels, as shown in Figure 2-8, *A.*

Statistical Characteristics of the "Gate" Concept The patch-clamping technique has made it possible to measure ionic currents through single membrane channels. The indi-

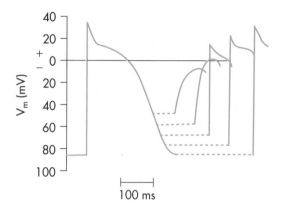

Figure 2-10 ■ **The changes in action potential amplitude and slope of the upstroke as action potentials are initiated at different stages of the relative refractory period of the preceding excitation.** (Redrawn from Rosen MR, Wit AL, Hoffman BF: *Am Heart J* 88:380, 1974.)

vidual channels open and close repeatedly in a quasirandom manner. This process is illustrated in Figure 2-11, which shows the current flow through single Na^+ channels in a myocardial cell. To the left of the arrow, the membrane potential was clamped at −85 mV. At the arrow, the potential was suddenly changed to −45 mV, at which value it was held for the remainder of the record.

Figure 2-11 indicates that immediately after the membrane potential was made less negative, one Na^+ channel opened three times in sequence. It remained open for about 2 or 3 ms each time and closed for about 4 or 5 ms between openings. In the open state, it allowed 1.5 pA of current to pass. During the first and second openings of this channel, a second channel also opened, but for periods of only 1 ms. During the brief times that both channels were open simultaneously, the total current was 3 pA. After the first channel closed for the third time, both channels remained closed for the rest of the recording, even though the membrane was held constant at −45 mV.

The overall change in ionic conductance of the entire cell membrane at any given time reflects the number of channels that are open at that time. Because the individual channels open and close in an irregular pattern, the overall membrane conductance represents the statisti-

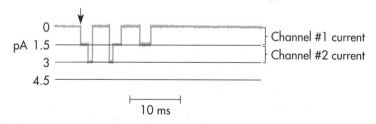

Figure 2-11 ■ **The current flow (in picoamperes) through two individual Na^+ channels in a cultured cardiac cell, recorded by the patch-clamping technique. The membrane potential had been held at −85 mV but was suddenly changed to −45 mV at the arrow and held at this potential for the remainder of the record.** (Redrawn from Cachelin AB, DePeyer JE, Kokubun S, et al: *J Physiol* 340:389, 1983.)

cal probability of the open or closed state of the individual channels. The temporal characteristics of the activation process then represent the time course of the increasing probability that the specific channels will be open, rather than the kinetic characteristics of the activation gates in the individual channels. Similarly, the temporal characteristics of inactivation reflect the time course of the decreasing probability that the channels will be open and not the kinetic characteristics of the inactivation gates in the individual channels.

Genesis of Early Repolarization In many cardiac cells that have a prominent plateau, phase 1 constitutes an early, brief period of limited repolarization between the end of the action potential upstroke and the beginning of the plateau (Figure 2-12). Phase 1 reflects the activation of a **transient outward current,** i_{to}, mostly carried by K^+. Activation of these K^+ channels during phase 1 leads to a brief efflux of K^+ from the cell because the interior of the cell is positively charged and because the internal K^+ concentration greatly exceeds the external

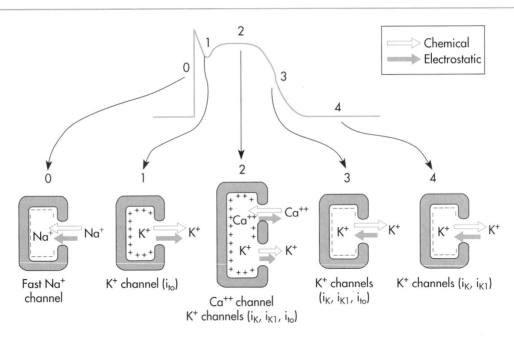

Figure 2-12 ■ **The principal ionic currents and channels that generate the action potential in a cardiac cell.** Phase 0, The chemical and electrostatic forces both favor the entry of Na^+ into the cell through fast Na^+ channels to generate the upstroke. Phase 1, The chemical and electrostatic forces both favor the efflux of K^+ through i_{to} channels to generate early, partial repolarization. Phase 2, During the plateau, the net influx of Ca^{++} through Ca^{++} channels is balanced by the efflux of K^+ through i_K, i_{K1}, and i_{to} channels. Phase 3, The chemical forces that favor the efflux of K^+ through i_K, i_{K1}, and i_{to} channels predominate over the electrostatic forces that favor the influx of K^+ through these same channels. Phase 4, The chemical forces that favor the efflux of K^+ through i_K and i_{K1} channels exceed very slightly the electrostatic forces that favor the influx of K^+ through these same channels.

concentration (Figure 2-12). This brief efflux of positively charged ions brings about the brief, limited repolarization (phase 1).

Phase 1 is prominent in Purkinje fibers (Figure 2-3) and in epicardial fibers from the ventricular myocardium (Figure 2-13); it is much less developed in endocardial fibers. When the basic cycle length at which the epicardial fibers are stimulated is increased from 300 to 2000 ms, phase 1 becomes more pronounced and the action potential duration is increased substantially. The same increase in basic cycle length has no effect on the early portion of the plateau in endocardial fibers, and it has a smaller effect on the action potential duration than it does in epicardial fibers (Figure 2-13).

Genesis of the Plateau During the plateau (phase 2) of the action potential, Ca^{++} enters the cell through calcium channels that activate and inactivate much more slowly than do the fast Na^+ channels. During the flat portion of phase 2 (Figure 2-12), this influx of positive charge (carried by Ca^{++}) is balanced by the efflux of an equal amount of positive charge (carried by K^+). The K^+ exits through various specific K^+ channels, as described in the next section.

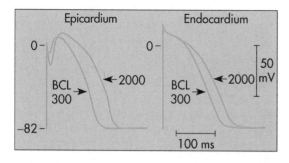

Figure 2-13 ■ **Action potentials recorded from canine epicardial and endocardial strips driven at basic cycle lengths of 300 and 2000 ms.** (From Litovsky SH, Antzelevitch C: *J Am Coll Cardiol* 14:1053, 1989.)

Ca^{++} Conductance During the Plateau The Ca^{++} channels are voltage-regulated channels that are activated as V_m becomes progressively less negative during the upstroke of the action potential. Two types of Ca^{++} channels (**L-type** and **T-type**) have been identified in cardiac tissues. Some of their important characteristics are illustrated in Figure 2-14, which displays the Ca^{++} currents generated by voltage-clamping an isolated atrial myocyte. Note that when V_m is suddenly increased to +30 mV from a holding potential of −30 mV *(lower panel),* an inward Ca^{++} current (denoted by a downward deflection) is activated. Note also that after the inward current reaches its maximal value (in the downward direction), it returns toward zero very gradually (i.e., the channel inactivates very slowly). Thus the current that passes through these channels is **long lasting,** and they have therefore been designated L-type channels. They are the predominant type of Ca^{++} channels in the heart, and they are activated during the action potential upstroke when V_m reaches about −10 mV. The L-type channels are blocked by the so-called **Ca^{++} channel antagonists,** such as verapamil, nifedipine, and diltiazem.

The T-type (transient) Ca^{++} channels are much less abundant in the heart. They are activated at more negative potentials (about −70 mV) than are the L-type channels. Note in Figure 2-14 *(upper panel)* that when V_m is suddenly increased to −20 mV from a holding potential of −80 mV, a Ca^{++} current is activated and then is inactivated very quickly.

Opening of the Ca^{++} channels is reflected by an increase in Ca^{++} conductance (g_{Ca}), which begins immediately after the upstroke of the action potential (Figure 2-15). Because the intracellular Ca^{++} concentration is much less than the extracellular Ca^{++} concentration (Table 2-1), when the Ca^{++} channels open, Ca^{++} enters the cell throughout the plateau. The Ca^{++} that enters the myocardial cell during the pla-

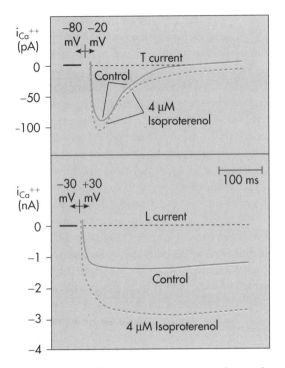

Figure 2-14 ■ **Effects of isoproterenol on the Ca^{++} currents conducted by T-type *(upper panel)* and L-type *(lower panel)* Ca^{++} channels in canine atrial myocytes.** *Upper panel,* Potential changed from −80 to −20 mV; *lower panel,* potential changed from −30 to +30 mV. (Redrawn from Bean BP: *J Gen Physiol* 86:1, 1985.)

teau is involved in **excitation-contraction coupling,** as described in Chapter 3.

Various factors may influence g$_{Ca}$. An increase in g$_{Ca}$ by **catecholamines,** such as **isoproterenol** and **norepinephrine,** is probably the principal mechanism by which catecholamines enhance cardiac muscle contractility. Catecholamines interact with β-**adrenergic receptors** located in the cardiac cell membranes. This interaction stimulates the membrane-bound enzyme, **adenylyl cyclase,** which raises the intracellular concentration of **cyclic AMP** (see Figure 3-5). This change enhances the activation of the L-type Ca^{++} channels in the cell membrane (see Figure 2-14, *lower panel*) and thus augments the influx of Ca^{++} into the cells from the interstitial fluid. However, catecholamines do not affect the Ca^{++} current through the T-type channels (see Figure 2-14, *upper panel*).

K$^+$ Conductance During the Plateau During the plateau of the action potential, the concentration gradient for K$^+$ between the inside and outside of the cell is virtually the same as it is during phase 4, but the V$_m$ is positive. Therefore the chemical and electrostatic forces greatly favor the efflux of K$^+$ from the cell during the plateau (see Figure 2-12). If g$_K$ were the

Figure 2-15 ■ **Changes in the conductances (B) of Na$^+$ *(gNa),* Ca^{++} *(gCa),* and K$^+$ *(gK)* during the various phases of the action potential (A) of a fast-response cardiac cell.** The conductance diagram shows directional changes only.

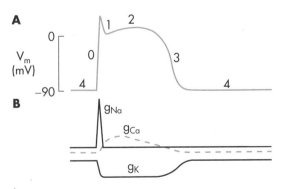

BOX 2-2

The Ca^{++} channel antagonists decrease g_{Ca}. By reducing the amount of Ca^{++} that enters the myocardial cells during phase 2, these drugs diminish the strength of the cardiac contraction (Figure 2-16). Despite this direct depressant effect of the Ca^{++} channel antagonists on the contractile strength of the heart, these agents are used widely in the treatment of **congestive heart failure,** a common clinical condition in which the heart is unable to generate enough blood flow to meet the needs of the tissues. These drugs also diminish the contraction of the vascular smooth muscle, and thereby induce generalized vasodilation. This reduces the counterforce **(afterload)** that opposes the propulsion of blood from the ventricles into the arterial system, as explained in Chapters 3 and 4. Hence vasodilator drugs, such as the Ca^{++} channel antagonists, are often referred to as **afterload reducing drugs.** This ability to diminish the counterforce enables the heart to provide a more adequate cardiac output, despite the direct depressant effect that these drugs exert on myocardial fibers.

same during the plateau as it is during phase 4, the efflux of K^+ during phase 2 would greatly exceed the influx of Ca^{++}, and a plateau could not be sustained. However, as V_m approaches and attains positive values near the end of phase 0, g_K suddenly decreases (see Figure 2-15).

The changes in g_K during the different phases of the action potential may be appreciated by examining the current-voltage relationship for the i_{K1} channels (the channels that mainly determine g_K during phase 4). An example of this relationship in an isolated ventricular myocyte is shown in Figure 2-5. Note that the current-voltage curve intersects the voltage axis at a V_m of about -70 mV. The absence of ionic current flow at the intersection indicates that the electrostatic forces must have been equal to the chemical (diffusional) forces (Figure 2-4) at this potential. Thus in this isolated ventricular cell, the Nernst equilibrium potential (E_K) for K^+ was -70 mV; in a myocyte in the intact ventricle, E_K is normally about -95 mV.

When the membrane potential was clamped at levels negative to -70 mV in this isolated cell (Figure 2-5), the electrostatic forces exceeded the chemical forces and an inward K^+ current was induced (as denoted by the negative values of K^+ current over this range of voltages). Note also that for V_m more negative than -70 mV, the curve has a steep slope. Thus when V_m equals or is negative to E_K, a small change in V_m induces a substantial change in K^+ current; that is, g_K is large. During phase 4, the V_m of a myocardial cell is slightly less negative than E_K (see Figure 2-6).

When the transmembrane potential of this isolated myocyte was clamped at levels less negative than -70 mV (see Figure 2-5), the chemical forces exceeded the electrostatic forces. Therefore the net K^+ currents were outward (as denoted by the positive values along the corresponding section of the Y axis).

During phase 4 of the cardiac cycle, the driving force for K^+ (the difference between V_m and E_K) favored the efflux of K^+, mainly through the i_{K1} channels. Note that for V_m values positive to -70 mV, the curve is relatively flat; this is especially pronounced for values of V_m positive to -40 mV. A given change in voltage causes only a small change in ionic current (i.e., g_K is small). Thus g_K is small for outwardly directed K^+ currents but substantial for inwardly directed K^+ currents; i.e., the i_{K1} current is **inwardly rectified.** The rectification is most marked over the plateau (phase 2) range of transmembrane potentials (see Figure 2-5). *This characteristic prevents excessive loss of K^+ during the prolonged plateau, during which the electrostatic and chemical forces both favor the efflux of K^+.*

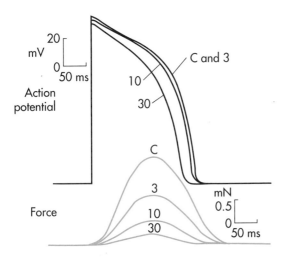

Figure 2-16 ■ **The effects of diltiazem, a Ca^{++} channel blocking drug, on the action potentials (in millivolts) and isometric contractile forces (in millinewtons) recorded from an isolated papillary muscle of a guinea pig. The tracings were recorded under control conditions (C) and in the presence of diltiazem, in concentrations of 3, 10, and 30 μmol/L.** (Redrawn from Hirth C, Borchard U, Hafner D: *J Mol Cell Cardiol* 15:799, 1983.)

The **delayed rectifier K$^+$ channels,** which conduct the i_K current, are also activated at voltages that prevail toward the end of phase 0. However, activation proceeds very slowly, over several hundreds of milliseconds. Hence activation of these channels tends to increase g_K very slowly and slightly during phase 2. These channels play only a minor role during phase 2, but they do contribute to repolarization (phase 3), as described in the next section. The action potential plateau persists as long as the efflux of charge carried by certain cations (mainly K$^+$) is balanced by the influx of charge carried by other cations (mainly Ca^{++}). The effects of altering this balance are demonstrated by administration of a calcium channel antagonist. Figure 2-16 shows that with increasing concentrations of diltiazem, the voltage of the plateau becomes less positive, and the duration of the plateau di-

minishes. Similarly, administration of certain K$^+$ channel antagonists prolongs the action potential substantially.

Genesis of Final Repolarization The process of final repolarization (phase 3) starts at the end of phase 2, when the efflux of K$^+$ from the cardiac cell begins to exceed the influx of Ca^{++}. At least three outward K$^+$ currents (i_{to}, i_K, and i_{K1}) bring about the rapid repolarization (phase 3) of the cardiac cell (see Figure 2-12).

The transient outward current (i_{to}) not only accounts for the brief, partial repolarization (phase 1), as previously described, but it also helps determine the duration of the plateau; hence it also helps initiate repolarization. For example, the transient outward current is much more pronounced in atrial than in ventricular myocytes. In atrial cells, therefore, the outward K$^+$ current exceeds the inward Ca^{++} current early in the plateau, whereas the outward and inward currents remain equal for a much longer time in ventricular myocytes. Hence the plateau of the action potential is much less pronounced in atrial than in ventricular myocytes (Figure 2-17).

The delayed rectifier K$^+$ current (i_K) is activated near the end of phase 0, but activation is very slow. Therefore the outward i_K current tends to increase gradually throughout the plateau. Concurrently, the Ca^{++} channels are inactivated after the beginning of the plateau, and therefore the inward Ca current decreases. As the efflux of K$^+$ begins to exceed the influx of Ca^{++}, V_m becomes progressively less positive, and repolarization is initiated. Two types of delayed rectifier K$^+$ currents, I_K, are present in cardiac myocytes. The distinction is based mainly on the speed of activation. The currents that activate more rapidly are designated I_{Kr}, whereas the currents that are activated more slowly are designated I_{Ks}. The action potentials recorded from myocytes in the endocardial, central, and epicardial regions of the left ventricle differ substantially in duration. Figure 2-13 illustrates

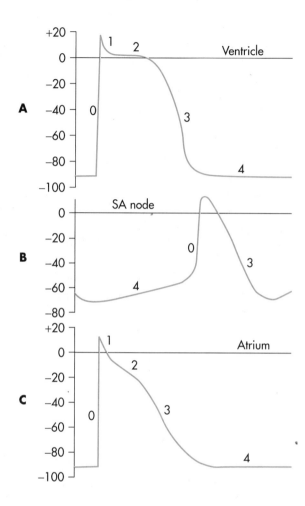

Figure 2-17 ▪ **Typical action potentials (in millivolts) recorded from cells in the ventricle** (A), **SA node** (B), **and atrium** (C). **Sweep velocity in** B **is one half that in** A **or** C.

some of the differences that prevail in the epicardial and endocardial layers of the ventricle. Such differences are induced, at least in part, by differences in the distributions of these two types of I_K channels.

The **inwardly rectified K+ current** (i_{K1}) contributes substantially to repolarization. As the net efflux of cations causes V_m to become more negative during phase 3, the conductance

of the channels that carry the i_{K1} current progressively increases. This is reflected by the hump that is evident in the flat portion of the current-voltage curve at V_m values between -20 and -70 mV in Figure 2-5. Thus as V_m passes through this range of values less negative than E_K, the outward K+ current increases and thereby accelerates repolarization.

Restoration of Ionic Concentrations The excess Na+ that entered the cell rapidly during phase 0 and more slowly throughout the action potential is removed from the cell by the action of the enzyme Na+,K+-ATPase. This enzyme ejects Na+ in exchange for the K+ that had exited mainly during phases 2 and 3.

Similarly, most of the excess Ca++ that had entered the cell during phase 2 is eliminated by an Na+/Ca++ exchanger, which exchanges 3 Na+ for 1 Ca++. However, a small fraction of the Ca++ is eliminated by an ATP-driven Ca++ pump (see Figure 3-5).

Ionic Basis of the Slow Response

Fast-response action potentials (see Figure 2-1, *A*) may be considered to consist of four principal components: an upstroke (phase 0), an early repolarization (phase 1), a plateau (phase 2), and a period of final repolarization (phase 3). In the slow response (see Figure 2-1, *B*), phase 0 is much less steep, phase 1 is absent, phase 2 is brief and not flat, and phase 3 is not separated very distinctly from phase 2. In the fast response, the upstroke is produced by the influx of Na+ through the fast channels (see Figure 2-15). These channels can be blocked by certain compounds, such as tetrodotoxin.

When the fast Na+ channels are blocked, slow responses may be generated in the same fibers under appropriate conditions. The Purkinje fiber action potentials shown in Figure 2-3 clearly exhibit the two response types. In the control tracing (panel *A*), a prominent notch (phase 1) separates the upstroke from the plateau. Action potential *A* in Figure 2-3 is a typical fast-response action potential. In action potentials B to E, progressively larger quantities of tetrodotoxin were added to the bathing solution to gradually block the fast Na^+ channels. It is evident that the sharp upstroke becomes progressively less prominent in action potentials B to D, and it disappears entirely in E. Thus the tetrodotoxin had a pronounced effect on the steep upstroke, and only a negligible influence on the plateau. With elimination of the steep upstroke (panel E), the action potential resembles a typical slow response.

Certain cells in the heart, notably those in the SA and AV nodes, are normally slow-response fibers. In such fibers, depolarization is achieved by the inward current of Ca^{++} through the Ca^{++} channels. These ionic events closely resemble those that occur during the plateau of fast-response action potentials.

■ CONDUCTION IN CARDIAC FIBERS DEPENDS ON LOCAL CIRCUIT CURRENTS

The propagation of an action potential traveling down a cardiac muscle fiber by local circuit currents is similar to the process that occurs in nerve and skeletal muscle fibers. In Figure 2-18, consider that the left half of the cardiac fiber has already been depolarized, whereas the right half

is still in the resting state. The fluids normally in contact with the external and internal surfaces of the membrane are essentially solutions of electrolytes and thus are good conductors of electricity. Hence current (in the abstract sense) flows from regions of higher potential to those of lower potential, denoted by the plus and minus signs, respectively. In the external fluid, current flows from right to left between the active and resting zones, and it flows in the reverse direction intracellularly. In electrolyte solutions, the true current is carried by a movement of cations in one direction and anions in the opposite direction. At the cell exterior, for example, cations will flow from right to left, and anions from left to right (Figure 2-18). In the cell interior, the opposite migrations occur. These local currents tend to depolarize the region of the resting fibers adjacent to the border. Repetition of this process constitutes propagation of the excitation wave along the length of the cardiac fiber.

Conduction of the Fast Response

In the fast response, the fast Na^+ channels are activated when the transmembrane potential is suddenly brought from a resting value of about −90 mV to the threshold value of about −70 mV. The inward Na^+ current then depolarizes the cell very rapidly at that site. This portion of the fiber becomes part of the depolarized zone, and the border is displaced accordingly (to the right in Figure 2-18). The same process then begins at the new border.

At any given point on the fiber, the greater the **amplitude** of the action potential and the greater the **rate of change of potential** (dV_m/dt) during phase 0, the more rapid is the conduction down the fiber. The amplitude of the action potential equals the difference in potential between the fully depolarized and the fully polarized regions of the cell interior (Figure 2-18). The magnitude of the local currents is proportional to this potential difference. Because these local currents shift the potential

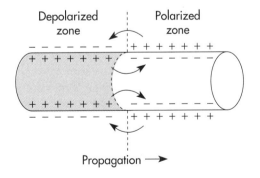

Figure 2-18 ■ The role of local currents in the propagation of a wave of excitation down a cardiac fiber.

of the resting zone toward the threshold value, they are the local stimuli that depolarize the adjacent resting portion of the fiber to its threshold potential. *The greater the potential difference between the depolarized and polarized regions* (i.e., the greater the amplitude of the action potential), *the more efficacious are the local stimuli, and the more rapidly the wave of depolarization is propagated down the fiber.*

The rate of change of potential (dV_m/dt) during phase 0 is also an important determinant of the conduction velocity. The reason can be appreciated by referring again to Figure 2-18. If the active portion of the fiber depolarized very gradually, the local currents across the border between the depolarized and polarized regions would be very small. Thus the resting region adjacent to the active zone would be depolarized very slowly, and consequently each new section of the fiber would require more time to reach threshold.

The level of the resting membrane potential is also an important determinant of conduction velocity. This factor operates through its influence on the amplitude and maximal slope of the action potential. The resting potential may vary for several reasons: (1) it can be altered experimentally by varying $[K^+]_o$ (see Figure 2-6); (2) in cardiac fibers that are intrinsically automatic, V_m becomes progressively less negative during phase 4 (see Figure 2-17, *B*); and (3) dur-

ing a premature contraction, repolarization may not have been completed when the next excitation arrives (Figure 2-10). In general, the less negative the level of V_m, the less is the velocity of impulse propagation, regardless of the reason for the change in V_m.

The results of an experiment in which the resting V_m of a bundle of Purkinje fibers was varied by altering the value of $[K^+]_o$ are shown in Figure 2-19. When $[K^+]_o$ was 3 mM (panels *A* and *F*), the resting V_m was −82 mV and the slope of phase 0 was steep. At the end of phase 0, the overshoot attained a value of 30 mV. Hence the amplitude of the action potential was 112 mV. The fiber bundle was stimulated at some distance from the impaled cell, and the stimulus artifact (St) appears as a diphasic deflection just before phase 0. The time from this artifact to the beginning of phase 0 is inversely proportional to the conduction velocity.

When $[K^+]_o$ was increased gradually to 16 mM (panels *B* to *E*), the resting V_m became progressively less negative. Concomitantly, the amplitudes and durations of the action potentials and the steepness of the upstrokes all diminished. As a consequence, the conduction velocity diminished progressively, as indicated by the distances from the stimulus artifacts to the upstrokes.

At the $[K^+]_o$ levels of 14 and 16 mM (panels *D* and *E*), the resting V_m had attained levels sufficient to inactivate all the fast Na^+ channels.

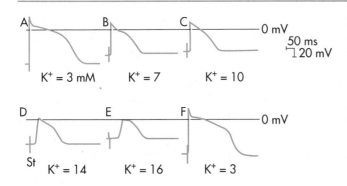

Figure 2-19 ■ **The effect of changes in external potassium concentration on the transmembrane action potentials recorded from a Purkinje fiber. The stimulus artifact *(St)* appears as a biphasic spike to the left of the upstroke of the action potential. The horizontal lines near the peaks of the action potentials denote 0 mV.** (From Myerburg RJ, Lazzara R. In Fisch E, editor: *Complex electrocardiography,* Philadelphia, 1973, FA Davis.)

BOX 2-3

Most of the experimentally induced changes in transmembrane potential shown in Figure 2-19 also take place in patients with **coronary artery disease.** When blood flow to a region of the myocardium is diminished, the supply of oxygen and metabolic substrates delivered to the ischemic tissues is insufficient. The Na^+,K^+-ATPase in the membrane of the cardiac myocytes requires considerable metabolic energy to maintain the normal transmembrane exchanges of Na^+ and K^+. When blood flow is inadequate, the activity of the Na^+,K^+-ATPase is impaired, and the ischemic myocytes gain excess Na^+ and lose K^+ to the surrounding interstitial space. Consequently, the K^+ concentration in the extracellular fluid surrounding the ischemic myocytes is elevated, and therefore the myocytes are affected by the elevated K^+ concentration in much the same way as was the myocyte depicted in Figure 2-19. Such changes may lead to serious aberrations of cardiac rhythm and conduction.

The action potentials in panels D and E are characteristic slow responses, presumably mediated by the inward current of Ca^{++}. When the $[K^+]_o$ concentration of 3 mM was reestablished (panel F), the action potential was again characteristic of the normal fast response (as in panel A).

Conduction of the Slow Response

Local circuits (see Figure 2-18) are also responsible for propagation of the slow response. However, the characteristics of the conduction process differ quantitatively from those of the fast response. The threshold potential is about -40 mV for the slow response, and conduction is much slower than for the fast response. The conduction velocities of the slow responses in the SA and AV nodes are about 0.02 to 0.1 m/s. The fast-response conduction velocities are about 0.3 to 1 m/s for myocardial cells and 1 to 4 m/s for the specialized conducting fibers in the atria and ventricles. Conduction in slow response fibers is more likely to be blocked than is conduction in fast response fibers. Also, impulses in slow response fibers cannot be conducted at such rapid repetition rates.

■ CARDIAC EXCITABILITY DEPENDS ON THE ACTIVATION AND INACTIVATION OF SPECIFIC CURRENTS

Currently, detailed knowledge of cardiac excitability is essential because of the rapid development of artificial pacemakers and other electrical devices for correcting serious disturbances of rhythm. The excitability characteristics of cardiac cells differ considerably, depending on whether the action potentials are fast or slow responses.

Fast Response

Once the fast response has been initiated, the depolarized cell will no longer be excitable until about the middle of the period of final repolarization (see Figure 2-1, A). The interval from the beginning of the action potential until the fiber is able to conduct another action potential is called the **effective refractory period.** In the fast response, this period extends from the beginning of phase 0 to a point in phase 3 where repolarization has reached about -50 mV (time c to time d in Figure 2-1, A). At about this value of V_m the fast channels have recovered sufficiently from inactivation to permit a feeble response to stimulation.

Full excitability is not regained until the cardiac fiber has been fully repolarized (time e in Figure 2-1, A). During period d to e in the figure, an action potential may be evoked, but only when the stimulus is stronger than that which could elicit a response during phase 4. Period d to e is called the **relative refractory period.**

When a fast response is evoked during the relative refractory period of a previous excitation, its characteristics vary with the membrane potential that exists at the time of stimulation. The nature of this voltage dependency is illustrated in Figure 2-10. As the fiber is stimulated later and later in the relative refractory period, the amplitude of the response and the rate of rise of the upstroke increase progressively. As a consequence of the greater amplitude and upstroke slope of the evoked response, the propagation velocity increases as the cell is stimulated later in the relative refractory period. Once the fiber is fully repolarized, the response is constant no matter what time in phase 4 the stimulus is applied. By the end of phase 3, the fast Na^+ channels have recovered fully from inactivation.

Slow Response

The relative refractory period during the slow response frequently extends well beyond phase 3 (see Figure 2-1, *B*). Even after the cell has completely repolarized, it may be difficult to evoke a propagated response for some time. This characteristic is called **postrepolarization refractoriness.**

Action potentials evoked early in the relative refractory period are small, and the upstrokes are not very steep (Figure 2-20). The amplitudes and upstroke slopes gradually improve as action potentials are elicited later and later in the relative refractory period. The recovery of full excitability is much slower than for the fast response. Impulses that arrive early in the relative refractory period are conducted much more slowly than those that arrive late in that period. The lengthy refractory periods also lead to conduction blocks. Even when slow responses recur at a low repetition rate, the fiber may be able to conduct only a fraction of those impulses.

Effects of Cycle Length

Changes in cycle length alter the action potential duration of cardiac cells and thus change their refractory periods. Consequently, the

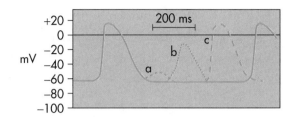

Figure 2-20 ■ **The effects of excitation at various times after the initiation of an action potential in a slow-response fiber. In this fiber, excitation very late in phase 3 (or early in phase 4) induces a small, nonpropagated (local) response** *(a)***. Later in phase 4, a propagated response** *(b)* **may be elicited; its amplitude is small and the upstroke is not very steep. This response, which displays postrepolarization refractoriness, will be conducted very slowly. Still later in phase 4, full excitability will be regained, and the response** *(c)* **will display its normal characteristics.** (Modified from Singer DH, Baumgarten CM, Ten Eick RE, et al: *Prog Cardiovasc Dis* 24:97, 1981.)

changes in cycle length are often important factors in the initiation or termination of certain dysrhythmias. The changes in action potential durations produced by stepwise reductions in cycle length from 2000 to 200 ms in a Purkinje fiber are shown in Figure 2-21. Note that as the cycle length is diminished, the action potential duration decreases.

This direct correlation between action potential duration and cycle length is ascribable mainly to changes in g_K that involve the delayed rectifier K^+ channels. The i_K current activates slowly, remains activated for hundreds of milliseconds before it is inactivated, and inactivates very slowly. Consequently, as the basic cycle length is diminished, each action potential tends to occur earlier in the inactivation period of the i_K current initiated by the preceding action potential. Therefore the shorter the basic cycle length, the greater the outward K^+ current will be during phase 2. Hence the action potential duration diminishes.

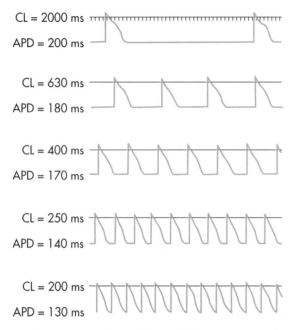

CL = 2000 ms
APD = 200 ms

CL = 630 ms
APD = 180 ms

CL = 400 ms
APD = 170 ms

CL = 250 ms
APD = 140 ms

CL = 200 ms
APD = 130 ms

Figure 2-21 ■ **The effect of changes in cycle length *(CL)* on the action potential duration *(APD)* of canine Purkinje fibers.** (Modified from Singer D, Ten Eick RE: *Am J Cardiol* 28:381, 1971.)

■ THE HEART GENERATES ITS OWN PACEMAKING ACTIVITY

The nervous system controls various aspects of cardiac behavior, including the frequency at which the heart beats and the vigor of each contraction. However, cardiac function certainly does not require intact nervous pathways. Indeed, a patient with a completely denervated heart (a cardiac transplant patient) can adapt well to stressful situations.

The properties of **automaticity** (the ability of the heart to initiate its own beat) and of **rhythmicity** (the regularity of such pacemaking activity) are intrinsic to cardiac tissue. *The heart continues to beat even when it is completely removed from the body.* If the coronary vasculature is artificially perfused, rhythmic cardiac contraction will persist for many hours. Apparently, at least some cells in the walls of all

four cardiac chambers are capable of initiating beats; such cells reside mainly in the nodal tissues or specialized conducting fibers of the heart.

The region of the mammalian heart that ordinarily generates impulses at the greatest frequency is the SA node; it is the **natural pacemaker** of the heart.

Detailed mapping of the electrical potentials on the surface of the right atrium has revealed that two or three sites of automaticity, located 1 or 2 cm from the SA node itself, serve along with the SA node as an **atrial pacemaker complex.** At times, all of these loci initiate impulses simultaneously. At other times, the site of earliest excitation shifts from locus to locus, depending on such conditions as the level of autonomic neural activity.

Ectopic pacemakers may serve as a safety mechanism when the normal pacemaking centers cease functioning. However, if an ectopic center fires while the normal pacemaking center still functions, the ectopic activity may induce either sporadic rhythm disturbances, such as **premature depolarizations,** or continuous rhythm disturbances, such as **paroxysmal tachycardias.** These **dysrhythmias** are discussed at the end of this chapter.

When the SA node and the other components of the atrial pacemaker complex are excised or destroyed, pacemaker cells in the AV node usually become the pacemakers for the entire heart. After some time, which may vary from minutes to days, automatic cells in the atria usually become dominant.

Purkinje fibers that comprise the specialized conduction system of the ventricles also possess automaticity. Characteristically, they fire at a very slow rate. When the AV junction is unable to conduct the cardiac impulse from the atria to the ventricles, **idioventricular pacemakers** in the Purkinje fiber network initiate the ventricular contractions. Such contractions occur at a frequency of only 30 to 40 beats per minute. These low frequencies are usually not sufficient to allow the heart to pump an adequate cardiac output.

Regions of the heart other than the SA node may initiate beats under special circumstances; such sites are called **ectopic foci,** or **ectopic pacemakers.** Ectopic foci may become pacemakers when (1) their own rhythmicity becomes enhanced, (2) the rhythmicity of the higher-order pacemakers becomes depressed, or (3) all conduction pathways are blocked between the ectopic focus and those regions with greater rhythmicity.

Sinoatrial Node

The SA node is the phylogenetic remnant of the sinus venosus of lower vertebrate hearts. In humans it is about 8 mm long and 2 mm thick. It lies in the groove where the superior vena cava joins the right atrium (Figure 2-22). The sinus node artery runs lengthwise through the center of the node.

The SA node contains two principal types of cells: (1) small, round cells, which have few organelles and myofibrils, and (2) slender, elongated cells, which are intermediate in appearance between the round and the ordinary atrial myocardial cells. The round cells are probably the pacemaker cells, whereas the transitional cells probably conduct the impulses within the node and to the nodal margins.

A typical transmembrane action potential recorded from a cell in the SA node is depicted in Figure 2-17, *B.* Compared with the transmembrane potential recorded from a ventricular myocardial cell (Figure 2-17, *A*), the resting potential of the SA node cell is usually less, the up-

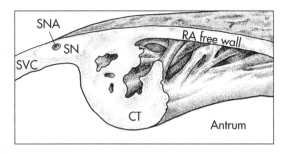

Figure 2-22 ■ **The location of the SA node** *(SN)* **near the junction between the superior vena cava** *(SVC)* **and right atrium** *(RA).* **SNA, Sinoatrial artery; CT, crista terminalis.** (Redrawn from James TN: *Am J Cardiol* 40:965, 1977.)

stroke of the action potential (phase 0) is less steep, a plateau is not sustained, and repolarization (phase 3) is more gradual. These are all characteristic of the slow response.

The transmembrane potential during phase 4 is much less negative in SA (and AV) nodal automatic cells than in atrial or ventricular myocytes because the i_{K1} type of K^+ channel is very sparse in the nodal cells. Therefore the ratio of g_K/g_{Na} during phase 4 is much less in the nodal cells than in the myocytes. Hence during phase 4, V_m approaches the K^+ equilibrium potential (E_K) much more closely in myocytes than it does in nodal cells.

Under ordinary conditions, tetrodotoxin has no influence on the SA nodal action potential. This indicates that the upstroke of the action potential is not produced by an inward current of Na^+ through the fast channels.

However, the principal distinguishing feature of a pacemaker fiber resides in phase 4. In nonautomatic cells the potential remains constant during this phase, whereas in a pacemaker fiber there is a slow depolarization, called the **pacemaker potential,** throughout phase 4. Depolarization proceeds at a steady rate until a threshold is attained, and then an action potential is triggered.

The discharge frequency of pacemaker cells may be varied either by a change in the rate of depolarization during phase 4 or the maximal diastolic potential (Figure 2-23). With a decrease in the rate of depolarization (*1* to *2* in Figure 2-23, *A*) the threshold potential is attained later, and the heart rate decreases. When the diastolic potential at the end of phase 3 becomes more negative (from *3* to *4* in Figure 2-23, *B*), more time is required to reach threshold, and the heart rate diminishes.

Changes in autonomic neural activity often also induce a **pacemaker shift,** where the site of initiation of the cardiac impulse may shift to a different locus within the SA node or to a different component of the atrial pacemaker complex.

Ionic Basis of Automaticity

Several ionic currents contribute to the slow depolarization that occurs during phase 4 in automatic cells in the heart. In the pacemaker cells of the SA node, the diastolic depolarization is mediated by at least three ionic currents: (1) an inward current, i_f, induced by hyperpolariza-

tion; (2) a calcium current, i_{Ca}; and (3) an outward K^+ current, i_K (Figure 2-24).

The inward hyperpolarization current, i_f, is carried mainly by Na^+; the current is conducted through specific channels that differ from the fast Na^+ channels. This hyperpolarization cur-

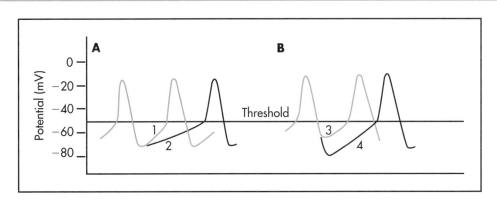

Figure 2-23 ■ **Mechanisms involved in changes of frequency of pacemaker firing. A, A reduction in the slope of the pacemaker potential from *1* to *2* will diminish the frequency.** B, **An increase in the maximum negativity at the end of repolarization (from *3* to *4*) will also diminish the frequency.**

rent becomes activated during the repolarization phase of the action potential, as the membrane potential becomes more negative than about −50 mV. The more negative the membrane potential becomes at the end of repolarization, the greater the activation of the i_f current becomes.

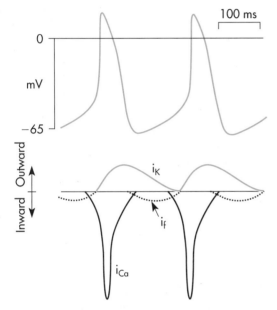

Figure 2-24 ■ **The transmembrane potential changes** *(top half)* **that occur in SA node cells are produced by three principal currents** *(bottom half):* **(1) the current, i_{Ca}; (2) a hyperpolarization-induced inward current, i_f; and (3) an outward K⁺ current, i_K.** (Redrawn from Brown HF: *Physiol Rev* 61:644, 1981.)

The second current responsible for diastolic depolarization is the calcium current i_{Ca}. This current becomes activated toward the end of phase 4, as the transmembrane potential reaches a value of about −55 mV (see Figure 2-24).

Once the Ca^{++} channels become activated, the influx of Ca^{++} into the cell increases. The influx of Ca^{++} accelerates the rate of diastolic depolarization, which then leads to the upstroke of the action potential. A decrease in the external Ca^{++} concentration (Figure 2-25) or the addition of a calcium channel antagonist (Figure 2-26) diminishes the amplitude of the action potential and the slope of the pacemaker potential in SA node cells.

The progressive diastolic depolarization mediated by the two inward currents, i_f and i_{Ca}, is opposed by a third current, an outward K⁺ current, i_K. This efflux of K⁺ tends to repolarize the cell after the upstroke of the action potential. The outward K⁺ current continues well beyond the time of maximal repolarization, but it diminishes throughout phase 4 (see Figure 2-24). Hence the opposition of i_K to the depolarizing effects of the two inward currents (i_{Ca} and i_f) gradually decreases.

The ionic basis for automaticity in the AV node pacemaker cells is identical to that in the SA node cells. Similar mechanisms also account for automaticity in Purkinje fibers, except that the calcium current is not involved. Hence the **slow diastolic depolarization** is mediated principally by the imbalance between the

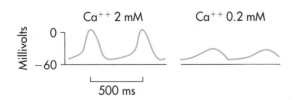

Figure 2-25 ■ **Transmembrane action potentials recorded from an SA node pacemaker cell in an isolated rabbit atrium preparation. The concentration of Ca^{++} in the bath was changed from 2 to 0.2 mM.** (Modified from Kohlhardt M, Figulla HR, Tripathi O: *Basic Res Cardiol* 71:17, 1976.)

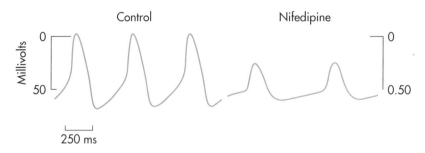

Figure 2-26 ■ **The effects of nifedipine (5.6×10^{-7} M), a Ca^{++} channel antagonist, on the transmembrane potentials recorded from a rabbit SA node cell.** (From Ning W, Wit AL: *Am Heart J* 106:345, 1983.)

hyperpolarization-induced inward current, i_f, and the outward K^+ current, i_K.

The autonomic neurotransmitters affect automaticity by altering the ionic currents across the cell membranes. The adrenergic transmitters increase all three currents involved in SA nodal automaticity. The adrenergically mediated increase in the slope of diastolic depolarization indicates that the augmentations of i_f and i_{Ca} must exceed the enhancement of i_K.

The hyperpolarization (Figure 2-27) induced by the acetylcholine released at the vagus endings in the heart is achieved by an increase in g_K. This change in conductance is mediated through activation of specific K^+ channels that are controlled by the cholinergic receptors. Acetylcholine also depresses the i_f and i_{Ca} currents.

Overdrive Suppression

The automaticity of pacemaker cells becomes depressed after a period of excitation at a high frequency. This phenomenon is known as **overdrive suppression.** Because of the greater intrinsic rhythmicity of the SA node than of the other latent pacemaking sites in the heart, the firing of the SA node tends to suppress the automaticity in the other loci.

The mechanism responsible for overdrive suppression appears to be based on the activity

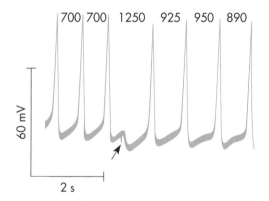

Figure 2-27 ■ **Effect of a brief vagal stimulus (*arrow*) on the transmembrane potential recorded from an SA node pacemaker cell in an isolated cat atrium preparation. The cardiac cycle lengths, in milliseconds, are denoted by the numbers at the top of the figure.** (Modified from Jalife J, Moe GK: *Circ Res* 45:595, 1979.)

of the membrane pump $(Na^+,K^+\text{-ATPase})$, which actively extrudes Na^+ from the cell, in partial exchange for K^+. During each depolarization, a certain quantity of Na^+ enters the cell; therefore the more frequently it is depolarized, the greater is the amount of Na^+ that enters the cell per minute. At high excitation frequencies the Na^+ pump becomes more active in extruding this larger quantity of Na^+ from the cell interior. The quantity of Na^+ extruded by the pump exceeds the quantity of K^+ that enters the cell; the ratio is 3:2. This enhanced activity of the pump hyperpolarizes the cell, because of the net loss of cations from the cell interior. Because of the hyperpolarization, the slow diastolic depolarization requires more time to reach the threshold, as shown in Figure 2-23, *B*. Furthermore, when the overdrive suddenly ceases, the Na^+ pump may not decelerate instantaneously but may continue to operate at an accelerated rate for some time. This excessive extrusion of Na^+ opposes the gradual depolarization of the pacemaker cell during phase 4 and thereby suppresses its intrinsic automaticity temporarily.

BOX 2-6

If an ectopic focus in one of the atria suddenly begins to fire at a high rate (e.g., 150 impulses per minute) in an individual with a normal heart rate of 70 beats per minute, the ectopic center would become the pacemaker for the entire heart. When that rapid ectopic focus suddenly stops firing, the SA node might remain quiescent briefly because of overdrive suppression. The interval from the end of the period of overdrive until the SA node resumes firing is called the **sinus node recovery time.** In patients with the so-called **sick sinus syndrome,** the sinus node recovery time may be markedly prolonged. The resultant period of asystole (cardiac standstill) might cause loss of consciousness.

Atrial Conduction

From the SA node, the cardiac impulse spreads radially throughout the right atrium (Figure 2-28) along ordinary atrial myocardial fibers, at a conduction velocity of approximately 1 m/s. A special pathway, the **anterior interatrial myocardial band** (or **Bachmann's bundle**), conducts the impulse from the SA node directly to the left atrium. Three tracts, the **anterior, middle, and posterior internodal pathways,** have been described. These tracts consist of a mixture of ordinary myocardial cells and specialized conducting fibers. Some authorities assert that these pathways constitute the principal routes for conduction of the cardiac impulse from the SA to the AV node.

The configuration of the atrial action potential is depicted in Figure 2-17, *C*. Compared with the potential recorded from a typical ventricular fiber (see Figure 2-17, *A*), the plateau (phase 2) is not as well developed, repolarization (phase 3) occurs as a slower rate, and the duration of the action potential is shorter.

Atrioventricular Conduction

The cardiac action potential proceeds along the internodal pathways in the atrium and ultimately reaches the AV node (see Figure 2-28). This node is approximately 22 mm long, 10 mm wide, and 3 mm thick in adult humans. The node is situated posteriorly on the right side of the interatrial septum near the ostium of the coronary sinus. The AV node contains the same two cell types as the SA node, but the round cells are more sparse and the elongated cells preponderate.

The AV node is divided into three functional regions: (1) the AN region, the transitional zone between the atrium and the remainder of the node; (2) the N region, the midportion of the AV node; and (3) the NH region, the zone in which nodal fibers gradually merge with the **bundle of His,** which is the upper portion of the specialized conducting system for the ventricles. Normally, the AV node and bundle of His constitute the only pathways for conduction from atria to ventricles.

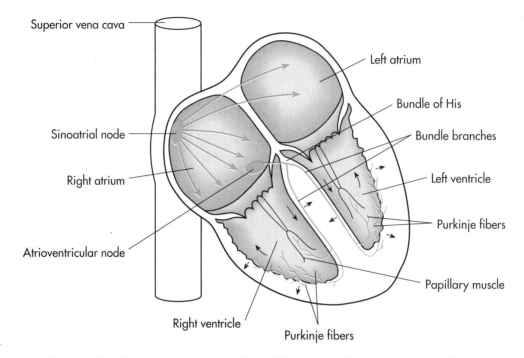

Superior vena cava

Left atrium

Bundle of His

Bundle branches

Sinoatrial node

Left ventricle

Right atrium

Purkinje fibers

Atrioventricular node

Papillary muscle

Right ventricle

Purkinje fibers

Figure 2-28 ▪ **Schematic representation of the conduction system of the heart.**

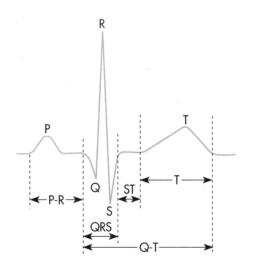

Figure 2-29 ▪ **Configuration of a typical scalar electrocardiogram, illustrating the important deflections and intervals.**

Several features of AV conduction are of physiological and clinical significance. The principal delay in the passage of the impulse from the atria to the ventricles occurs in the AN and N regions of the AV node. The conduction velocity is actually less in the N region than in the AN region. However, the path length is substantially greater in the AN region than in the N region. The conduction times through the AN and N zones account for the delay between the onsets of the **P wave** (the electrical manifestation of the spread of atrial excitation) and the **QRS complex** (spread of ventricular excitation) in the electrocardiogram (Figure 2-29). *Functionally, this delay between atrial and ventricular excitation permits optimal ventricular filling during atrial contraction.*

In the N region, slow-response action potentials prevail. The resting potential is about −60

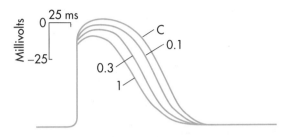

Figure 2-30 ■ **Transmembrane potentials recorded from a rabbit AV node cell under control conditions *(C)* and in the presence of the calcium channel blocking drug diltiazem in concentrations of 0.1, 0.3, and 1.0 μmol/L.** (Redrawn from Hirth C, Borchard U, Hafner D: *J Mol Cell Cardiol* 15:799, 1983.)

mV, the upstroke velocity is very low (about 5 V/s), and the conduction velocity is about 0.05 m/s. Tetrodotoxin, which blocks the fast Na^+ channels, does not affect the action potentials in this region. Conversely, the Ca^{++} channel antagonists decrease the amplitude and duration of the action potentials (Figure 2-30) and depress AV conduction. The shapes of the action potentials in the AN region are intermediate between those in the N region and atria. Similarly, the action potentials in the NH region are transitional between those in the N region and bundle of His. The relative refractory period of the cells in the N region extends well beyond

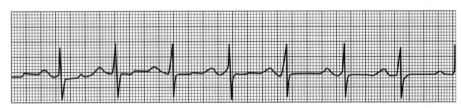

A, First-degree heart block; P-R interval is 0.28 s.

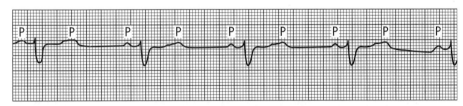

B, Second-degree heart block (2:1).

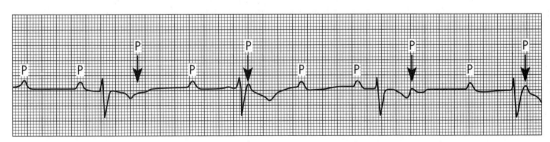

C, Third-degree heart block; note the dissociation between the P waves and the QRS complexes.

Figure 2-31 ■ **Atrioventricular (AV) blocks.**

the period of complete repolarization; i.e., these cells display postrepolarization refractoriness (see Figure 2-20).

As the repetition rate of atrial depolarizations is increased, conduction through the AV junction slows. An abnormal prolongation of AV conduction time is called **first-degree AV block** (Figure 2-31, *A*). Most of the prolongation of AV conduction induced by an increase in repetition rate takes place in the N region.

Impulses tend to be blocked in the AV node at stimulus repetition rates that are easily conducted in other regions of the heart. If the atria are depolarized at a high frequency, only a fraction (e.g., one half) of the atrial impulses might be conducted through the AV junction to the ventricles. The conduction pattern in which only a fraction of the atrial impulses are conducted to the ventricles is called **second-degree AV block** (see Figure 2-31, *B*). This type of block may protect the ventricles from excessive contraction frequencies, wherein the filling time between successive ventricular contractions might be inadequate, and therefore the ventricles would be unable to deliver an adequate cardiac output.

Retrograde conduction can occur through the AV node. However, the propagation time is significantly longer, and the impulse tends to be blocked at lower repetition rates during conduction in the retrograde than during conduction in the antegrade direction. Finally, the AV node is a common site for reentry; the underlying mechanisms are explained on pp 35 and 40.

The autonomic nervous system regulates AV conduction. Weak vagal activity may simply prolong the AV conduction time. Stronger vagal activity may cause some or all of the impulses arriving from the atria to be blocked in the node. The conduction pattern in which none of the atrial impulses reach the ventricles over a substantial number of atrial depolarizations is called

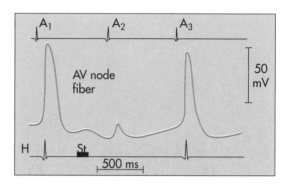

Figure 2-32 ■ **Effects of a brief vagal stimulus** *(St)* **on the transmembrane potential recorded from an AV nodal fiber from a rabbit. Note that shortly after vagal stimulation, the membrane of the fiber was hyperpolarized. The atrial excitation** *(A$_2$)* **that arrived at the AV node when the cell was hyperpolarized failed to be conducted, as denoted by the absence of a depolarization in the His electrogram** *(H)*. **The atrial excitations that preceded** *(A$_1$)* **and followed** *(A$_3$)* **excitation A$_2$ were conducted to the His bundle region.** (Redrawn from Mazgalev T, Dreifus LS, Michelson EL, et al: *Am J Physiol* 251:H631, 1986.)

third-degree, or **complete, AV block** (see Figure 2-31, *C*). The delayed conduction or block induced by vagal stimulation occurs largely in the N region of the node.

The acetylcholine released by the vagus nerve fibers hyperpolarizes the conducting fibers in the N region (Figure 2-32). The greater the hyperpolarization at the time of arrival of the atrial impulse, the more impaired the AV conduction will be. In the experiment shown in Figure 2-32, vagus nerve fibers were stimulated intensely (at St) shortly before the second atrial depolarization (A$_2$). This atrial impulse arrived at the AV node cell when its cell membrane was maximally hyperpolarized. The absence of a corresponding depolarization of the bundle of His (H) shows that the second atrial impulse was not conducted through the AV node. Only a

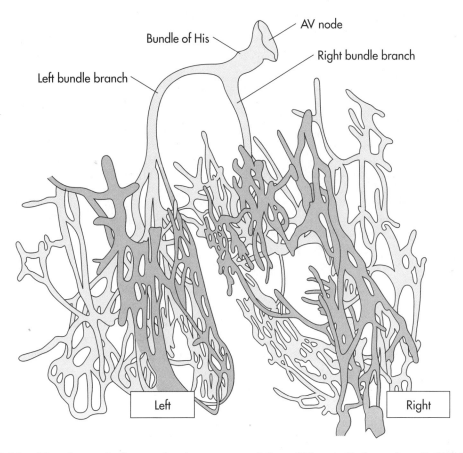

Bundle of His

AV node

Left bundle branch

Right bundle branch

Left

Right

Figure 2-33 ■ **AV and ventricular conduction system of the calf heart.** (Redrawn from DeWitt LM: *Anat Rec* 3:475, 1909.)

small, nonpropagated response to the second atrial impulse is evident in the recording from the conducting fiber.

The cardiac sympathetic nerves, on the other hand, facilitate AV conduction. They decrease AV conduction time and enhance the rhythmicity of the latent pacemakers in the AV junction. The norepinephrine released at the sympathetic nerve terminals increases the amplitude and slope of the upstroke of the AV nodal action potentials, principally in the AN and N regions of the node.

BOX 2-7

First- and second-degree AV blocks are most frequently caused by inflammatory processes (acute rheumatic fever), drugs (calcium channel antagonists), or rapid atrial rates (supraventricular tachycardias). Third-degree AV block is most often caused by a degenerative process of unknown cause or by severe myocardial ischemia (inadequate coronary blood supply).

Third-degree AV block is often referred to as **complete heart block** because the impulse is unable to traverse the AV conduction pathway from atria to ventricles. His bundle electrograms reveal that the most common sites of complete block are distal to the bundle of His. Because of the slow ventricular rhythm (32 beats per minute in this example), circulation of blood is often inadequate, especially during muscular activity. Third-degree block is often associated with syncope (so-called **Stokes-Adams attacks**) caused principally by insufficient cerebral blood flow. Third-degree block is one of the most common conditions requiring treatment by artificial pacemakers.

Impulse conduction in the right bundle branch, the main left bundle branch, or either division of the left bundle branch may be impaired as a consequence of a degenerative process or of coronary artery disease. Conduction blocks in one or more of these pathways give rise to characteristic electrocardiographic patterns. Block of either of the main bundle branches is known as right or left **bundle branch block.** Block of either division of the left bundle branch is called **left anterior hemiblock** or **left posterior hemiblock.**

Ventricular Conduction

The bundle of His passes subendocardially down the right side of the interventricular septum for about 1 cm and then divides into the right and left **bundle branches** (Figures 2-28 and 2-33). The right bundle branch is a direct continuation of the bundle of His and proceeds down the right side of the interventricular septum. The left bundle branch, which is considerably thicker than the right, arises almost perpendicularly from the bundle of His and perforates the interventricular septum. On the subendocardial surface of the left side of the interventricular septum, the main left bundle branch splits into a thin **anterior division** and a thick **posterior division.**

The right bundle branch and the two divisions of the left bundle branch ultimately subdivide into a complex network of conducting fibers called *Purkinje fibers,* which ramify over the subendocardial surfaces of both ventricles. In certain mammalian species, such as cattle, the Purkinje fiber network is arranged in discrete, encapsulated bundles (see Figure 2-33).

Purkinje fibers are the broadest cells in the heart, 70 to 80 μm in diameter, compared with 10 to 15 μm for ventricular myocytes. The large diameter accounts in part for the greater conduction velocity in Purkinje than in myocardial fibers. Purkinje cells have abundant, linearly arranged sarcomeres, just as do myocardial cells. However, the T-tubular system is absent in the Purkinje cells of many species but is well developed in the myocardial cells.

The conduction of the action potential over the Purkinje fiber system is faster than in any other of conduction velocity tissue within the heart; estimates of conduction velocity vary from 1 to 4 m/s. This permits a rapid activation of the entire endocardial surface of the ventricles.

The action potentials recorded from Purkinje fibers resemble those of ordinary ventricular myocardial fibers (see Figure 2-17, *A*). In general, phase 1 is more prominent in Purkinje fiber action potentials (see Figure 2-3) than in those recorded from ventricular fibers (especially endocardial fibers), and the duration of the plateau (phase 2) is longer.

Because of the long refractory period of the Purkinje fibers, many premature activations of the atria are conducted through the AV junc-

tion but are blocked by the Purkinje fibers. Therefore they fail to evoke a premature contraction of the ventricles. This function of protecting the ventricles against the effects of premature atrial depolarizations is especially pronounced at slow heart rates, because the action potential duration, and hence the effective refractory period of the Purkinje fibers, vary inversely with the heart rate (see Figure 2-21). At slow heart rates, the effective refractory period of the Purkinje fibers is especially prolonged; as the heart rate increases, the refractory period diminishes. Similar rate-dependent changes in the refractory period also occur in most of the other cells in the heart. However, in the AV node, the effective refractory period does not change appreciably over the normal range of heart rates, and it actually increases at very rapid heart rates. Therefore *at high heart rates, it is the AV node that protects the ventricles when atrial impulses arrive at excessive repetition rates.*

The first portions of the ventricles to be excited are the interventricular septum (except its basal portion) and the papillary muscles. The wave of activation spreads into the substance of the septum from both its left and its right endocardial surfaces. Early contraction of the septum tends to make it more rigid and allows it to serve as an anchor point for the contraction of the remaining ventricular myocardium. Also, early contraction of the papillary muscles prevents eversion of the AV valves during ventricular systole.

The endocardial surfaces of both ventricles are activated rapidly, but the wave of excitation spreads from endocardium to epicardium at a slower velocity (about 0.3 to 0.4 m/s). Because the right ventricular wall is appreciably thinner than the left, the epicardial surface of the right ventricle is activated earlier than the epicardial surface of the left ventricle. Also, apical and central epicardial regions of both ventricles are activated somewhat earlier than are their respec-

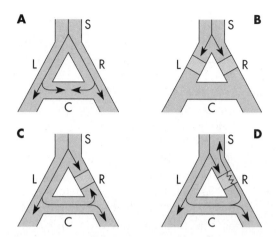

Figure 2-34 ■ **The role of unidirectional block in reentry. In panel A, an excitation wave traveling down a single bundle (S) of fibers continues down the left (L) and right (R) branches. The depolarization wave enters the connecting branch (C) from both ends and is extinguished at the zone of collision. In panel B, the wave is blocked in the L and R branches. In panel C, bidirectional block exists in branch R. In panel D, unidirectional block exists in branch R. The antegrade impulse is blocked, but the retrograde impulse is conducted through and reenters bundle S.**

tive basal regions. The last portions of the ventricles to be excited are the posterior basal epicardial regions and a small zone in the basal portion of the interventricular septum.

■ AN IMPULSE CAN TRAVEL AROUND A REENTRY LOOP

Under certain conditions, a cardiac impulse may reexcite some region through which it had passed previously. This phenomenon, known as **reentry,** is responsible for many clinical disturbances of cardiac rhythm. The reentry may be **ordered** or **random.** In the ordered variety, the impulse traverses a fixed anatomic path, whereas in the random type the path continues to change. The principal example of random reentry is **fibrillation** (p 49).

The conditions necessary for reentry are illustrated in Figure 2-34. In each of the four panels, a single bundle *(S)* of cardiac fibers splits into a left *(L)* and a right *(R)* branch. A connecting bundle *(C)* runs between the two branches. Normally, the impulse coming down bundle *S* is conducted along the *L* and *R* branches (panel *A*). As the impulse reaches connecting link *C,* it enters link *C* from both sides and becomes extinguished at the point of collision. The impulse from the left side cannot proceed further because the tissue beyond had just been depolarized from the other direction, and therefore it is absolutely refractory. The impulse cannot pass through bundle *C* from the right either, for the same reason.

Panel *B* of Figure 2-34 shows that the impulse cannot make a complete circuit if antegrade block exists in the two branches (*L* and *R*) of the fiber bundle. Furthermore, if bidirectional block exists at any point in the loop (e.g., branch *R* in panel *C*), the impulse will not be able to reenter.

A necessary condition for reentry is that at some point in the loop the impulse can pass in one direction but not in the other. This phenomenon is called **unidirectional block.** As shown in panel *D*, the impulse may travel down branch *L* normally and may be blocked in the antegrade direction in branch *R*. The impulse that had been conducted down branch *L* and through the connecting branch *C* may be able to penetrate the depressed region in branch *R* from the retrograde direction, even though the antegrade impulse had been blocked previously at this same site. The antegrade impulse arrives at the depressed region in branch *R* earlier than the impulse that traverses a longer path and enters branch *R* from the opposite direction. The antegrade impulse may be blocked simply because it arrives at the depressed region during its effective refractory period. If the retrograde impulse is delayed sufficiently, the refractory period may have ended, and the impulse will be conducted back into bundle *S.*

Unidirectional block is a necessary condition for reentry, but not a sufficient one. *The effective refractory period of the reentered region must also be less than the propagation time around the loop.* In panel *D,* if the retrograde impulse is conducted through the depressed zone in branch *R* and if the tissue just beyond is still refractory from the antegrade depolarization, branch *S* will not be reexcited. Therefore the conditions that promote reentry are those that prolong conduction time or shorten the effective refractory period.

The functional components of reentry loops responsible for specific dysrhythmias in intact hearts are diverse. Some loops are very large and involve entire specialized conduction bundles; other loops are microscopic. The loop may include myocardial fibers, specialized conducting fibers, nodal cells, and junctional tissues, in almost any conceivable arrangement. Also, the cardiac cells in the loop may be normal or deranged.

■ AFTERDEPOLARIZATIONS LEAD TO TRIGGERED ACTIVITY

Triggered activity is so named because it is always coupled to a preceding action potential. Consequently, dysrhythmias induced by triggered activity are difficult to distinguish from those induced by reentry, which is also always coupled to a previous action potential. Triggered activity is caused by **afterdepolarizations.** Two types of afterdepolarizations are recognized: **early afterdepolarizations (EADs)** and **delayed afterdepolarizations (DADs).** EADs occur at the end of the plateau (phase 2) of an action potential or about midway through repolarization (phase 3), whereas DADs occur near the very end of repolarization or just after full repolarization (phase 4).

Accessory AV pathways are present in some people. Such pathways often serve as a part of a reentry loop (Figure 2-34), which could lead to serious cardiac rhythm disturbances in these patients. The **Wolff-Parkinson-White syndrome,** a congenital disturbance, is the most common clinical disorder in which a bypass tract of myocardial fibers serves as an accessory pathway between atria and ventricles. Ordinarily, the syndrome causes no functional abnormality. It is easily detected in the electrocardiographic reading, because a portion of the ventricular myocardium is preexcited via the bypass tract. Slightly later, the normal excitation of the remainder of the ventricular myocardium via the AV node and His-Purkinje system imparts a bizarre configuration to the ventricular (QRS) complex of the **electrocardiogram.** Occasionally, however, a reentry loop develops in which the atrial impulse travels to the ventricle via one of the two AV pathways (AV node or bypass tract), and then the impulse travels back to the atria through the other of the two pathways. Continuous circling around the loop leads to a very rapid rhythm **(supraventricular tachycardia),** which may be incapacitating because the rapid rate may not allow sufficient time for ventricular filling.

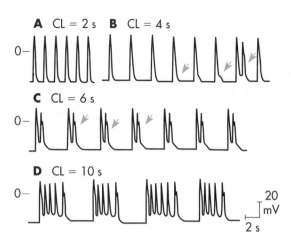

Figure 2-35 ■ **Effect of pacing at different cycle lengths *(CL)* on cesium-induced early afterdepolarizations *(EADs)* in a canine Purkinje fiber.** A, EADs not evident. B, EADs first appear *(arrows).* The third EAD reaches threshold and triggers an action potential *(third arrow).* C, EADs that appear after each driven depolarization trigger an action potential. D, **Triggered action potentials occur in salvos.** (Modified from Damiano BP, Rosen M: *Circulation* 69:1013, 1984.)

Early Afterdepolarizations

EADs are more likely to occur when the prevailing heart rate is slow; rapid pacing suppresses EADs. In the experiment shown in Figure 2-35, EADs were induced by cesium in an isolated Purkinje fiber preparation. No afterdepolarizations were evident when the preparation was driven at a cycle length of 2 s. When the cycle length was increased to 4 s, EADs appeared. Most were subthreshold (first two arrows), but one of the EADs did reach threshold and triggered an action potential. When the cycle length was increased to 6 s, each driven

action potential generated an EAD that triggered a second action potential. Furthermore, when the cycle length was increased to 10 s, each driven action potential triggered a salvo of four or five additional action potentials.

EADs may be produced experimentally by interventions that prolong the action potential. Because EADs may be initiated at either of two distinct levels of transmembrane potential, namely, at the end of the plateau and about midway through repolarization, two different mechanisms may be involved in generating them.

Considerable information has been obtained about the mechanism responsible for those EADs that appear at the end of the plateau. The more prolonged the action potential, the more likely are EADs to occur. For those action potentials that trigger EADs, the plateau appears to be prolonged enough so that those Ca^{++} channels that were activated at the beginning of the plateau and then inactivated would have sufficient time to be activated again before the plateau had expired. This secondary activation would trigger an afterdepolarization. Less information is available about the cellular mechanisms responsible for those EADs that appear midway through repolarization.

Delayed Afterdepolarizations

In contrast to EADs, DADs tend to appear when the heart rate is high. The salient characteristics of DADs are shown in Figure 2-36. The trans-

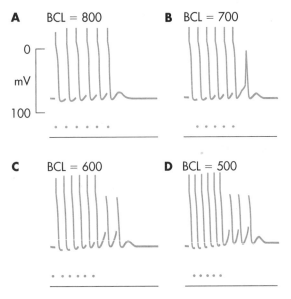

Figure 2-36 ■ Transmembrane action potentials recorded from isolated canine Purkinje fibers. Acetylstrophanthidin was added to the bath, and sequences of six driven beats (denoted by the dots) were produced at basic cycle lengths *(BCL)* of 800, 700, 600, and 500 ms. Note that delayed afterpotentials occurred after the driven beats, and that these afterpotentials reached threshold after the last driven beat in panels B to D, **but not in panel** A. (From Ferrier GR, Saunders JH, Mendez C: *Circ Res* 32:600, 1973.)

membrane potentials were recorded from Purkinje fibers that were exposed to a high concentration of **acetylstrophanthidin,** a digitalis-like substance. In the absence of driving stimuli, these fibers were quiescent. In each panel, a sequence of six driven depolarizations was induced at various basic cycle lengths.

When the cycle length was 800 ms (panel *A*), the last driven depolarization was followed by a brief DAD that did not reach threshold. Once that afterdepolarization had subsided, the transmembrane potential remained constant until another driving stimulus was given. The upstroke of a DAD can be detected after each of the first five driven depolarizations.

When the basic cycle length was diminished to 700 ms (panel *B*), the DAD that followed the last driven beat did reach threshold, and a nondriven depolarization (or **extrasystole**) ensued. This extrasystole was itself followed by an afterpotential that was subthreshold. Diminution of the basic cycle length to 600 ms (panel *C*) also evoked an extrasystole after the last driven depolarization. The afterpotential that followed the extrasystole did reach threshold, however, and a second extrasystole occurred. A sequence of three extrasystoles followed the six driven depolarizations that were separated by intervals of 500 ms (panel *D*). Slightly shorter basic cycle lengths or slightly greater concentrations of acetylstrophanthidin evoked a continuous sequence of nondriven beats, resembling a paroxysmal tachycardia (described on p 48).

DADs are associated with elevated intracellular Ca^{++} concentrations. The amplitudes of the DADs are increased by interventions that raise intracellular Ca^{++} concentrations. Such interventions include elevated extracellular Ca^{++} concentrations and toxic levels of digitalis glycosides. The elevated levels of intracellular Ca^{++} provoke the oscillatory release of Ca^{++} from the sarcoplasmic reticulum. Hence in myocardial cells, the DADs are accompanied by small changes in developed force. The high intracellular Ca^{++} concentrations also activate certain membrane channels that permit the passage of Na^+ and K^+. The net flux of these cations constitutes a **transient inward current,** i_{ti}, that is at least partly responsible for the afterdepolarization of the cell membrane.

■ ELECTROCARDIOGRAPHY DISPLAYS THE SPREAD OF CARDIAC EXCITATION

The electrocardiograph is a valuable instrument, because it enables the physician to infer the course of the cardiac impulse simply by recording the variations in electrical potential at various loci on the surface of the body. By analyzing the details of these potential fluctuations, the physician gains valuable insight concerning (1) the anatomical orientation of the heart, (2) the relative sizes of its chambers, (3) a variety of disturbances of rhythm and conduction, (4) the extent, location, and progress of ischemic damage to the myocardium, (5) the effects of altered electrolyte concentrations, and (6) the influence of certain drugs (notably digitalis derivatives and antidysrhythmic agents). The science of electrocardiography is extensive and complex, but only the elementary basis of electrocardiography is considered here.

Scalar Electrocardiography

The systems of leads used to record routine electrocardiograms are oriented in certain planes of the body. The diverse electromotive forces that exist in the heart at any moment can be represented by a three-dimensional vector. A system of recording leads oriented in a given plane detects the projection of the three-dimensional vector on that plane. Furthermore, the potential difference between two recording electrodes represents the projection of the vector on the line between the two leads. Components of vectors projected on such lines are not vectors but **scalar quantities** (having magnitude but not di-

rection). Hence, a recording of the changes with time of the differences of potential between two points on the surface of the skin is called a **scalar electrocardiogram.**

Configuration of the Scalar Electrocardiogram The scalar electrocardiogram detects the changes with time of the electrical potential between some point on the skin surface and an indifferent electrode or between pairs of points on the skin surface. The cardiac impulse progresses through the heart in a complex three-dimensional pattern. Hence the precise configuration of the electrocardiogram varies from individual to individual, and in any given individual the pattern varies with the anatomical location of the leads.

In general, the pattern consists of P, QRS, and T waves (see Figure 2-29). The P-R interval (or more precisely, the P-Q interval) is a measure of the time from the onset of atrial activation to the onset of ventricular activation; it normally ranges from 0.12 to 0.20 s. A considerable fraction of this time involves passage of the impulse through the AV conduction system. Pathological prolongations of this interval are associated with disturbances of AV conduction produced by inflammatory, circulatory, pharmacological, or nervous mechanisms.

The configuration and amplitude of the QRS complex vary considerably among individuals. The duration is usually between 0.06 and 0.10 s. Abnormal prolongation may indicate a block in the normal conduction pathways through the ventricles (such as a block of the left or right bundle branch). During the ST interval the entire ventricular myocardium is depolarized. Therefore the ST segment lies on the **isoelectric line,** under normal conditions. Any appreciable deviation from the isoelectric line is noteworthy and may indicate ischemic damage of the myocardium. The Q-T interval is sometimes referred to as the period of "electrical systole" of the ventricles. Its duration is about 0.4 s, but it varies inversely with the heart rate, mainly because the myocardial cell action potential duration varies inversely with the heart rate (see Figure 2-21).

In most leads the T wave is deflected in the same direction from the isoelectric line as the major component of the QRS complex, although biphasic or oppositely directed T waves are perfectly normal in certain leads. When the T wave and QRS complex deviate in the same direction from the isoelectric line, it indicates that the repolarization process proceeds in a direction counter to the depolarization process. T waves that are abnormal in either direction or amplitude may indicate myocardial damage, electrolyte disturbances, or cardiac hypertrophy.

Standard Limb Leads The original electrocardiographic lead system was devised by Einthoven. In his lead system the **resultant cardiac vector** (the vector sum of all electrical activity occurring in the heart at any given moment) was considered to lie in the center of a triangle (assumed to be equilateral) formed by the left and right shoulders and the pubic region (Figure 2-37). This triangle, called the **Einthoven triangle,** is oriented in the frontal plane of the body. Hence only the projection of the resultant cardiac vector on the frontal plane is detected by this system of leads. For convenience, the electrodes are connected to the right and left forearms rather than to the corresponding shoulders because the arms represent simple extensions of the leads from the shoulders. Similarly, the leg is taken as an extension of the lead system from the pubis, and the third electrode is connected to the left leg (by convention).

Certain conventions dictate the manner in which these **standard limb leads** are connected to the galvanometer. Lead I records the potential difference between the left arm (LA) and right arm (RA). The galvanometer connections are such that when the potential at LA (V_{LA}) exceeds the potential at RA (V_{RA}), the gal-

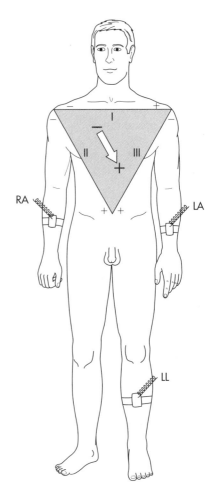

Figure 2-37 ■ Einthoven triangle, illustrating the galvanometer connections for standard limb leads I, II, and III.

vanometer is deflected upward from the isoelectric line. In Figures 2-37 and 2-38 this arrangement of the galvanometer connections for lead I is designated by a ($+$) at LA and by a ($-$) at RA. Lead II records the potential difference between RA and LL (left leg) and yields an upward deflection when V_{LL} exceeds V_{RA}. Finally, lead III registers the potential difference between LA and LL and yields an upward deflection when V_{LL} exceeds V_{LA}. These galvanometer connections

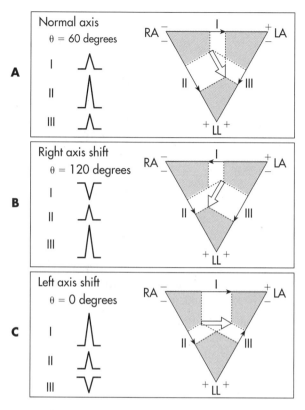

Figure 2-38 ■ **Magnitude and direction of the QRS complexes in limb leads I, II, and III, when the mean electrical axis (θ) is 60 degrees** (A), **120 degrees** (B), **and 0 degrees** (C).

were arbitrarily chosen so that the QRS complexes will be upright in all three standard limb leads in most normal individuals.

Let the frontal projection of the resultant cardiac vector at some moment be represented by an arrow (tail negative, head positive), as in Figure 2-37. Then, the potential difference, $V_{LA} - V_{RA}$, recorded in lead I will be represented by the component of the vector projected along the horizontal line between LA and RA, as shown in Figure 2-38. If the cardiac vector makes an angle, θ, of 60 degrees with the horizontal (as in panel A of Figure 2-38), the magnitude of the potential recorded by lead I will equal the vector magnitude times cosine 60 degrees. The deflection recorded in lead I will be upward, because the positive arrowhead lies closer to LA than to RA. The deflection in lead II will also be upright, because the arrowhead lies closer to LL than to RA. The magnitude of the lead II deflection will be greater than that in lead I because in this example the direction of the vector parallels that of lead II; therefore the magnitude of the projection on lead II exceeds that on lead I. Similarly, in lead III the deflection will be upright, and in this example, where θ = 60 degrees, its magnitude will equal that in lead I.

If the vector in panel A of Figure 2-38 is the resultant of the electrical events occurring during the peak of the QRS complex, the orientation of this vector is said to represent the **mean electrical axis** of the heart in the frontal plane. The positive direction of this axis is taken in the clockwise direction from the horizontal plane (contrary to the usual mathematical convention). For normal individuals, the average mean electrical axis is approximately +60 degrees (as in panel A of Figure 2-38). Therefore the QRS complexes are usually upright in all three leads and largest in lead II.

With appreciable shift of the mean electrical axis to the right (panel B of Figure 2-38, where θ = 120 degrees), the displacements of the QRS complexes in the standard leads changes considerably. In this case the largest upright deflection is in lead III and the deflection in lead I is inverted, because the arrowhead is closer to RA than to LA. With left axis shift (panel C of Figure 2-38, where θ = 0 degrees), the largest upright deflection is in lead I, and the QRS complex in lead III is inverted.

As is evident from this discussion, the standard limb leads I, II, and III are oriented in the frontal plane at 0, 60, and 120 degrees, respectively, from the horizontal plane. Other limb leads, which are also oriented in the frontal plane, are usually recorded in addition to the standard leads. These "unipolar limb leads" lie along axes at angles of $+90$, -30, and -150 degrees from the horizontal plane. Such lead systems are described in all textbooks on electrocardiography and are not considered further here.

To obtain information concerning the projections of the cardiac vector on the sagittal and transverse planes of the body in scalar electrocardiography, the **precordial leads** are usually recorded. Most commonly, each of six selected points on the anterior and lateral surfaces of the chest in the vicinity of the heart is connected in turn to the galvanometer. The other galvanometer terminal is usually connected to a **central terminal,** which is composed of a junction of three leads from LA, RA, and LL, each in series with a 5000-ohm resistor. The voltage of this central terminal remains at a theoretical zero potential throughout the cardiac cycle.

include those that arise from the SA node and those that originate from various ectopic foci.

Altered Sinoatrial Rhythms

The frequency of pacemaker discharge varies by the mechanisms described earlier in this chapter (see Figure 2-23). Changes in SA nodal discharge frequency are usually produced by the cardiac autonomic nerves. Examples of electrocardiograms of sinus tachycardia and sinus bradycardia are shown in Figure 2-39. The P, QRS, and T deflections are all normal, but the duration of the cardiac cycle (the **P-P interval**) is altered. Characteristically, when sinus bradycardia or tachycardia develops, the cardiac frequency changes gradually and requires several beats to attain its new steady-state value. Electrocardiographic evidence of **respiratory cardiac dysrhythmia is common and is manifested as a rhythmic variation in the**

BOX 2-11

Changes in the mean electrical axis may occur with alterations in the anatomical position of the heart or with changes in the relative preponderance of the right and left ventricles. For example, the axis tends to shift toward the left (more horizontal) in short, stocky individuals and toward the right (more vertical) in tall, thin persons. Also, with left or right **ventricular hypertrophy** (increased myocardial mass), the axis will shift toward the hypertrophied side.

■ DYSRHYTHMIAS OCCUR FREQUENTLY AND CONSTITUTE IMPORTANT CLINICAL PROBLEMS

Cardiac dysrhythmias reflect disturbances of either **impulse propagation** or **impulse initiation.** The principal disturbances of impulse propagation are conduction blocks and reentrant rhythms. Disturbances of impulse initiation

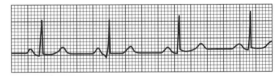

A, Normal sinus rhythm.

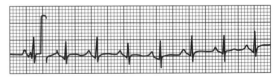

B, Sinus tachycardia.

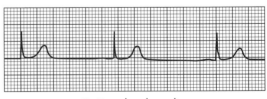

C, Sinus bradycardia.

Figure 2-39 ■ Sinoatrial rhythms.

P-P interval at the respiratory frequency (see Figure 4-11).

Atrioventricular Transmission Blocks

Various physiological, pharmacological, and pathological processes can impede impulse transmission through the AV conduction tissue. The site of block can be localized more precisely by recording the **His bundle electrogram** (Figure 2-40). To obtain such tracings, an electrode catheter is introduced into a peripheral vein and threaded centrally until the tip containing the electrodes lies in the AV junctional region between the right atrium and ventricle. When the electrodes are properly positioned, a distinct deflection (Figure 2-40, *H*) is registered, which represents the passage of the cardiac impulse down the bundle of His. The time intervals required for propagation from the atrium to the bundle of His (**A-H interval**) and from the bundle of His to the

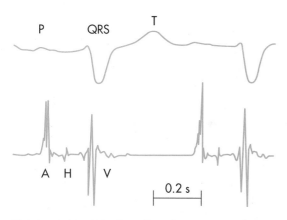

Figure 2-40 ■ **His bundle electrogram (*lower tracing*, retouched) and lead II of the scalar electrocardiogram (*upper tracing*). The deflection, *H*, which represents the impulse conduction over the bundle of His, is clearly visible between the atrial, *A,* and ventricular, *V,* deflections. The conduction time from the atria to the bundle of His is denoted by the A-H interval; that from the bundle of His to the ventricles, by the H-V interval.**

ventricles (**H-V interval**) may be measured accurately. Abnormal prolongation of the former or latter interval indicates block above or below the bundle of His, respectively.

Premature Depolarizations

Premature depolarizations occur at times in most normal individuals but are more common under certain abnormal conditions. They may originate in the atria, AV junction, or ventricles. One type of premature depolarization is coupled to a normally conducted depolarization by a constant **coupling interval.** If the normal depolarization is suppressed temporarily (e.g., by vagal stimulation), the premature depolarization will also be suppressed. Such premature depolarizations are called **coupled extrasystoles,** or simply extrasystoles, and they probably reflect a reentry phenomenon (see Figure 2-34). A second type of premature depolarization occurs as the result of enhanced automaticity in some ectopic focus. This ectopic center may fire regularly and be protected from depolarization by the normal cardiac impulse. If this premature depolarization occurs at a regular interval or at a simple multiple of that interval, the disturbance is called **parasystole.**

A **premature atrial depolarization** is shown in the electrocardiogram in Figure 2-41, *A.* The normal interval between beats was 0.89 s (heart rate, 68 beats/min). The premature atrial depolarization (second P wave in the figure) followed the preceding P wave by only 0.56 s. The configuration of the premature P wave differs from the configuration of the other, normal P waves because the course of atrial excitation, originating at some ectopic focus in the atrium, is different from the normal spread of excitation that originates in the SA node. The QRS complex of the premature depolarization is usually normal in configuration because the spread of ventricular excitation occurs over the usual pathways.

A

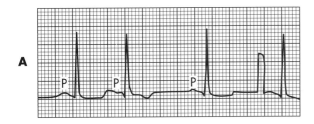

B

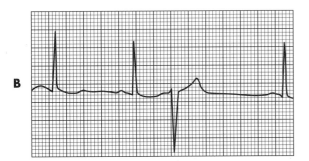

Figure 2-41 ■ A premature atrial depolarization (A) and a premature ventricular depolarization (B). The premature atrial depolarization (second beat in the top tracing) is followed by normal QRS and T waves. The interval after the premature depolarization is not much longer than the usual interval between beats. The brief rectangular deflection just before the last depolarization is a standardization signal. The premature ventricular depolarization (B) is characterized by bizarre QRS and T waves and is followed by a compensatory pause.

A **premature ventricular depolarization** appears in Figure 2-41, *B.* Because the premature excitation originated at some ectopic focus in the ventricles, the impulse spread was aberrant, and the configurations of the QRS and T waves were entirely different from the normal deflections. The premature QRS complex followed the preceding normal QRS complex by only 0.47 s. The interval after the premature excitation was 1.28 s, considerably longer than the normal interval between beats (0.89 s). The interval (1.75 s), which was from the QRS complex just before the premature excitation to the QRS complex

just after it, was virtually equal to the duration of two normal cardiac cycles (1.78 s).

The prolonged interval that usually follows a premature ventricular depolarization is called a **compensatory pause.** The reason for the compensatory pause after a premature ventricular depolarization is that the ectopic ventricular impulse does not disturb the natural rhythm of the SA node. Either the ectopic ventricular impulse is not conducted retrograde through the AV conduction system, or if it is, the time required is such that the SA node has already fired at its natural interval before the ectopic impulse could have reached it. Likewise, the SA nodal impulse that was generated between the second and third QRS complexes in Figure 2-41, *B* did not affect the ventricle because the AV junction and perhaps also the ventricles were still refractory from the premature excitation. In Figure 2-41, *B,* the P wave that originated in the SA node at the time of the premature depolarization occurred at the same time as the T wave of the premature cycle and therefore cannot easily be identified in the tracing.

Ectopic Tachycardias

When a tachycardia originates from some ectopic site in the heart, the onset and termination are typically abrupt, in contrast to the more gradual changes in heart rate in sinus tachycardia. Because of the sudden appearance and abrupt cessation, such ectopic tachycardias are usually called **paroxysmal tachycardias.**

Such tachycardias may cause lightheadedness or even transient loss of consciousness (syncope), because the very rapid contraction frequency does not permit adequate time for ventricular filling between heartbeats.

Paroxysmal tachycardias that originate in the atria or in the AV junctional tissues (Figure 2-42, *A*) are usually indistinguishable, and therefore both are included in the term **paroxysmal supraventricular tachycardia.** The

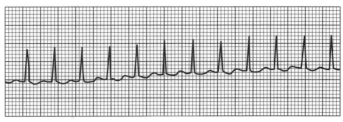

A, Supraventricular tachycardia.

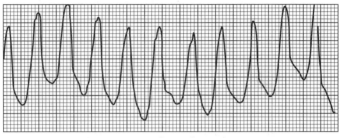

B, Ventricular tachycardia.

Figure 2-42 ■ **Paroxysmal tachycardias.**

tachycardia often results from an impulse repetitively circling a reentry loop that includes atrial tissue, the AV junction, or both. The QRS complexes are often normal because ventricular activation proceeds over the normal pathways.

Paroxysmal ventricular tachycardia originates from an ectopic focus in the ventricles. The electrocardiogram is characterized by repeated, bizarre QRS complexes that reflect the aberrant intraventricular impulse conduction (Figure 2-42, *B*). Paroxysmal ventricular tachycardia is much more ominous than supraventricular tachycardia because it is frequently a precursor of ventricular fibrillation, a lethal dysrhythmia described in the next section.

Fibrillation

Under certain conditions, cardiac muscle undergoes an irregular type of contraction that is entirely ineffectual in propelling blood. Such a dysrhythmia is termed **fibrillation** and may in-

---

BOX 2-12

Episodes of ectopic tachycardia may persist for only a few beats or for many hours or days, and the episodes often recur. Paroxysmal tachycardias may occur as the result of (1) the rapid firing of an ectopic pacemaker, (2) triggered activity secondary to afterpotentials that reach threshold, or (3) an impulse circling a reentry loop repetitively.

---

volve either the atria or the ventricles. Fibrillation probably represents a reentry phenomenon in which the reentry loop fragments into multiple, irregular circuits.

The tracing in Figure 2-43, *A,* illustrates the electrocardiographic changes in **atrial fibrillation.** This condition occurs in various types of chronic heart disease. The atria do not contract and relax sequentially during each cardiac cycle and hence do not contribute to ventricular filling. Instead, the atria undergo a continuous, uncoordinated, rippling type of activity. In the electrocardiogram there are no P waves; they are replaced by continuous irregular fluctuations of potential, called **f waves.**

Although atrial fibrillation and flutter are compatible with life and even with full physical activity, the onset of **ventricular fibrillation** leads to loss of consciousness within a few seconds. The irregular, continuous, uncoordinated twitchings of the ventricular muscle fibers pump no blood. In the electrocardiogram (Figure 2-43, *B*), irregular fluctuations of potential are manifest.

Fibrillation is often initiated when a premature impulse arrives during the **vulnerable period.** In the ventricles, this period coincides with the downslope of the T wave. During this period, the excitability of the cardiac cells varies. Some fibers are still in their effective refractory periods, others have almost fully recovered their excitability, and still others are able to conduct impulses, but only at very slow conduction velocities. As a consequence, the action potentials are propagated over the chambers in multiple wavelets that travel along circuitous paths and at various conduction velocities. As a region of cardiac cells becomes excitable again, it will ultimately be reentered by one of the wave fronts traveling about the chamber. The process is self-sustaining.

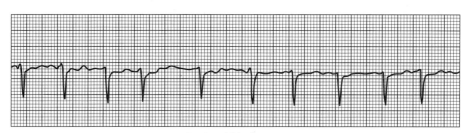

A, Atrial fibrillation.

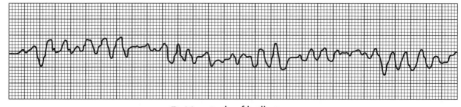

B, Ventricular fibrillation.

Figure 2-43 ■ **Atrial and ventricular fibrillation.**

Electric shock is sometimes also used to treat ventricular fibrillation, and sometimes also atrial fibrillation, especially when the disturbance does not respond optimally to drugs. The timing of the shock is coordinated with the absolute refractory period of the ventricles (i.e., during or shortly after the QRS deflection of the electrocardiogram), so that the shock does not affect ventricular excitation. However, the shock will render all the atrial myocytes temporarily refractory, and thereby interrupt the prevailing reentry circuits.

Summary

- The transmembrane action potentials that can be recorded from cardiac myocytes comprise the following five phases (0 to 4):
  - Phase 0, upstroke. A suprathreshold stimulus rapidly depolarizes the membrane by activating the fast Na^+ channels.
  - Phase 1, early partial repolarization. Achieved by the efflux of K^+ through channels that conduct the transient outward current, i_{to}.
  - Phase 2, plateau. Achieved by a balance between the influx of Ca^{++} through Ca^{++} channels and the efflux of K^+ through several types of K^+ channels.
  - Phase 3, final repolarization. Initiated when the efflux of K^+ exceeds the influx of Ca^{++}. The resulting partial repolarization rapidly increases the K^+ conductance and rapidly restores full repolarization.
  - Phase 4, resting potential. The transmembrane potential of the fully repolarized cell is determined mainly by the conductance of the cell membrane to K^+.
- Two principal types of action potentials may be recorded from cardiac cells:
  - Fast-response action potentials may be recorded from atrial and ventricular myocardial fibers and from specialized conducting (Purkinje) fibers. The action potential is characterized by a large-amplitude, steep upstroke, which is produced by the activation of the fast Na^+ channels. The effective refractory period begins at the upstroke of the action potential and persists until about midway through phase 3.
  - Slow-response action potentials may be recorded from normal SA and AV nodal cells and from abnormal myocardial cells that have been partially depolarized. The action potential is characterized by a less negative resting potential, a smaller amplitude, and a less steep upstroke than is the fast-response action potential. The upstroke is produced by the activation of Ca^{++} channels.
- Automaticity is characteristic of certain cells in the heart, notably those in the SA and AV nodes and in the specialized conducting system. Automaticity is achieved by a slow depolarization of the membrane during phase 4.
- The SA node initiates the impulse that induces cardiac contraction. This impulse is propagated from the SA node to the atria, and the wave of excitation ultimately reaches the AV node.
- The AV node cells are slow-response fibers and the impulse travels very slowly through the AV node. The consequent delay between atrial and ventricular depolarization provides adequate time for atrial contraction to help fill the ventricles.
- Impulses may be initiated abnormally (1) by slow diastolic depolarization of automatic cells in ectopic sites or (2) by afterdepolarizations that reach threshold.

- Ectopic foci. Automatic cells in the atrium, AV node, or His-Purkinje system may initiate propagated cardiac impulses either because the ordinarily more rhythmic, normal pacemaker cells are suppressed, or because the rhythmicity of the ectopic foci is abnormally enhanced.
- Afterdepolarizations. Under abnormal conditions, afterdepolarizations may appear early in phase 3 of a normally initiated beat, or they may be delayed until near the end of phase 3 or the beginning of phase 4. Such afterdepolarizations may themselves trigger propagated impulses.
- Disturbances of impulse conduction consist mainly of simple conduction block and reentry.
  - Simple conduction block. Failure of propagation in a cardiac fiber as the result of a disease process (e.g., ischemia, inflammation) or a drug.
  - Reentry. A cardiac impulse may traverse a loop of cardiac fibers and reenter previously excited tissue when the impulse is conducted slowly around the loop and the impulse is blocked unidirectionally in some section of the loop.
- The electrocardiogram is recorded from the surface of the body and traces the conduction of the cardiac impulse through the heart. The component waves of the electrocardiogram are
  - P wave. Spread of excitation over the atria.
  - QRS interval. Spread of excitation over the ventricles.
  - T wave. Spread of repolarization over the ventricles.

■ BIBLIOGRAPHY

1. Armour JA, Ardell JL: *Neurocardiology,* New York, 1994, Oxford University Press.
2. Beaumont J, Michaels DC, Delmar M, et al: A model study of changes in excitability of ventricular muscle cells: inhibition, facilitation, and hysteresis. *Am J Physiol* 268:H1181, 1995.
3. Billette J, Nattel S: Dynamic behavior of the atrioventricular node: a functional model of interaction between recovery, facilitation, and fatigue. *J Cardiovasc Electrophysiol* 5:90, 1994.
4. Demir SS, Clark JW, Giles WR: Parasympathetic modulation of sinoatrial node pacemaker activity in rabbit heart: a unifying model. *Am J Physiol* 276:H2221, 1999.
5. Fozzard JA, Hanck DA: Structure and function of voltage-dependent sodium channels: comparison of brain II and cardiac isoforms. *Physiol Rev* 76:887, 1996.
6. Irisawa H, Brown HF, Giles W: Cardiac pacemaking in the sinoatrial node. *Physiol Rev* 73:197, 1993.
7. Jalife J, Delmar M, Davidenko JM, et al: *Basic cardiac electrophysiology for the clinician,* Armonk, NY, 1999, Futura.
8. Levy MN, Schwartz PJ: *Vagal control of the heart: experimental basis and clinical implications,* Armonk, NY, 1994, Futura.
9. Meijler FL, Janse MJ: Morphology and electrophysiology of the mammalian atrioventricular node. *Physiol Rev* 68:608, 1988.
10. Sicouri S, Antzelevitch C: Electrophysiologic characteristics of M cells in the canine left ventricular free wall. *J Cardiovasc Electrophysiol* 6:591, 1995.
11. Spach MS, Josephson ME: Initiating reentry: the role of nonuniform anisotropy in small circuits. *J Cardiovasc Electrophysiol* 5:182, 1994.
12. Sperelakis N: *Physiology and pathophysiology of the heart,* ed 3, Boston, 1995, Kluwer Academic.
13. Spooner PM, Brown AM, Catterall WA, et al: *Ion channels in the cardiovascular system: function and dysfunction,* Armonk, NY, 1994, Futura.
14. Wit AL, Janse MJ: *Ventricular arrhythmias of ischemia and infarction: electrophysiological mechanisms,* Armonk, NY, 1993, Futura.
15. Zipes DP, Jalife J: *Cardiac electrophysiology: from cell to bedside,* ed 3, Philadelphia, 1999, WB Saunders.

■ CASE 2

HISTORY

A 63-year-old man suddenly felt a crushing pain beneath his sternum. He became weak, he was sweating profusely, and he noticed his heart was beating rapidly. He called his physician, who made the diagnosis of myocardial infarction. The tests made at the hospital confirmed his doctor's suspicion that the patient had suffered a "heart attack"; that is, a major coronary artery to the left ventricle had suddenly become occluded. An electrocardiogram indicated that the SA node was the source of the rapid heart rate. Two hours after admission to the hospital, the patient suddenly became much weaker. His arterial pulse rate was only about 40 beats/min. An electrocardiogram at this time revealed that the atrial rate was about 90 beats/min, and that conduction through the AV junction was completely blocked, undoubtedly because the infarct affected the AV conduction system. Electrodes of an artificial pacemaker were inserted into the patient's right ventricle, and the ventricle was placed at a frequency of 75 beats/min. The patient felt stronger and more comfortable almost immediately.

QUESTIONS

1. Soon after coronary artery occlusion, the interstitial fluid K^+ concentration rose substantially in the flow-deprived region. In this region, the high extracellular K^+ concentration
   a. Increased the propagation velocity of the myocardial action potentials
   b. Decreased the postrepolarization refractoriness of the myocardial cells
   c. Increased the resting (phase 4) transmembrane potential to a less negative value
   d. Diminished the automaticity of the myocardial cells
   e. Decreased the likelihood of reentry dysrhythmias
2. The mechanism by which the SA node generated impulses at a rapid rate during the early stages of the coronary artery occlusion involves
   a. An increased slope of the action potential upstroke (phase 0) of the automatic cells
   b. An increased slope of the slow diastolic depolarization of the automatic cells
   c. An increased firing threshold of the automatic cells

   d. An increased negativity (hyperpolarization) of the initial portion of the slow diastolic depolarization
   e. An increased action potential amplitude of the automatic cells
3. The most likely mechanism responsible for the patient's arterial pulse rate of about 40 beats/min after impulse conduction through the AV junction was blocked is
   a. Excitation of the ventricles via an AV bypass tract
   b. Conversion of ventricular myocardial fibers to automatic cells
   c. Firing of ventricular ectopic cells that have the same electrophysiological characteristics as SA node cells
   d. Firing of automatic cells (Purkinje fibers) in the specialized conduction system of the ventricles
   e. Excitation of ventricular cells by the rhythmic activity in the autonomic neurons that innervate the heart
4. While the heart was being paced, the cardiologist discontinued ventricular pacing periodically to test the patient's cardiac status. The cardiologist found that the ventricles did not begin beating spontaneously until about 5 to 10 sec after cessation of pacing, because the preceding period of pacing led to
   a. Overdrive suppression of the automatic cells in the ventricles
   b. Release of norepinephrine from the cardiac sympathetic nerves
   c. Release of neuropeptide Y from the cardiac sympathetic nerves
   d. Fatigue of the ventricular myocytes
   e. Release of acetylcholine from the cardiac parasympathetic nerves

CHAPTER 3

The Cardiac Pump

Objectives

1. Indicate how the microscopic and gross anatomy of the heart enable it to pump blood through the systemic and pulmonary circulations.

2. Indicate how electrical excitation of the heart is coupled to its contractions.

3. Elucidate the main factors that determine cardiac contractile force.

4. Describe and explain the pressure changes in the heart chambers and great vessels during a complete cardiac cycle.

THE HEART EXHIBITS A WIDE RANGE of activity and functional capacity, and performs a staggering amount of work over the lifetime of an individual. The heart can function independently of extra-cardiac stimuli, but its performance is influenced by humoral and neural factors. In this chapter we consider some of the basic intrinsic mechanisms that affect cardiac activity; the effects of extra-cardiac factors are discussed in subsequent chapters.

■ THE GROSS AND MICROSCOPIC STRUCTURES OF THE HEART ARE UNIQUELY DESIGNED FOR OPTIMAL FUNCTION

Myocardial Cell

Several important morphological and functional differences exist between myocardial and skeletal muscle cells. However, the contractile elements within the two types of cells are quite similar; each skeletal and cardiac muscle cell is made up of **sarcomeres** (from Z line to Z line) that contain thick filaments composed of myosin (in the A band) and thin filaments containing actin. The thin filaments extend from the point where they are anchored to the Z line (through the I band) to interdigitate with the thick filaments. As in the case of skeletal muscle, shortening occurs by the sliding filament mechanism. Actin filaments slide along adjacent myosin filaments by cycling of the intervening crossbridges, thereby bringing the Z lines closer together.

A striking difference in the appearance of cardiac and skeletal muscle is the semblance of a syncytium in cardiac muscle with branching in-

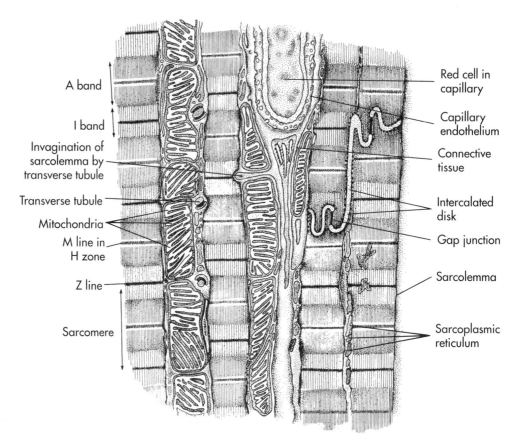

A band

I band

Invagination of
sarcolemma by
transverse tubule

Transverse tubule

Mitochondria

M line in
H zone

Z line

Sarcomere

Red cell in
capillary

Capillary
endothelium

Connective
tissue

Intercalated
disk

Gap junction

Sarcolemma

Sarcoplasmic
reticulum

Figure 3-1 ■ **Diagram of an electron micrograph of cardiac muscle showing large numbers of mito-chondria and the intercalated disks with nexi (gap junctions), transverse tubules, and longitudinal tubules.**

terconnecting fibers (Figures 3-1 and 3-2). How-ever, the myocardium is not a true anatomical syncytium, because laterally the myocardial fibers are separated from adjacent fibers by their respective sarcolemmas, and the end of each fi-ber is separated from its neighbor by dense structures, **intercalated disks,** that are con-tinuous with the sarcolemma (Figures 3-1 to 3-3). Nevertheless, *cardiac muscle functions as a syncytium, because a wave of depolarization followed by contraction of the entire myocar-dium (an all-or-none response) occurs when a*

suprathreshold stimulus is applied to any one focus.

As the wave of excitation approaches the end of a cardiac cell, the spread of excitation to the next cell depends on the electrical conductance of the boundary between the two cells. **Gap junctions (nexi)** with high conductances are present in the intercalated disks between adja-cent cells (see Figures 3-1 to 3-3). These gap junctions, which facilitate the conduction of the cardiac impulse from one cell to the next, are made up of **connexons,** hexagonal structures

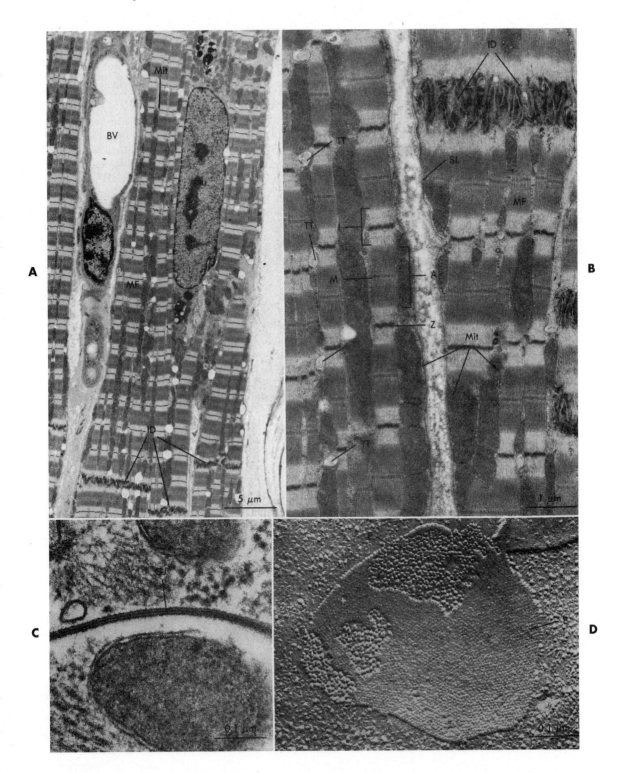

Figure 3-2 ▪ A, Low-magnification electron micrograph of a monkey heart (ventricle). Typical features of myocardial cells include the elongated nucleus *(Nu)*, striated myofibrils *(MF)* with columns of mitochondria *(Mit)* between the myofibrils, and intercellular junctions (intercalated disks, *ID)*. A blood vessel *(BV)* is located between two myocardial cells. B, Medium-magnification electron micrograph of monkey ventricular cells showing details of ultrastructure. The sarcolemma *(SL)* is the boundary of the muscle cells and is thrown into multiple folds where the cells meet at the intercalated disk region *(ID)*. The prominent myofibrils *(MF)* show distinct banding patterns, including the A band *(A)*, dark Z lines *(Z)*, I band regions *(I)*, and M lines *(M)* at the center of each sarcomere unit. Mitochondria *(Mit)* occur either in rows between myofibrils or in masses just underneath the sarcolemma. Regularly spaced transverse tubules *(TT)* appear at the Z line levels of the myofibrils. C, High-magnification electron micrograph of a specialized intercellular junction between two myocardial cells of the mouse. Called a gap junction *(GJ)* or nexus, this attachment consists of very close apposition of the sarcolemmal membranes of the two cells and appears in thin section to consist of seven layers. D, Freeze-fracture replica of mouse myocardial gap junction, showing distinct arrays of characteristic intramembranous particles. Large particles *(P)* belong to the inner half of the sarcolemma of one myocardial cell, whereas the "pitted" membrane face *(E)* is formed by the outer half of the sarcolemma of the cell above.

Figure 3-3 ▪ A, Low-magnification electron micrograph of the right ventricular wall of a mouse heart. Tissue was fixed in a phosphate-buffered glutaraldehyde solution and postfixed in ferrocyanide-reduced osmium tetroxide. This procedure has resulted in the deposition of electron-opaque precipitate in the extracellular space, thus outlining the sarcolemmal borders *(SL)* of the muscle cells and delineating the intercalated disks *(ID)* and transverse tubules *(TT)*. *Nu,* Nucleus of the myocardial cell. B, Mouse cardiac muscle in longitudinal section, treated as in A. The path of the extracellular space is traced through the intercalated disk region *(ID)*, and sarcolemmal invaginations that are oriented transverse to the cell axis (transverse tubules, *TT)* or parallel to it (axial tubules, *AT)* are clearly identified. Gap junctions *(GJ)* are associated with the intercalated disk. Mitochondria are large and elongated and lie between the myofibrils. C, Mouse cardiac muscle. Tissue treated with ferrocyanide-reduced osmium tetroxide to identify the internal membrane system (sarcoplasmic reticulum, SR). Specific staining of the SR reveals its architecture as a complex network of small-diameter tubules that are closely associated with the myofibrils and mitochondria.

that connect the cytosol of adjacent cells. Each connexon consists of six polypeptides surrounding a core channel approximately 1.6 to 2.0 nm wide, which serves as a low-resistance pathway for cell-to-cell conductance.

Impulse conduction in cardiac tissues progresses more rapidly in a direction parallel to the long axes of the constituent fibers than in a direction perpendicular to the long axes of those fibers. Gap junctions exist in the borders between myocardial fibers that are in contact with each other longitudinally; they are very sparse or absent in the borders between myocardial fibers that lie side by side.

Another difference between cardiac and fast skeletal muscle fibers is in the number of mito-

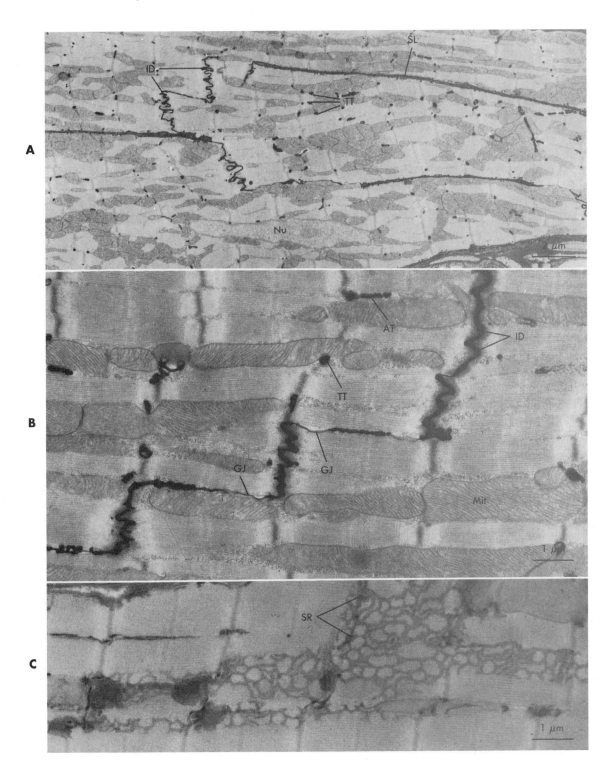

chondria (**sarcosomes**) in the two tissues. Fast skeletal muscle, which is called on for relatively short periods of repetitive or sustained contractions and which can metabolize anaerobically and build up a substantial oxygen debt, has relatively few mitochondria in the muscle fibers. In contrast, cardiac muscle, which contracts repetitively for a lifetime and requires a continuous supply of oxygen, is very rich in mitochondria (see Figures 3-1 to 3-3). Rapid oxidation of substrates with the synthesis of adenosine triphosphate (ATP) can keep pace with the myocardial energy requirements because of the large numbers of mitochondria containing the respiratory enzymes necessary for oxidative phosphorylation.

To provide adequate oxygen and substrate for its metabolic machinery, the myocardium is also endowed with a rich capillary supply, about one capillary per fiber. Thus diffusion distances are short, and oxygen, carbon dioxide, substrates, and waste material can move rapidly between myocardial cell and capillary. With respect to exchange of substances between the capillary blood and the myocardial cells, electron micrographs of myocardium show deep invaginations of the sarcolemma into the fiber at the Z lines (see Figures 3-1 to 3-3). These sarcolemmal invaginations constitute the **transverse-tubular, or T-tubular, system.** The lumina of these T tubules are continuous with the bulk interstitial fluid, and they play a key role in excitation-contraction coupling.

In mammalian ventricular cells, adjacent T tubules are interconnected by longitudinally running or axial tubules that form an extensively interconnected lattice of "intracellular" tubules (Figure 3-3). This T-tubular system is open to the interstitial fluid, is lined with a basement membrane continuous with that of the surface sarcolemma, and contains micropinocytotic vesicles. Thus in ventricular cells the myofibrils and mitochondria have ready access to a space that is continuous with the interstitial fluid. The T-tubular system is absent or poorly developed in atrial cells of many mammalian hearts.

A network of **sarcoplasmic reticulum** (see Figure 3-3) consisting of small-diameter sarcotubules is also present surrounding the myofibrils; these sarcotubules are believed to be "closed" because colloidal tracer particles (2 to 10 nm in diameter) do not enter them. They do not contain basement membrane. Flattened elements of the sarcoplasmic reticulum are often found in close proximity to the T-tubular system, as well as to the surface sarcolemma, forming "diads."

The Force of Cardiac Contraction Is Largely Determined by the Resting Length of the Myocardial Fibers

Skeletal and cardiac muscle show similar length-force relationships. The sarcomere length has been determined with electron microscopy in papillary muscles and intact ventricles rapidly fixed during systole or diastole. The developed force is maximal when the muscle begins its contractions at resting sarcomere lengths of 2 to 2.4 mm. At such lengths, there is optimal overlap of thick and thin filaments, and a maximal number of crossbridge attachments. Stretch of the myocardium and increases in load enhance the sensitivity of the myofilaments to Ca^{++} and the force of contraction, presumably by increasing the affinity of troponin C for Ca^{++}. The mechanism responsible for this greater affinity of troponin C for Ca^{++} remains to be determined. One concept is that the thick and thin filaments are brought closer to each other as the diameter of the muscle fiber narrows during stretch.

Developed force of cardiac muscle is less than the maximal value when the sarcomeres are stretched beyond the optimal length, because of less overlap of the filaments, and hence less cycling of the crossbridges. At resting sarcomere lengths shorter than the optimal value,

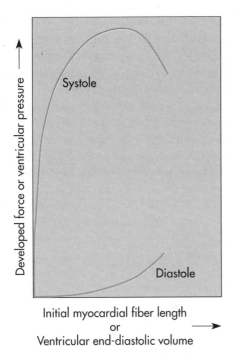

Figure 3-4 ■ Relationship of myocardial resting fiber length (sarcomere length) or end-diastolic volume to developed force or peak systolic ventricular pressure during ventricular contraction in the intact dog heart. (Redrawn from Patterson SW, Piper H, Starling EH: *J Physiol* 48:465, 1914.)

the thin filaments that extend from adjacent Z lines overlap each other in the central region of the sarcomere. This arrangement of the thick and thin filaments diminishes contractile force.

In general, the fiber length-force relationship for the papillary muscle also holds true for fibers in the intact heart. This relationship may be expressed graphically, as in Figure 3-4, by substituting ventricular systolic pressure for force and end-diastolic ventricular volume for myocardial resting fiber (and hence sarcomere) length. The lower curve in Figure 3-4 represents the increment in pressure produced by each increment in volume when the heart is in diastole. The up-

per curve represents the peak pressure developed by the ventricle during systole at each degree of filling and illustrates the **Frank-Starling relationship** of initial myocardial fiber length (or initial volume) to force (or pressure) development by the ventricle.

Note that the pressure-volume curve in diastole is initially quite flat, indicating that large increases in volume can be accommodated with only small increases in pressure, yet systolic pressure development is considerable at the lower filling pressures. However, the ventricle becomes much less distensible with greater filling, as evidenced by the sharp rise of the diastolic curve at large intraventricular volumes. In the normal intact heart, peak force may be attained at a filling pressure of 12 mm Hg. At this intraventricular diastolic pressure, which is about the upper limit observed in the normal heart, the sarcomere length is 2.2 μm. However, developed force peaks at filling pressures as high as 30 mm Hg in the isolated heart; even at higher diastolic pressures (>50 mm Hg), the sarcomere length is not greater than 2.6 μm. This resistance to stretch of the myocardium at high filling pressures probably resides in the noncontractile constituents of the tissue (connective tissue) and may serve as a safety factor against overloading the heart in diastole. Usually, ventricular diastolic pressure is about 0 to 7 mm Hg, and the average diastolic sarcomere length is about 2.2 μm. Thus *the normal heart operates on the ascending portion of the Frank-Starling curve* depicted in Figure 3-4.

Excitation-Contraction Coupling Is Mediated Mainly by Calcium

The heart requires optimal concentrations of Na^+, K^+, and Ca^{++} to function normally. In the absence of Na^+, the heart is not excitable and will not beat because the action potential depends on extracellular Na ions. In contrast, the resting membrane potential is independent

If the heart becomes greatly distended with blood during diastole, as may occur in cardiac failure, it is less efficient; more energy is required (greater wall tension) for the distended heart to eject the same volume of blood per beat than for the normal undilated heart. This is an example of Laplace's law (p 158), which states that the tension in the wall of a vessel (in this case the ventricles) equals the transmural pressure (pressure across the wall, or distending pressure) times the radius of the vessel or chamber. The Laplace relationship applies to infinitely thin-walled vessels but can be applied to the heart if correction is made for wall thickness. The equation is $\tau = Pr/w$ where τ = wall stress, P = transmural pressure, r = radius, and w = wall thickness.

of the Na ion gradient across the membrane (see Figure 2-7). Under normal conditions, the extracellular K^+ concentration is about 4 mM. A moderate reduction in extracellular K^+ has little effect on myocardial excitation and contraction, but it flattens the T-wave of the electrocardiogram. A severe reduction in extracellular (K^+) produces weakness, paralysis, and cardiac arrest. Large increases in extracellular K^+ produce dysrhythmias, depolarization, loss of excitability of the myocardial cells, and cardiac arrest in diastole. *Ca^{++} is also essential for cardiac contraction;* removal of Ca^{++} from the extracellular fluid results in decreased contractile force and eventual arrest in diastole. Conversely, an increase in extracellular Ca^{++} enhances contractile force, and very high Ca^{++} concentrations induce cardiac arrest in systole (rigor). *The free intracellular Ca^{++} is the agent responsible for the contractile state of the myocardium.*

Initially, a wave of excitation spreads rapidly along the myocardial sarcolemma from cell to cell via gap junctions. Excitation also spreads into the interior of the cells via the T tubules (see Figures 3-1 to 3-3), which invaginate the cardiac fibers at the Z lines. Electrical stimulation at the Z line or the application of ionized Ca to the Z lines in the skinned (sarcolemma removed) cardiac fiber elicits a localized contraction of adjacent myofibrils. During the plateau (phase 2) of the action potential, Ca^{++} permeability of the sarcolemma increases. Ca^{++} enters the cell through voltage-dependent L-type Ca^{++} channels in the sarcolemma and in the T tubules. The channel protein is called the dihydropyridine receptor because of its high affinity binding for this group of Ca^{++} channel antagonists (Figure 3-5). Opening of the Ca^{++} channels is facilitated by phosphorylation of the channel proteins by a cyclic AMP (cAMP)–dependent protein kinase. The primary source of extracellular Ca^{++} is the interstitial fluid (10^{-3}M Ca^{++}). Some Ca^{++} also may be bound to the sarcolemma and to the **glycocalyx,** a mucopolysaccharide that covers the sarcolemma. The amount of calcium that enters the cell interior from the extracellular space is not sufficient to induce contraction of the myofibrils, but it serves as a trigger (**trigger Ca^{++}**) to release Ca^{++} from the intracellular Ca^{++} stores in the sarcoplasmic reticulum (Figure 3-5). The Ca^{++} leaves the sarcoplasmic reticulum (SR) through calcium release channels, which are called **ryanodine receptors** because the channel protein, also called **foot protein** or **junctional processes** of the SR, binds ryanodine (Figures 3-5 and 3-6). The cytosolic free Ca^{++} increases from a resting level of about 10^{-7}M to levels of 10^{-6} to 10^{-5}M during excitation, and the Ca^{++} binds to the protein troponin C. The Ca^{++}-troponin complex interacts with tropomyosin to unblock active sites between the actin and myosin filaments, which allows crossbridge cycling and hence contraction of the myofibrils (systole).

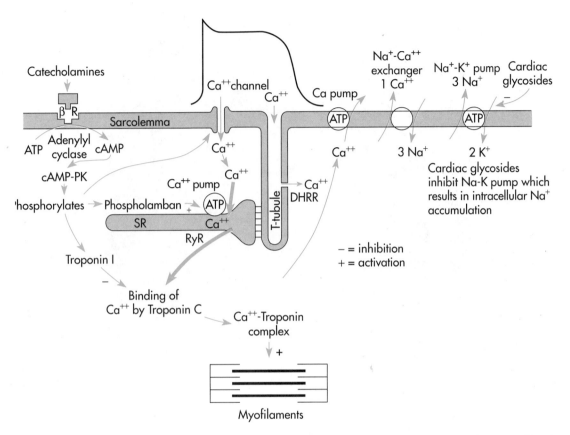

Figure 3-5 ■ Schematic diagram of the movements of calcium in excitation-contraction coupling in cardiac muscle. The influx of Ca^{++} from the interstitial fluid during excitation triggers the release of Ca^{++} from the sarcoplasmic reticulum *(SR)*. The free cytosolic Ca^{++} activates contraction of the myofilaments (systole). Relaxation (diastole) occurs as a result of uptake of Ca^{++} by the sarcoplasmic reticulum, by extrusion of intracellular Ca^{++} by $Na - Ca^{++}$ exchange, and to a limited degree by the Ca pump. *βR*, β-adrenergic receptor; *cAMP*, cyclic adenosine monophosphate; *cAMP-PK*, cyclic AMP-dependent protein kinase; *DHRR*, dihydropyridine receptor; *RyR*, ryanodine receptor.

Mechanisms that raise systolic Ca^{++} increase the developed force, and those that lower Ca^{++} decrease the developed force. For example, catecholamines increase the movement of Ca^{++} into the cell by phosphorylation of the Ca^{++} channels via a cAMP-dependent protein kinase. In addition, catecholamines, like other agonists, enhance myocardial contractile force by increasing the sensitivity of the contractile machinery to Ca^{++}. An increase in systolic Ca^{++} is also achieved by increasing extracellular Ca^{++} or decreasing the Na^+ gradient across the sarcolemma.

The sodium gradient can be reduced by increasing intracellular Na^+ or decreasing extracellular Na^+. Cardiac glycosides increase intra-

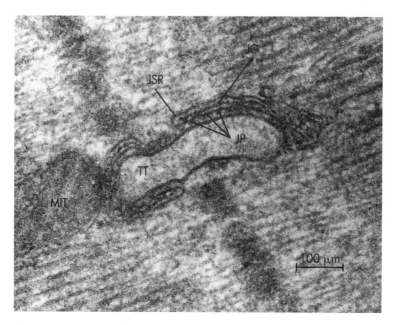

Figure 3-6 ■ **An electron micrograph of mammalian myocardium that shows a cross section of a transverse tubule *(TT)* adjacent to junctional sarcoplasmic reticulum *(JSR)*. Junctional processes *(JP)* extend from the JSR into the cell cytoplasm. The JPs are proteins that make up the calcium release channels from the SR and are also called *ryanodine receptors* because they bind the insecticide ryanodine. *MIT,* Mitochondrion;*JG,* junctional gap.** (Courtesy Joachim R. Sommer.)

cellular Na^+ by poisoning the Na-K pump, which results in an accumulation of Na^+ in the cells. The elevated cytosolic Na^+ reverses the Na-Ca exchanger so that less Ca^{++} is removed from the cell. A lowered extracellular Na^+ results in a reduction in Na^+ entry into the cell and hence less exchange of Na^+ for Ca^{++} (Figure 3-5).

Developed tension is diminished by a reduction in extracellular Ca^{++}, by an increase in the Na^+ gradient across the sarcolemma, or by administration of Ca^{++} blockers that prevent Ca^{++} from entering the myocardial cell (see Figure 2-16).

At the end of systole the Ca^{++} influx ceases and the sarcoplasmic reticulum is no longer stimulated to release Ca^{++}. In fact, the sarcoplasmic reticulum avidly takes up Ca^{++} by

Box 3-2

A patient in heart failure with a dilated heart, low cardiac output, fluid retention, high venous pressure, an enlarged liver, and peripheral edema is often treated with digitalis and a diuretic. The digitalis increases cardiomyocyte intracellular calcium, thereby enhancing contractile force, and the diuretic reduces extracellular fluid volume, thereby lessening the volume load (preload) on the heart and reducing venous pressure, liver congestion, and edema.

means of an ATP-energized calcium pump that is stimulated by **phospholamban** after the phospholamban is phosphorylated by cAMP-dependent protein kinase (Figure 3-5). Phosphorylation of troponin I inhibits the Ca^{++} binding of troponin C, which permits tropomyosin to again block the sites for interaction between the actin and myosin filaments, and relaxation (diastole) occurs (Figure 3-5). Cardiac contraction and relaxation are both accelerated by catecholamines and adenylyl cyclase activation. The resulting increase in cAMP activates the cAMP-dependent protein kinase, which phosphorylates the Ca channel in the sarcolemma. This allows a greater influx of Ca^{++} into the cell and thereby accelerates contraction. However, it also accelerates relaxation by phosphorylating phospholamban, which enhances Ca^{++} uptake by the sarcoplasmic reticulum, and by phosphorylating troponin I, which inhibits the Ca^{++} binding of troponin C. Thus the phosphorylations by cAMP-dependent protein kinase serve to increase both the speed of contraction and the speed of relaxation.

Mitochondria also take up and release Ca^{++}, but the process is too slow to be involved in excitation-contraction coupling. Only at very high intracellular Ca^{++} levels (pathological states) do the mitochondria take up a significant amount of Ca^{++}.

The Ca^{++} that enters the cell to initiate contraction must be removed during diastole. The removal is primarily accomplished by the exchange of 3 Na^+ for 1 Ca^{++} (Figure 3-5). Ca^{++} is also removed from the cell by an electrogenic pump that utilizes ATP to transport Ca^{++} across the sarcolemma (Figure 3-5).

Preload and Afterload Are Important in Determining Cardiac Performance

Figure 3-7 shows the sequence of events that occurs during the contraction of a preloaded and afterloaded papillary muscle. In Figure 3-7, A, the muscle is relaxed and bears no weight. For the intact left ventricle, this situation is analogous to the point in the cardiac cycle when the ventricle has relaxed after ejection has terminated, the aortic valve is closed, and the mitral valve is about to open (the end of isovolumic

relaxation—see Figure 3-11). In Figure 3-7, B, the resting muscle is stretched by a preload, which in the intact heart represents the end of filling of the left ventricle during ventricular diastole (in other words, it represents the **end-diastolic volume**). In Figure 3-7, C, the resting muscle is still stretched by the preload, but a supported afterload has been added without allowing the muscle to be stretched further. In the intact heart, this arrangement is analogous to the point in the cardiac cycle at which ventricular contraction starts and the mitral valve closes. The aortic valve has not yet opened because the ventricle has not developed enough intraventricular pressure to force it open (isovolumic contraction phase—see Figure 3-11). In Figure 3-7, D, the muscle contracts and lifts the afterload. In the intact heart, this situation represents left ventricular ejection into the aorta. During ejection, the afterload is represented by aortic and intraventricular pressures, which are virtually equal to each other.

The preload can be increased by greater filling of the left ventricle during diastole (Figure 3-4). At lower end-diastolic volumes, incremental increases in filling pressure during diastole elicit a greater systolic pressure during the subsequent contraction. Systolic pressure increases until a maximal systolic pressure is reached at the optimal preload (Figure 3-4). If diastolic filling continues beyond this point, no further increase in developed pressure will occur. At very high filling pressures, peak pressure development in systole is reduced.

At a constant preload, a higher systolic pressure can be reached during ventricular contractions by raising the afterload (e.g., increasing aortic pressure by restricting the runoff of blood to the peripheral vessels). Incremental increases in afterload produce progressively higher peak systolic pressures (Figure 3-8). If the afterload continues to increase, it becomes so great that the ventricle can no longer generate enough force to open the aortic valve (Figure 3-8). At

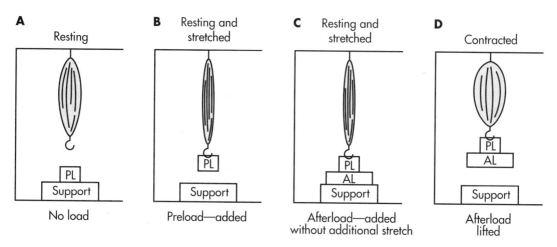

Figure 3-7 ■ **Preload and afterload in a papillary muscle.** A, Resting stage—in the intact heart just before opening of the AV valves. B, Preload—in the intact heart at the end of ventricular filling. C, Supported preload plus afterload—in the intact heart just before opening of the aortic valve. D, Lifting preload plus afterload—in the intact heart ventricular ejection with a decrease in ventricular volume. *PL*, Preload; *AL*, afterload; *PL + AL = total load.*

this point, ventricular systole is totally isometric; there is no ejection of blood and thus no change in volume of the ventricle during systole. The maximal pressure developed by the left ventricle under these conditions is the maximal isometric force the ventricle is capable of generating at a given preload. At preloads below the optimal filling volume, an increase in preload can yield a greater maximal isometric force.

Force and velocity are functions of the intracellular concentration of free calcium ions. When velocity is constant, force equals the afterload during contraction of the muscle. *Force and velocity are inversely related. With no load, the velocity of the muscle contraction is maximal, whereas with a maximal load (when contraction can no longer shorten the muscle), velocity is zero* (Figure 3-9).

Preloads and afterloads depend on certain characteristics of the vascular system and the behavior of the heart. With respect to the vasculature, the degree of venomotor tone and peripheral resistance influence preload and afterload. With respect to the heart, a change in rate or stroke volume can also alter preload and afterload. Hence cardiac and vascular factors interact to produce effects on preload and afterload (see Chapters 4 and 9 for a full explanation).

Box 3-3

In **heart failure,** the preload can be increased substantially because of the poor ventricular ejection and an increased blood volume caused by fluid retention. In **essential hypertension,** the high peripheral resistance augments the afterload by decreasing the peripheral runoff of the blood from the arterial system.

Contractility represents the performance of the heart at a given preload and afterload. *Contractility may be expressed experimentally as*

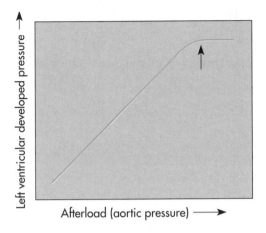

Figure 3-8 ■ **Effect of increasing afterload on developed pressure at constant preload. At the arrow, maximal developed pressure is reached. Further increments in afterload prevent opening of the aortic valve.**

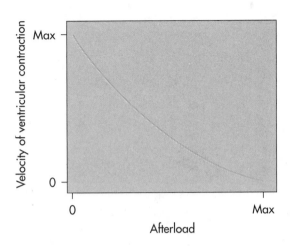

Figure 3-9 ■ **Effect of increasing afterload on the velocity of contraction at constant preload.**

the change in peak isometric force (isovolumic pressure) at a given initial fiber length (end-diastolic volume). Contractility can be augmented by certain drugs, such as norepinephrine or digitalis, and by an increase in contraction frequency **(tachycardia).** The increase in contractility **(positive inotropic effect)** produced by any of these interventions is reflected by incremental increases in developed force and velocity of contraction.

A reasonable index of myocardial contractility can be obtained from the contour of ventricular pressure curves (3-10). A hypodynamic heart is characterized by an elevated end-diastolic pressure, a slowly rising ventricular pressure, and a somewhat reduced ejection phase (curve *C,* Figure 3-10). A hyperdynamic heart (such as a heart stimulated by norepinephrine) shows reduced end-diastolic pressure, fast-rising ventricular pressure, and a brief ejection phase (curve *B,* Figure 3-10). The slope of the ascending limb of the ventricular pressure curve

Box 3-4

In rare instances, asthmatic patients accidentally received excessive doses of epinephrine subcutaneously. The patients develop marked tachycardia and increases in myocardial contractility, cardiac output, and total peripheral resistance. The result is dangerously high blood pressure. Treatment consists of a tourniquet on the injected limb, with intermittent brief releases of the tourniquet, and the use of adrenergic blocking drugs.

indicates the maximal rate of force development by the ventricle (maximal rate of change in pressure with time, **maximal dP/dt,** as illustrated by the tangents to the steepest portion of the ascending limbs of the ventricular pressure curves in Figure 3-10). The slope is maximal during the isovolumic phase of systole (Figure 3-11). At any given degree of ventricular filling, the slope pro-

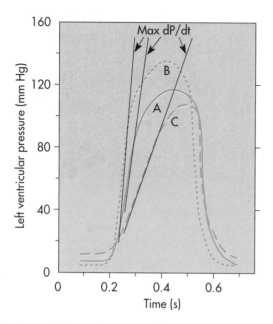

Figure 3-10 ▪ Left ventricular pressure curves with tangents drawn to the steepest portions of the ascending limbs to indicate maximal dP/dt values. A, Control; B, hyperdynamic heart, as with norepinephrine administration; C, hypodynamic heart, as in cardiac failure.

vides an index of the initial contraction velocity, and hence of contractility.

A similar indication of the contractile state of the myocardium can be obtained from the maximum velocity of blood flow in the ascending aorta during the cardiac cycle (i.e., the initial slope of the aortic flow curve) (see Figure 3-11). Also, the **ejection fraction,** which is the ratio of the volume of blood ejected from the left ventricle per beat **(stroke volume)** to the volume of blood in the left ventricle at the end of diastole (end-diastolic volume), is widely used clinically as an index of contractility. Other measurements (or combinations of measurements) that reflect the magnitude or velocity of the ventricular contraction have been used to assess the contractile state of the cardiac muscle. No index is entirely

satisfactory at present, which undoubtedly accounts for the several indices currently in use.

▪ THE CARDIAC CHAMBERS CONSIST OF TWO ATRIA, TWO VENTRICLES, AND FOUR VALVES

The atria are thin-walled, low-pressure chambers that function more as large reservoir conduits of blood for their respective ventricles than as important pumps for the forward propulsion of blood. The ventricles are formed by a continuum of muscle fibers that take origin from the fibrous skeleton at the base of the heart (chiefly around the aortic orifice). These fibers sweep toward the apex at the epicardial surface, and also pass toward the endocardium as they gradually undergo a 180-degree change in direction to lie parallel to the epicardial fibers and form the endocardium and papillary muscles (Figure 3-12). At the apex of the heart the fibers twist and turn inward to form papillary muscles, whereas at the base and around the valve orifices they form a thick powerful muscle that not only decreases ventricular circumference for ejection of blood but also narrows the AV valve orifices as an aid to valve closure. In addition to a reduction in circumference, ventricular ejection is accomplished by a decrease in the longitudinal axis with descent of the base of the heart. The earlier contraction of the apical part of the ventricles, coupled with approximation of the ventricular walls, propels the blood toward the outflow tracts. The right ventricle, which develops a mean pressure about one-seventh of that developed by the left ventricle, is considerably thinner than the left.

Cardiac Valves

The cardiac valves consist of thin flaps of flexible, tough, endothelium-covered fibrous tissue firmly attached at the base to the fibrous valve rings. Movements of the valve leaflets are essentially passive, and the orientation of the cardiac

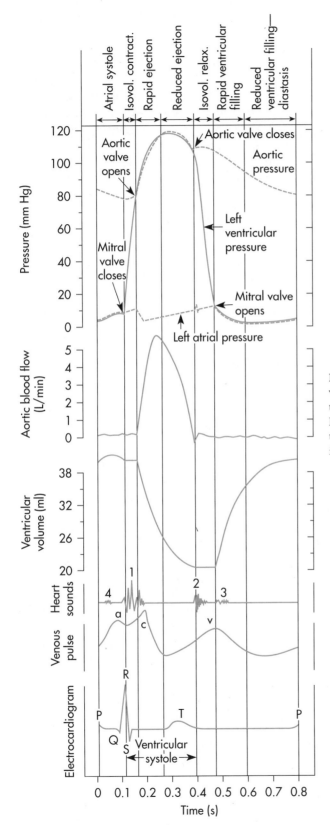

Figure 3-11 ■ Left atrial, aortic, and left ventricular pressure pulses correlated in time with aortic flow, ventricular volume, heart sounds, venous pulse, and the electrocardiogram for a complete cardiac cycle in the dog.

Endocardium

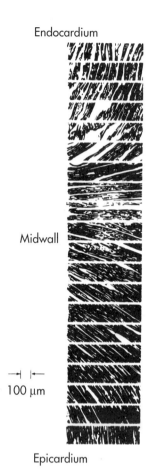

Midwall

—| |←—
100 μm

Epicardium

Figure 3-12 ▪ Sequence of photomicrographs showing fiber angles in successive sections taken from the middle of the free wall of the left ventricle from a heart in systole. The sections are parallel to the epicardial plane. The fiber angle is 90 degrees at the endocardium, running through 0 degrees at the midwall to −90 degrees at the epicardium. (From Streeter DD Jr, Spotnitz HM, Patel DP, et al: *Circ Res* 24:339, 1969.)

valves is responsible for unidirectional flow of blood through the heart. There are two types of valves in the heart—the **atrioventricular (AV) valves** and the **semilunar valves** (Figures 3-13 and 3-14).

Atrioventricular Valves The valve between the right atrium and right ventricle is made up of three cusps **(tricuspid valve)**, whereas that between the left atrium and left ventricle has two cusps **(mitral valve).** The total area of the cusps of each AV valve is approximately twice that of the respective AV orifice so that there is considerable overlap of the leaflets in the closed position (see Figures 3-13 and 3-14). Attached to the free edges of these valves are fine, strong ligaments **(chordae tendineae),** which arise from the powerful papillary muscles of the respective ventricles and prevent eversion of the valves during ventricular systole.

In the normal heart, the valve leaflets are relatively close during ventricular filling and provide a funnel for the transfer of blood from atrium to ventricle. This partial approximation of the valve surfaces during diastole is caused by eddy currents behind the leaflets and also by some tension on the free edges of the valves, exerted by the chordae tendineae and papillary muscles that are stretched by the filling ventricle. Movements of the mitral valve leaflets throughout the cardiac cycle are shown in an **echocardiogram** (Figure 3-15). Echocardiography consists of sending short pulses of high-frequency sound waves (ultrasound) through the chest tissues and the heart and recording the echoes reflected from the various structures. The timing and pattern of the reflected waves provide such information as the diameter of the heart, the ventricular wall thickness, and the magnitude and direction of the movements of various components of the heart.

In Figure 3-15 the echocardiograph is positioned to depict movement of the anterior leaflet of the mitral valve. The posterior leaflet moves in a pattern that is a mirror image of the anterior leaflet, but in the projection shown in Figure 3-15 the excursions appear much smaller. At

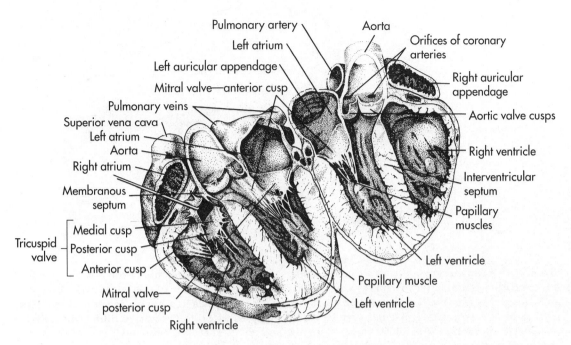

Pulmonary artery

Aorta

Left atrium

Orifices of coronary arteries

Left auricular appendage

Right auricular appendage

Mitral valve—anterior cusp

Pulmonary veins

Aortic valve cusps

Superior vena cava

Right ventricle

Left atrium

Aorta

Interventricular septum

Right atrium

Papillary muscles

Membranous septum

Medial cusp

Tricuspid valve

Posterior cusp

Anterior cusp

Left ventricle

Mitral valve—posterior cusp

Papillary muscle

Left ventricle

Right ventricle

Figure 3-13 ▪ **Drawing of a heart split perpendicular to the interventricular septum illustrates the anatomical relationships of the leaflets of the atrioventricular and aortic valves.**

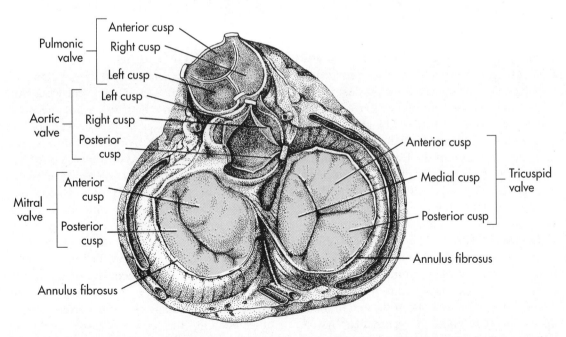

Anterior cusp

Pulmonic valve

Right cusp

Left cusp

Left cusp

Aortic valve

Right cusp

Posterior cusp

Anterior cusp

Anterior cusp

Medial cusp

Tricuspid valve

Mitral valve

Posterior cusp

Posterior cusp

Annulus fibrosus

Annulus fibrosus

Figure 3-14 ▪ **Four cardiac valves as viewed from the base of the heart. Note how the leaflets overlap in the closed valves.**

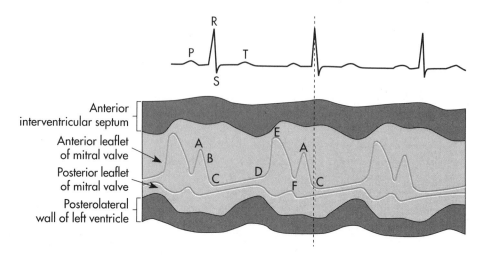

Figure 3-15 ■ **Drawing made from an echocardiogram showing movements of the mitral valve leaflets (particularly the anterior leaflet) and the changes in the diameter of the left ventricular cavity and the thickness of the left ventricular walls during cardiac cycles in a normal person.** *D to C,* **Ventricular diastole;** *C to D,* **ventricular systole;** *D to E,* **rapid filling;** *E to F,* **reduced filling (diastasis);** *F to A,* **atrial contraction. The mitral valve closes at** *C* **and opens at** *D.* **Simultaneously recorded electrocardiogram at top.**

point *D* the mitral valve opens, and during rapid filling (*D* to *E*) the anterior leaflet moves toward the ventricular septum. During the reduced filling phase (*E* to *F*) the valve leaflets float toward each other, but the valve does not close. The ventricular filling contributed by atrial contraction (*F* to *A*) forces the leaflets apart, and a second approximation of the leaflets follows (*A* to *C*). At point *C* the valve is closed by ventricular contraction. The valve leaflets, which bulge toward the atrium, stay pressed together during ventricular systole (*C* to *D*).

Semilunar Valves The valves between the right ventricle and the pulmonary artery and between the left ventricle and the aorta consist of three cuplike cusps attached to the valve rings (see Figures 3-13 and 3-14). At the end of the reduced ejection phase of ventricular systole, there is a brief reversal of blood flow toward the

ventricles (shown as a negative flow in the phasic aortic flow curve in Figure 3-11) that snaps the cusps together and prevents regurgitation of blood into the ventricles. During ventricular systole the cusps do not lie back against the walls of the pulmonary artery and aorta but float in the bloodstream approximately midway between the vessel walls and their closed position. Behind the semilunar valves are small outpocketings of the pulmonary artery and aorta (**sinuses of Valsalva**), where eddy currents develop that tend to keep the valve cusps away from the vessel walls. The orifices of the right and left coronary arteries are behind the right and the left cusps, respectively, of the aortic valve. Were it not for the presence of the sinuses of Valsalva and the eddy currents developed therein, the coronary ostia could be blocked by the valve cusps.

The Pericardium Is an Epithelized Fibrous Sac That Invests the Heart

The pericardium consists of a visceral layer that adheres to the epicardium and a parietal layer that is separated from the visceral layer by a thin layer of fluid. This fluid provides lubrication for the continuous movement of the enclosed heart. The distensibility of the pericardium is small, so that it strongly resists a large, rapid increase in cardiac size. Because of this characteristic, the pericardium plays a role in preventing sudden overdistension of the chambers of the heart. However, in congenital absence of the pericardium or after its surgical removal, cardiac function is within physiological limits. Nevertheless, with the pericardium intact, an increase in diastolic pressure in one ventricle increases the pressure and decreases the compliance of the other ventricle.

Box 3-5

With slow, progressive, and sustained enlargement of the heart, as occurs in cardiac hypertrophy, or with a slow progressive increase in pericardial fluid, as occurs in pericarditis with pericardial effusion, the intact pericardium is gradually stretched.

The Two Major Heart Sounds Are Mainly Produced by Closure of the Cardiac Valves

Four sounds are usually produced by the heart, but only two are ordinarily audible through a stethoscope. With electronic amplification the less intense sounds can be detected and recorded graphically as a **phonocardiogram.** This means of registering heart sounds that may be inaudible to the human ear helps to delineate the precise timing of the heart sounds relative to other events in the cardiac cycle.

The first heart sound is initiated at the onset of ventricular systole (Figure 3-11) and consists of a series of vibrations of mixed, unrelated, low frequencies (a noise). It is the loudest and longest of the heart sounds, has a crescendo-decrescendo quality, and is heard best over the apical region of the heart. The tricuspid valve sounds are heard best in the fifth intercostal space just to the left of the sternum; the mitral sounds are heard best in the fifth intercostal space at the cardiac apex.

The first heart sound is chiefly caused by oscillation of blood in the ventricular chambers and vibration of the chamber walls. The vibrations are engendered in part by the abrupt rise of ventricular pressure with acceleration of blood back toward the atria, but primarily by sudden tension and recoil of the AV valves and adjacent structures with deceleration of the blood resulting from closure of the AV valves. The vibrations of the ventricles and the contained blood are transmitted through surrounding tissues and reach the chest wall, where they may be heard or recorded. The intensity of the first sound is a function of the force of ventricular contraction and of the distance between the valve leaflets. The first sound is loudest when the leaflets are farthest apart, as occurs when the interval between atrial and ventricular systoles is prolonged (AV valve leaflets float apart) or when ventricular systole immediately follows atrial systole.

The second heart sound, which occurs with closure of the semilunar valves (Figure 3-11), is composed of higher-frequency vibrations (higher pitch), is of shorter duration and lower intensity, and has a more snapping quality than the first heart sound. The second sound is caused by abrupt closure of the semilunar valves, which initiates oscillations of the columns of blood and the tensed vessel walls by the stretch and recoil of the closed valve. The second sound caused by closure of the pulmonic valve is heard best in the second thoracic interspace just to the left of the sternum, whereas that caused by closure of the aortic valve is heard best in the same intercostal space but to the right of the sternum. Conditions that bring about a more rapid closure of the semilunar valves, such as increases in pulmonary artery or aortic pressure (e.g., pulmonary or systemic hypertension), increase the intensity of the second heart sound. In adults the aortic valve sound is usually louder than the pulmonic, but in cases of pulmonary hypertension the reverse is often true.

A normal phonocardiogram taken simultaneously with an electrocardiogram is illustrated in Figure 3-16. Note that the first sound, which starts just beyond the peak of the R wave, is composed of irregular waves and is of greater intensity and duration than the second sound, which appears at the end of the T wave. A third and fourth heart sound do not appear on this record.

The third heart sound, which is sometimes heard in children with thin chest walls or in patients with left ventricular failure, consists of a few low-intensity, low-frequency vibrations heard best in the region of the apex. It occurs in early diastole and is believed to be the result of vibrations of the ventricular walls caused by abrupt cessation of ventricular distension and deceleration of blood entering the ventricles.

Box 3-6

In overloaded hearts, as in congestive heart failure, when the ventricular volume is very large and the ventricular walls are stretched to the point where distensibility abruptly decreases, a third heart sound may be heard. A third heart sound in patients with heart disease is usually a grave sign.

A fourth, or atrial, sound, consisting of a few low-frequency oscillations, is occasionally heard in normal individuals. It is caused by oscillation of blood and cardiac chambers created by atrial contraction (Figure 3-11).

Because the onset and termination of right and left ventricular systoles are not precisely synchronous, differences in the time of vibration of the two AV valves or two semilunar valves can sometimes be detected with the stethoscope. Such asynchrony of valve vibrations, which may sometimes indicate abnormal cardiac function, is manifested as **a split sound** over the apex of the heart for the AV valves and over the base of the heart for the semilunar valves.

■ THE SEQUENTIAL CONTRACTION AND RELAXATION OF THE ATRIA AND VENTRICLES CONSTITUTE THE CARDIAC CYCLE

Ventricular Systole

Isovolumic Contraction   The onset of ventricular contraction coincides with the peak of the R wave of the electrocardiogram and the initial vibration of the first heart sound. It is indi-

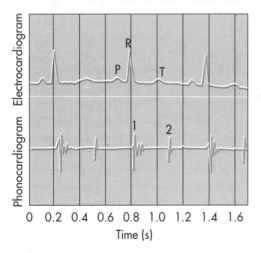

Figure 3-16 ■ Phonocardiogram illustrating the first and second heart sounds and their relationship to the P, R, and T waves of the electrocardiogram. (Time lines = 0.04 s.)

cated on the ventricular pressure curve as the
earliest rise in ventricular pressure after atrial
contraction. The interval of time between the
start of ventricular systole and the opening of
the semilunar valves (when ventricular pressure
rises abruptly) is termed **isovolumic contraction** because ventricular volume is constant during this brief period (Figure 3-11).

The increment in ventricular pressure during isovolumic contraction is transmitted across
the closed valves. Isovolumic contraction has
also been referred to as *isometric contraction.* However, some fibers shorten and others
lengthen, as evidenced by changes in ventricular shape; it is therefore not a true isometric
contraction.

Ejection Opening of the semilunar valves
marks the onset of the ejection phase, which
may be subdivided into an earlier, shorter phase
(rapid ejection) and a later, longer phase **(reduced ejection).** The rapid ejection phase is
distinguished from the reduced ejection phase

by (1) the sharp rise in ventricular and aortic
pressures that terminates at the peak ventricular
and aortic pressures, (2) a more abrupt decrease
in ventricular volume, and (3) a greater aortic
blood flow (Figure 3-11). The sharp decrease in
the left atrial pressure curve at the onset of ejection results from the descent of the base of the
heart and stretch of the atria. During the
reduced ejection period, runoff of blood from
the aorta to the periphery exceeds ventricular
output, and therefore aortic pressure declines.
Throughout ventricular systole the blood returning to the atria produces a progressive increase
in atrial pressure. Note that during approximately the first third of the ejection period, left
ventricular pressure slightly exceeds aortic pressure and flow accelerates (continues to increase), whereas during the last two thirds of
ventricular ejection the reverse holds true. This
reversal of the ventricular-aortic pressure gradient in the presence of continued flow of blood
from the left ventricle to the aorta (caused by
the momentum of the forward blood flow) is
the result of the storage of potential energy in
the stretched arterial walls, which produces a
deceleration of blood flow into the aorta (see
Chapter 6). The peak of the flow curve coincides in time with the point at which the left
ventricular pressure curve intersects the aortic
pressure curve during ejection. Thereafter flow
decelerates (continues to decrease) because the
pressure gradient has been reversed.

With right ventricular ejection, there is shortening of the free wall of the right ventricle (descent of the tricuspid valve ring) in addition to
lateral compression of the chamber. However,
with left ventricular ejection, there is very little
shortening of the base-to-apex axis, and ejection
is accomplished chiefly by compression of the
left ventricular chamber.

The effect of ventricular systole on left ventricular diameter is shown in an echocardiogram
(see Figure 3-15). During ventricular systole (see

Figure 3-15, *C* to *D*) the septum and the free wall of the left ventricle become thicker and move closer to each other.

The venous pulse curve shown in Figure 3-11 has been taken from a jugular vein. The **a wave** is caused by atrial contraction, the **c wave** by the impact of the adjacent common carotid artery and to some extent by transmission of a pressure wave produced by the abrupt closure of the tricuspid valve in early ventricular systole, and the **v wave** by the pressure of blood returning from the peripheral vessels and the abrupt opening of the tricuspid valve. Note that except for the c wave, the venous pulse closely follows the atrial pressure curve.

At the end of ejection, a volume of blood approximately equal to that ejected during systole remains in the ventricular cavities. This **residual volume** is fairly constant in normal hearts but is smaller with increased heart rate or reduced outflow resistance and larger when the opposite conditions prevail.

In addition to serving as a small adjustable blood reservoir, the residual volume to a limited degree can permit transient disparities between the outputs of the two ventricles.

Box 3-8

An increase in myocardial contractility, as produced by catecholamines or by digitalis in a patient with a depressed heart, may decrease residual volume and increase stroke volume and ejection fraction. With severely hypodynamic and dilated hearts, as in **heart failure,** the residual volume can become many times greater than the stroke volume.

Ventricular Diastole

Isovolumic Relaxation Closure of the aortic valve produces the **incisura** on the descending limb of the aortic pressure curve and the

second heart sound (with some vibrations evident on the atrial pressure curve), and marks the end of ventricular systole. The period between the closure of the semilunar valves and the opening of the AV valves is termed **isovolumic relaxation** and is characterized by a precipitous fall in ventricular pressure without a change in ventricular volume.

Rapid Filling Phase The major part of the ventricular filling occurs immediately on opening of the AV valves when the blood that had returned to the atria during the previous ventricular systole is abruptly released into the relaxing ventricles. This period of ventricular filling is called the **rapid filling phase.** In Figure 3-11 the onset of the rapid filling phase is indicated by the decrease in left ventricular pressure below left atrial pressure, resulting in the opening of the mitral valve. The rapid flow of blood from atria to relaxing ventricles produces a decrease in atrial and ventricular pressures and a sharp increase in ventricular volume.

Diastasis The rapid filling phase is followed by a phase of slow filling, called **diastasis.** During diastasis, blood returning from the periphery flows into the right ventricle and blood from the lungs into the left ventricle. This small, slow addition to ventricular filling is indicated by a gradual rise in atrial, ventricular, and venous pressures and in ventricular volume (see Figure 3-11).

Atrial Systole The onset of atrial systole occurs soon after the beginning of the P wave of the electrocardiogram (curve of atrial depolarization) and the transfer of blood from atrium to ventricle made by the peristalsis-like wave of atrial contraction completes the period of ventricular filling. Atrial systole is responsible for the small increases in atrial, ventricular, and venous (a wave) pressures, as well as in ventricular volume shown in Figure 3-11. Throughout ventricular diastole, atrial pressure barely exceeds ventricular pressure, indicating a low-

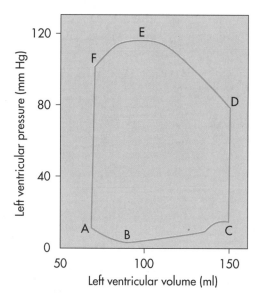

Figure 3-17 ■ **Pressure-volume loop of the left ventricle for a single cardiac cycle (ABCDEF).**

resistance pathway across the open AV valves during ventricular filling.

Because there are no valves at the junctions of the venae cavae and right atrium or of the pulmonary veins and left atrium, atrial contraction can force blood in both directions. Actually, little blood is pumped back into the venous tributaries during the brief atrial contraction, mainly because of the inertia of the inflowing blood.

Atrial contraction is not essential for ventricular filling, as can be observed in atrial fibrillation or complete heart block. However, its contribution is governed to a great extent by the heart rate and the structure of the AV valves. At slow heart rates, filling practically ceases toward the end of diastasis, and atrial contraction contributes little additional filling. During tachycardia, diastasis is abbreviated and the atrial contribution can become substantial, especially if it occurs immediately after the rapid filling phase when the AV pressure gradient is maximal.

Should tachycardia become so great that the rapid filling phase is encroached on, atrial contraction assumes great importance in rapidly propelling blood into the ventricle during this brief period of the cardiac cycle. Of course, if the period of ventricular relaxation is so brief that filling is seriously impaired, even atrial contraction cannot prevent inadequate ventricular filling. The consequent reduction in cardiac output may result in syncope. Obviously, if atrial contraction occurs simultaneously with ventricular contraction, no atrial contribution to ventricular filling can occur.

> **Box 3-9**
>
> In certain disease states, the AV valves may be markedly narrowed **(stenotic).** Under such conditions, atrial contraction plays a much more important role in ventricular filling than it does in the normal heart.

The Pressure-Volume Graph Illustrates the Sequential Dynamic Changes in a Single Cardiac Cycle The changes in left ventricular pressure and volume throughout the cardiac cycle are summarized in Figure 3-17. The element of time is not considered in this **pressure-volume loop.** Diastolic filling starts at *A* and terminates at *C,* when the mitral valve closes. The initial decrease in left ventricular pressure (*A* to *B*), despite the rapid inflow of blood from the atrium, is attributed to progressive ventricular relaxation and distensibility. During the remainder of diastole (*B* to *C*) the increase in ventricular pressure reflects ventricular filling and the passive elastic characteristics of the ventricle. Note that only a small increase in pressure occurs with the increase in ventricular volume during diastole (*B* to *C*). The small increase in pressure just to the left of *C* is caused by the contribution of atrial contraction to ventricular filling. With isovolumic contraction (*C* to *D*), there is a steep rise in pressure and no change in ventricular volume. At *D* the aortic valve opens, and during the first phase of ejection (rapid ejection, *D* to *E*), the large reduction in volume is associated with a continued but less steep increase in ventricular pressure than that which occurred during isovolumic contraction. This volume reduction is followed by reduced ejection (*E* to *F*) and a small decrease in ventricular pressure. The aortic valve closes at *F*, and this event is followed by isovolumic relaxation (*F* to *A*), characterized by a sharp drop in pressure and no change in volume. The mitral valve opens at *A* to complete one cardiac cycle.

■ THE FICK PRINCIPLE IS USED TO DETERMINE CARDIAC OUTPUT

In 1870 the German physiologist Adoph Fick contrived the first method for measuring cardiac output in intact animals and people. The basis for this method, called the **Fick principle,** is simply an application of the law of conservation of mass. It is derived from the fact that the quantity of oxygen (O_2) delivered to the pulmonary capillaries via the pulmonary artery, plus the quantity of O_2 that enters the pulmonary capillaries from the alveoli, must equal the quantity of O_2 that is carried away by the pulmonary veins.

This is depicted schematically in Figure 3-18. The rate, q_1, of O_2 delivery to the lungs equals the O_2 concentration in the pulmonary arterial blood, $[O_2]_{pa}$, times the pulmonary arterial blood flow, Q, which equals the cardiac output; that is,

$$q_1 = Q[O_2]_{pa} \tag{1}$$

Let q_2 be the net rate of O_2 uptake by the pulmonary capillaries from the alveoli. At equilibrium, q_2 equals the O_2 consumption of the body. The rate q_3, at which O_2 is carried away by the pulmonary venous blood, $[O_2]_{pv}$, is multiplied by the total pulmonary venous flow, which is virtually equal to the pulmonary arterial blood flow, Q; that is,

$$q_3 = Q[O_2]_{pv} \tag{2}$$

From conservation of mass,

$$q_1 + q_2 = q_3 \tag{3}$$

Therefore

$$Q[O_2]_{pa} + q_2 = Q[O_2]_{pv} \tag{4}$$

Solving for cardiac output,

$$Q = q_2/([O_2]_{pv} - [O_2]_{pa}) \tag{5}$$

Equation 5 is the statement of Fick's principle.

Box 3-10

In the clinical determination of cardiac output, O_2 consumption is computed from measurements of the volume and O_2 content of expired air over a given interval of time. Because the O_2 concentration of peripheral arterial blood is essentially identical to that in the pulmonary veins, $[O_2]_{pv}$ is determined by a sample of peripheral arterial blood withdrawn by needle puncture. Pulmonary arterial blood actually represents mixed systemic venous blood. Samples for O_2 analysis are obtained from the pulmonary artery or right ventricle through a catheter.

An example of calculation of cardiac output in a normal, resting adult is illustrated in Figure 3-18. With an O_2 consumption of 250 ml/min, an arterial (pulmonary venous) O_2 content of 0.20 ml O_2/ml blood, and a mixed venous (pulmonary arterial) O_2 content of 0.15 ml O_2/ml blood, the cardiac output would equal 250 ÷ (0.20 − 0.15) = 5000 ml/min.

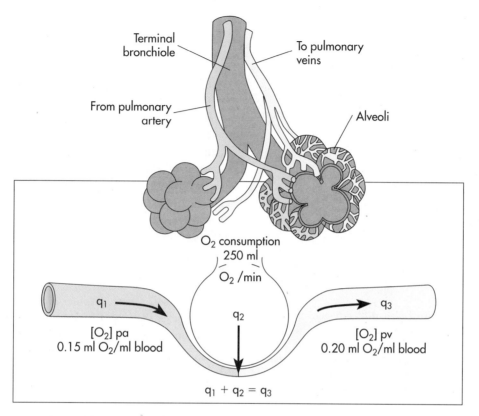

Figure 3-18 ■ Schema illustrates the Fick principle for measuring cardiac output. The change in color from pulmonary artery to pulmonary vein represents the change in color of the blood as venous blood becomes fully oxygenated.

The Fick principle is also used for estimating the O_2 consumption of organs in situ, when blood flow and the O_2 contents of the arterial and venous blood can be determined. Algebraic rearrangement reveals that O_2 consumption equals the blood flow times the arteriovenous O_2 concentration difference. For example, if the blood flow through one kidney is 700 ml/min, arterial O_2 content is 0.20 ml O_2/ml blood, and renal venous O_2 content is 0.18 ml O_2/ml blood, the rate of O_2 consumption by that kidney must be 700 (0.20 − 0.18) = 14 ml O_2/min.

The Indicator Dilution Technique is a Useful Method for Measuring Cardiac Output

The indicator dilution technique for measuring cardiac output is also based on the law of conservation of mass and is illustrated by the model in Figure 3-19. Let a liquid flow through a tube at a rate of Q ml/s, and let q mg of dye be injected as a slug into the stream at point *A*. Let mixing occur at some point downstream. If a small sample of liquid is continually withdrawn from point *B* farther downstream and passed through a den-

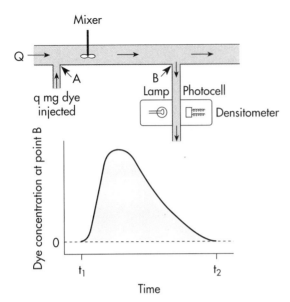

Figure 3-19 ▪ Indicator dilution technique for measuring cardiac output. In this model, in which there is no recirculation, q mg of dye are injected instantaneously at point A into a stream flowing at Q ml/min. A mixed sample of the fluid flowing past point B is withdrawn at a constant rate through a densitometer. The resulting dye concentration curve at point B has the configuration shown in the lower section of the figure.

sitometer, a curve of the dye concentration, c, may be recorded as a function of time, t, as shown in the lower half of Figure 3-19.

If no dye is lost between points A and B, the amount of dye, q, passing point B between times t_1 and t_2 will be

$$q = \bar{c}Q\,(t_2 - t_1) \qquad (6)$$

where $\bar{c}$ is the mean concentration of dye. The value of $\bar{c}$ may be computed by dividing the area of the dye concentration by the duration $(t_2 - t_1)$ of that curve; that is

$$\bar{c} = \int_{t_1}^{t_2} cdt/(t_2 - t_1) \qquad (7)$$

Substituting this value of $\bar{c}$ into equation 6 and solving for Q yields

$$Q = \frac{q}{\int_{t_1}^{t_2} cdt} \qquad (8)$$

Thus flow may be measured by dividing the amount of indicator injected upstream by the area under the downstream concentration curve.

This technique has been widely used to estimate cardiac output in humans. A measured quantity of some indicator (a dye or isotope that remains within the circulation) is injected rapidly into a large central vein or into the right side of the heart through a catheter. Arterial blood is continuously drawn through a detector (densitometer or isotope rate counter), and a curve of indicator concentration is recorded as a function of time.

Presently the most popular indicator dilution technique is **thermodilution.** The indicator is cold saline. The temperature and volume of the saline are measured accurately before injection. A flexible catheter is introduced into a peripheral vein and advanced so that the tip lies in the pulmonary artery. A small thermistor at the catheter tip records the changes in temperature. The opening in the catheter lies a few inches proximal to the tip. When the tip is in the pulmonary artery, the opening lies in or near the right atrium. The cold saline is injected rapidly into the right atrium through the catheter. The resultant change in temperature downstream is recorded by the thermistor in the pulmonary artery.

The thermodilution technique has the following advantages: (1) an arterial puncture is not necessary; (2) the small volumes of saline used in each determination are innocuous, allowing repeated determinations to be made; and (3) recirculation is negligible. Temperature equilibration takes place as the cooled blood flows through the pulmonary and systemic capillary beds, before it flows by the thermistor in the pulmonary artery the second time.

Summary

- Although the myocardium is made up of individual cells with discrete membrane boundaries, the cardiac myocytes that comprise the ventricles contract almost in unison, as do those of the atria. The myocardium functions as a syncytium with an all-or-none response to excitation. Cell-to-cell conduction occurs through gap junctions that connect the cytosol of adjacent cells.

- An increase in myocardial fiber length, as occurs with an augmented ventricular filling during diastole (preload), produces a more forceful ventricular contraction. This relation between fiber length and strength of contraction is known as Starling's law of the heart.

- On excitation, voltage-gated calcium channels open to admit extracellular Ca^{++} into the cell. The influx of Ca^{++} triggers the release of Ca^{++} from the sarcoplasmic reticulum. The elevated intracellular Ca^{++} produces contraction of the myofilaments.

- Relaxation is accomplished via restoration of the resting cytosolic Ca^{++} level by pumping it back into the sarcoplasmic reticulum and exchanging it for extracellular Na^+ across the sarcolemma.

- Velocity and force (afterload) of contraction are functions of the intracellular concentration of free Ca ions. Afterload and velocity are inversely related, so that with no load, velocity is maximal. In an isometric contraction, where no external shortening occurs, total load is maximal and velocity is zero.

- In ventricular contraction the preload is the stretch of the fibers by the blood during ventricular filling and the afterload is the aortic pressure against which the left ventricle ejects the blood.

- Contractility is an expression of cardiac performance at a given preload and afterload. Contractility is increased mainly by interventions that raise intracellular Ca^{++} and decreased by interventions that lower intracellular Ca^{++}.

- Simultaneous recording of left atrial, left ventricular, and aortic pressures; ventricular volume; heart sounds; and electrocardiogram graphically portray the sequential and related electrical and cardiodynamic events throughout a cardiac cycle. The first heart sound is caused mainly by abrupt closure of the AV valves; the second heart sound is caused by abrupt closure of the semilunar valves.

- Cardiac output can be determined, according to the Fick principle, by measuring the oxygen consumption of the body (MVO_2) and the oxygen content of arterial $[O_2]_a$ and mixed venous $[O_2]_v$ blood. Cardiac output = $MVO_2/([O_2]_a - [O_2]_v)$. It can also be measured by dye dilution or thermodilution techniques. The greater the cardiac output, the greater is the dilution of the injected dye or cold saline by the arterial blood.

■ BIBLIOGRAPHY

1. Alvarez BV, Pérez NG, Ennis IL, et al: Mechanisms underlying the increase in force and Ca^{++} transient that follow stretch of cardiac muscle: a possible explanation of the Anrep effect. *Circ Res* 85:716, 1999.
2. Bers DM, Lederer WJ, Berlin JR: Intracellular Ca transients in rat cardiac myocytes: role of Na-Ca exchange in excitation-contraction coupling. *Am J Physiol* 258:C944, 1990.
3. Blaustein MP, Lederer WJ: Sodium/calcium exchange: its physiological implications. *Physiol Rev* 79:763, 1999.
4. Carafoli E: Calcium pump of the plasma membrane. *Physiol Rev* 71:129, 1991.
5. Elzinga G, Westerhof N: Matching between ventricle and arterial load. *Circ Res* 68:1495, 1991.
6. Frank GB, Bianchi CP, ten Keurs HEDJ, editors: *Excitation-contraction coupling in skeletal cardiac and smooth muscle,* New York, 1992, Plenum Press.

7. Gaughan JP, Furukawa S, Jecranandam V, et al: Sodium/calcium exchange contributes to contraction and relaxation in failed human ventricular myocytes. *Am J Physiol* 277:H714, 1999.

8. Katz AM: Interplay between inotropic and lusitropic effects of cyclic adenosine monophosphate on the myocardial cell. *Circulation* 82:1-7, 1990.

9. Katz AM: *Physiology of the heart,* ed 2, New York, 1992, Raven Press.

10. Lakatta EG: Length modulation of muscle performance: Frank-Starling law of the heart. In Fozzard HA, et al, editors: *The heart and cardiovascular system,* ed 2, New York, 1991, Raven Press.

11. Lorenz JN, Kranias EG: Regulatory effects of phospholamban on cardiac function in intact mice. *Am J Physiol* 273:H2826, 1997.

12. Luo W, Grupp IL, Harrer J, et al: Targeted ablation of the phospholamban gene is associated with markedly enhanced myocardial contractility and loss of β-agonist stimulation. *Circ Res* 75:401,1994.

13. Niggi E: Ca^{++} sparks in cardiac muscle: is there life without them? *News Physiol Sci* 14:129, 1999.

14. Pieske B, Maier LS, Bers DM, et al: Ca^{++} handling and sarcoplasmic reticulum Ca^{++} content in isolated failing and nonfailing human myocardium. *Circ Res* 85:38, 1999.

15. Wier WG, Balke CW: Ca^{++} release mechanisms, Ca^{++} sparks, and local control of excitation-contraction coupling in normal heart muscle. *Circ Res* 85:770, 1999.

■ **CASE 3**

HISTORY

A 60-year-old woman entered the hospital complaining of shortness of breath, fatigue, and swelling of her ankles and lower legs. She had these symptoms for about 3 years but refused medical treatment until they became severe. As a child she had rheumatic fever and developed a murmur, which was diagnosed as mitral stenosis. Physical examination revealed a dyspneic, slightly cyanotic woman with ankle and pretibial edema, distended neck veins, an enlarged tender liver, ascites, and rales at the lung bases. Electrocardiogram showed atrial fibrillation and right axis deviation. A chest x-ray showed an enlarged heart and shadows at the lung basis that were compatible with pulmonary edema. A cardiac workup showed a low cardiac output. After a week of treatment for her congestive heart failure, her symptoms abated and she was sent home on medication.

QUESTIONS

1. Auscultation of the heart revealed a
   a. Harsh systolic murmur heard best at the cardiac apex
   b. Harsh systolic murmur heard best in the 2nd interspace to the left of the sternum
   c. Soft high pitched diastolic murmur heard best in the 2nd interspace to the left of the sternum
   d. Rumbling low pitched diastolic murmur heard best at the cardiac apex
   e. High pitched systolic murmur heard best in the 2nd interspace to the right of the sternum

2. Which of the following is not observed in atrial fibrillation?
   a. Irregular heart beat
   b. The heart rate measured by auscultation over the precordium is greater than that measured by palpation of the radial artery
   c. A very rapid regular rate
   d. Variation in the strength of the heart beats as palpated at the wrist
   e. No P waves in the electrocardiogram

3. Which of the following therapeutic measures would help this patient?
   a. Insertion of a pacemaker to correct the dysrhythmia
   b. Phlebotomy (blood removal via a peripheral vein)
   c. Saline infusion to increase preload and cardiac rhythm
   d. Intravenous adenosine to restore normal cardiac output
   e. Administration of a calcium uptake blocker such as diltiazem

4. Which of the following findings would be true for this patient?

a. Increased serum albumin
b. Increased pulmonary wedge pressure (obtained by threading a catheter via a peripheral vein as far as it will go into a branch of the pulmonary artery)
c. Increased sodium excretion
d. Reduced peripheral resistance
e. Increased pulse pressure

5. Which of the following drugs would <u>not</u> be prescribed for this patient?
   a. Dicumarol
   b. Digoxin
   c. Procainamide
   d. Hydrochlorothiazide
   e. Nitroglycerin

6. The patient's whole body oxygen consumption was 300 ml/min and the pulmonary artery and the brachial artery blood oxygen content were 8 ml/dl and 18 ml/dl, respectively. What was the patient's cardiac output?
   a. 2.0 L/min
   b. 4.8 L/min
   c. 3.0 L/min
   d. 1.3 L/min
   e. 1.2 L/min

CHAPTER 4

Regulation of the Heartbeat

Objectives

1. Describe the neural control of heart rate.

2. Explain the role of preload in the regulation of myocardial contraction.

3. Describe the neural regulation of myocardial contraction.

4. Explain the effects of hormones on myocardial contraction.

5. Explain the effects of blood gases on myocardial contraction.

THE QUANTITY OF BLOOD PUMPED BY the heart each minute (i.e., the **cardiac output, CO**) may be varied by changing the frequency of its beats (i.e., **heart rate, HR**) or the volume ejected per stroke (i.e., **stroke volume, SV**). Cardiac output is the product of heart rate and stroke volume; that is,

$$CO = HR \times SV$$

A discussion of the control of cardiac activity may therefore be subdivided into a consideration of the regulation of pacemaker activity and the regulation of myocardial performance. However, in the intact organism, a change in the behavior of one of these features of cardiac activity almost invariably alters the other.

Certain local factors, such as temperature changes and tissue stretch, can affect the dis-charge frequency of the sinoatrial (SA) node. However, the principal control of heart rate is relegated to the autonomic nervous system, and the discussion is restricted to this aspect of heart rate control. Also considered are the intrinsic and extrinsic factors that regulate myocardial performance.

■ HEART RATE IS CONTROLLED MAINLY BY THE AUTONOMIC NERVES

In normal adults the average heart rate at rest is approximately 70 beats per minute, but the rate is significantly greater in children. During sleep the heart rate diminishes by 10 to 20 beats per minute, but during emotional excitement or muscular activity it may accelerate to rates considerably above 100. In well-trained athletes at rest, the rate is usually only about 50 beats per minute.

The SA node is usually under the tonic influence of both divisions of the autonomic nervous system. The sympathetic system enhances automaticity, whereas the parasympathetic system inhibits it. Changes in heart rate usually involve a reciprocal action of the two divisions of the autonomic nervous system. Thus an increased heart rate is produced by a diminution of parasympathetic activity and concomitant increase in sympathetic activity; deceleration is usually achieved by the opposite mechanisms. Under certain conditions the heart rate may change by selective action of just one division of the autonomic nervous system, rather than by reciprocal changes in both divisions.

Ordinarily, in healthy, resting individuals, parasympathetic tone predominates. Abolition of parasympathetic influences by administration of **atropine** usually increases heart rate substantially, whereas abrogation of sympathetic effects by administration of **propranolol** usually decreases heart rate only slightly (Figure 4-1). When both divisions of the autonomic nervous system are blocked, the heart rate of young adults averages about 100 beats per minute. The rate that prevails after complete autonomic blockade is called the **intrinsic heart rate.**

Parasympathetic Pathways

The cardiac parasympathetic fibers originate in the medulla oblongata, in cells that lie in the **dorsal motor nucleus of the vagus** or in the **nucleus ambiguus.** The precise location varies from species to species. Efferent vagal fibers pass inferiorly through the neck as the cervical vagus nerves (Figure 4-2), which lie close to the common carotid arteries. They then pass through the mediastinum to synapse with postganglionic cells on the epicardial surface or within the walls of the heart itself. Most of the cardiac ganglion cells are located near the SA node and atrioventricular (AV) conduction tissue.

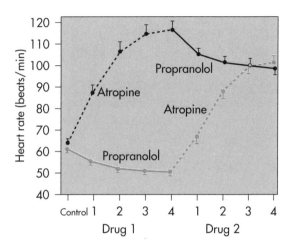

Figure 4-1 ■ **Effects of four equal doses of atropine (0.04 mg/kg total) and of propranolol (0.2 mg/kg total) on the heart rate of 10 healthy young men (mean age, 21.9 years). In half of the trials, atropine was given first** *(top curve);* **in the other half, propranolol was given first** *(bottom curve).* (Redrawn from Katona PG, McLean M, Dighton DH, et al: *J Appl Physiol* 52:1652, 1982.)

The right and left vagi are distributed differentially to the various cardiac structures. The right vagus nerve affects the SA node predominantly. Stimulation slows SA nodal firing or may even stop it for several seconds. The left vagus nerve mainly inhibits AV conduction tissue, to produce various degrees of AV block. However, the distributions of the efferent vagal fibers overlap, such that left vagal stimulation also depresses the SA node and right vagal stimulation impedes AV conduction.

The SA and AV nodes are rich in **cholinesterase.** Hence the effects of any given vagal impulse are ephemeral because the acetylcholine released at the nerve terminals is rapidly hydrolyzed. Furthermore, the effects of vagal activity on SA and AV nodal function have a very short latency (about 50 to 100 ms), because the released acetylcholine activates special K^+ channels in the cardiac cells. The opening of these

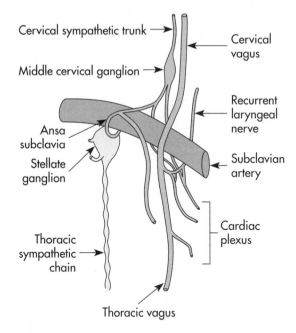

Figure 4-2 ■ **The cardiac autonomic nerves on the right side of the human body.**

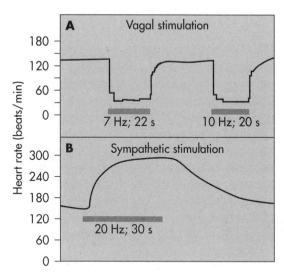

Figure 4-3 ■ **Changes in heart rate evoked by stimulation (horizontal bars) of the vagus (A) and sympathetic (B) nerves in an anesthetized dog.** (Modified from Warner HR, Cox AJ: *J Appl Physiol* 17:349, 1962.)

channels is so prompt because it does not require the operation of a second messenger system, such as the adenylyl cyclase system.

When the vagus nerves are stimulated at a constant frequency for several seconds, the heart rate decreases abruptly and attains a steady-state value within one or two cardiac cycles (Figure 4-3, *A*). Also, when stimulation is discontinued, the heart rate returns very quickly to its basal level. The combination of the brief latency and rapid decay of the response (because of the abundance of cholinesterase) provides the opportunity for the vagus nerves to exert a beat by beat control of SA and AV nodal function.

Parasympathetic influences preponderate over sympathetic effects at the SA node, as

shown in Figure 4-4. As the frequency of sympathetic stimulation in an anesthetized dog was increased from 0 to 4 Hz, the heart rate increased by about 80 beats per minute in the absence of vagal stimulation (Vag = 0 Hz). However, when the vagi were stimulated at 8 Hz, increasing the sympathetic stimulation frequency from 0 to 4 Hz had a negligible influence on heart rate. This vagal preponderance in the regulation of heart rate is mediated mainly by an effective throttling of the release of norepinephrine from the sympathetic nerve endings by the acetylcholine released from neighboring vagus nerve endings. This type of interaction between the two divisions of the autonomic nervous system is discussed more fully in association with Figure 4-5.

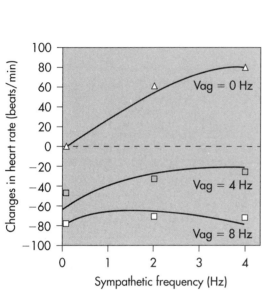

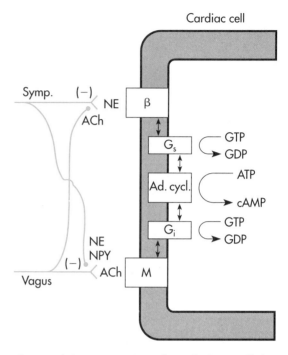

Figure 4-4 ■ **Changes in heart rate in an anesthetized dog when the vagus and cardiac sympathetic nerves were stimulated simultaneously. The sympathetic nerves were stimulated at 0, 2, and 4 Hz; the vagus nerves at 0, 4, and 8 Hz. The symbols represent the observed changes in heart rate; the curves were derived from a computed regression equation.** (Modified from Levy MN, Zieske H: *J Appl Physiol* 27:465, 1969.)

Figure 4-5 ■ **Interneuronal and intracellular mechanisms responsible for the interactions between the sympathetic and parasympathetic systems in the neural control of cardiac function.** (From Levy MN: In Kulbertus HE, Franck G, editors: *Neurocardiology,* Mt Kisco, NY, 1988, Futura.)

Sympathetic Pathways

The cardiac sympathetic fibers originate in the intermediolateral columns of the upper five or six thoracic and lower one or two cervical segments of the spinal cord. They emerge from the spinal column through the white communicating branches and enter the paravertebral chains of ganglia. The preganglionic and postganglionic neurons synapse mainly in the stellate and middle cervical ganglia (see Figure 4-2). The middle cervical ganglia lie close to the vagus nerves in the superior portion of the mediasti-

num. Sympathetic and parasympathetic fibers then join to form a complex plexus of mixed efferent nerves to the heart (see Figure 4-2).

The postganglionic cardiac sympathetic fibers approach the base of the heart along the adventitial surface of the great vessels. On reaching the base of the heart, these fibers are distributed to the various chambers as an extensive epicardial plexus. They then penetrate the myocardium, usually along the coronary vessels. *The adrenergic receptors in the nodal regions and in the myocardium are predominantly of*

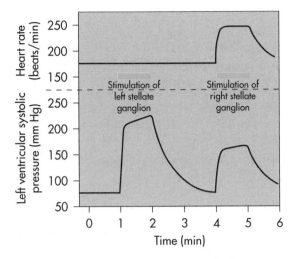

Figure 4-6 ■ **In the dog, stimulation of the left stellate ganglion has a greater effect on ventricular contractility than does right-sided stimulation, but it has a lesser effect on heart rate. In this example, traced from an original record, left stellate ganglion stimulation had no detectable effect at all on heart rate but had a considerable effect on ventricular performance in an isovolumic left ventricle preparation.** (From Levy MN: Unpublished tracing.)

the beta type; that is, they are responsive to β-adrenergic agonists, such as **isoproterenol,** and are inhibited by β-adrenergic blocking agents, such as **propranolol.**

As with the vagus nerves, the left and right sympathetic fibers are distributed differentially. In the dog, for example, the fibers on the left side have more pronounced effects on myocardial contractility than do fibers on the right side, whereas the fibers on the left side have much less effect on heart rate than do the fibers on the right side (Figure 4-6). In some dogs, left cardiac sympathetic nerve stimulation may not affect heart rate at all. This bilateral asymmetry probably also exists in humans. In a group of patients, right stellate ganglion blockade caused a mean reduction in heart rate of 14 beats per minute, whereas left-sided blockade decreased heart rate by only 2 beats per minute.

Figures 4-3, *B* and 4-6 show that the effects of sympathetic stimulation decay very gradually after the cessation of stimulation, in contrast to the abrupt termination of the response after vagal activity (see Figure 4-3, *A*). Most of the norepinephrine released during sympathetic stimulation is taken up again by the nerve terminals, and much of the remainder is carried away by the bloodstream. These processes are relatively slow. Furthermore, at the beginning of sympathetic stimulation, the facilitatory effects on the heart attain steady-state values much more slowly than do the inhibitory effects of vagal stimulation (see Figure 4-3).

At least two factors are responsible for the more gradual onset of the heart rate response to sympathetic activity than to vagal activity. First, the response to sympathetic activity depends mainly on the intracellular buildup of second messengers, mainly **cyclic AMP (cAMP),** in the automatic cells in the SA node. This is a slower process than that which transduces the response to vagal activity. The **muscarinic receptors** that respond to the acetylcholine released from the vagal terminals are coupled directly to the acetylcholine-regulated K^+ channels by a G protein; this direct coupling allows a prompt response. Second, the neurotransmitters are released at different rates from the postganglionic nerve endings of each of the two autonomic divisions. Enough acetylcholine can be released during a brief period (e.g., 1 second) of intense vagal activity to stop the heartbeat entirely. Conversely, even during intense sympathetic activity, enough **norepinephrine** is released during each cardiac cycle to change cardiac behavior by only a small increment. Thus the vagus nerves are able to exert beat-by-beat control of heart rate, whereas the sympathetic nerves are not able to alter cardiac behavior very much within one cardiac cycle.

Higher Centers Also Influence Cardiac Performance

Dramatic alterations in cardiac rate, rhythm, and contractility have been induced experimentally by stimulation of various regions of the brain. In the cerebral cortex the centers that regulate cardiac function are mostly in the anterior half of the brain, principally in the frontal lobe, the orbital cortex, the motor and premotor cortex, the anterior part of the temporal lobe, the insula, and the cingulate gyrus. In the thalamus, tachycardia may be induced by stimulation of the midline, ventral, and medial groups of nuclei. Variations in heart rate also may be evoked by stimulating the posterior and posterolateral regions of the hypothalamus.

Stimuli applied to the H_2 fields of Forel in the diencephalon elicit a variety of cardiovascular responses, including tachycardia; such changes simulate closely those observed during muscular exercise. Undoubtedly the cortical and diencephalic centers are responsible for initiating the cardiac reactions that occur during excitement, anxiety, and other emotional states. The hypothalamic centers are also involved in the cardiac response to alterations in environmental temperature. Localized temperature changes in the preoptic anterior hypothalamus alter heart rate and peripheral resistance.

Stimulation of the parahypoglossal area of the medulla activates the cardiac sympathetic and inhibits the cardiac parasympathetic pathways. In certain dorsal regions of the medulla, distinct cardiac accelerator and augmentor sites have been detected in animals with transected vagi. Stimulation of accelerator sites increases heart rate, whereas stimulation of augmentor sites increases cardiac contractility. The accelerator regions were found to be more abundant on the right and the augmentor sites more prevalent on the left. A similar distribution also exists in the hypothalamus. Therefore it appears that for the most part the sympathetic fibers descend the brainstem ipsilaterally.

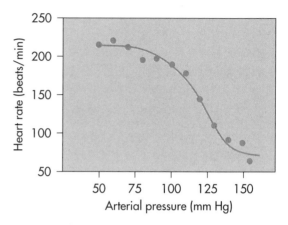

Figure 4-7 ■ Heart rate as a function of mean arterial pressure in a group of five conscious, chronically instrumented monkeys. The mean control arterial pressure was 114 mm Hg. Pressure was increased above the control value by infusing phenylephrine, and was decreased below the control value by infusing nitroprusside. (Adapted from Cornish KG, Barazanji MW, Yong T, et al: *Am J Physiol* 257:R595, 1989.)

Heart Rate Can Be Regulated Via the Baroreceptor Reflex

Acute changes in arterial blood pressure reflexly elicit inverse changes in heart rate (Figure 4-7) via the baroreceptors located in the aortic arch and carotid sinuses (see also Chapter 8). The inverse relation between heart rate and arterial blood pressure is usually most pronounced over an intermediate range of arterial blood pressures. In an experiment conducted on conscious, chronically instrumented monkeys (Figure 4-7), this range varied between about 70 and 160 mm Hg. Below the intermediate range of pressures, the heart rate maintains a constant, high value, whereas above this pressure range, it maintains a constant, low value.

The effects of changes in carotid sinus pressure on the activity in the cardiac autonomic nerves of an anesthetized dog are shown in Figure 4-8. Over an intermediate range of arterial pressures (from about 100 to 200 mm Hg), the

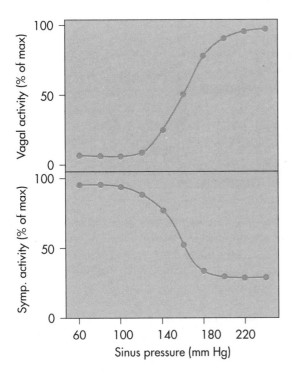

Figure 4-8 ■ Changes in neural activity in cardiac vagal and sympathetic nerve fibers induced by changes in pressure in the isolated carotid sinuses in an anesthetized dog. (Adapted from Kollai M, Koizumi K: *Pflugers Arch Ges Physiol* 413:365, 1989.)

alterations in heart rate are achieved by reciprocal changes in vagal and sympathetic neural activity. Below this range of arterial blood pressures, the high heart rate is achieved by intense sympathetic activity and the virtual absence of vagal activity. Conversely, above the intermediate range of arterial blood pressures, the low heart rate is achieved by intense vagal activity and a constant low level of sympathetic activity.

The Bainbridge Reflex and Atrial Receptors Regulate Heart Rate

In 1915 Bainbridge reported that infusions of blood or saline accelerated the heart rate in dogs. This increase in heart rate occurred

whether arterial blood pressure did or did not rise. Acceleration was observed whenever central venous pressure rose sufficiently to distend the right side of the heart, and the effect was abolished by bilateral transection of the vagi.

The magnitude and direction of the heart rate changes evoked by the Bainbridge reflex depend on the prevailing heart rate. When the heart rate is slow, intravenous infusions usually accelerate the heart. At more rapid heart rates, however, infusions ordinarily slow the heart. Increases in blood volume not only evoke the Bainbridge reflex, but they also activate other reflexes (notably the baroreceptor reflex) that tend to change the heart rate in the opposite direction. The actual change in heart rate evoked by an alteration of blood volume is therefore the result of these antagonistic reflex effects (Figure 4-9).

In unanesthetized dogs, infusions of blood increased heart rate and cardiac output proportionately (Figure 4-10); consequently, stroke volume remained virtually constant. Conversely, reductions in blood volume diminished the cardiac output but increased heart rate. Undoubtedly, the Bainbridge reflex was prepotent over the baroreceptor reflex when the blood volume was raised, but the baroreceptor reflex prevailed over the Bainbridge reflex when the blood volume was diminished.

Receptors that influence heart rate exist in both atria. They are located principally in the venoatrial junctions—in the right atrium at its junctions with the venae cavae and in the left atrium at its junctions with the pulmonary veins. Distension of these atrial receptors sends impulses centripetally in the vagi. The efferent impulses are carried by fibers from both autonomic divisions to the SA node. The cardiac response is highly selective. Even when the reflex increase in heart rate is large, changes in ventricular contractility have been negligible. Furthermore, the increase in heart rate is unat-

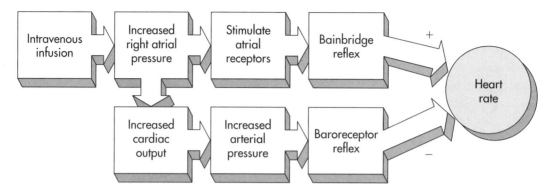

Figure 4-9 ■ **Intravenous infusions of blood or electrolyte solutions tend to increase heart rate via the Bainbridge reflex and to decrease heart rate via the baroreceptor reflex. The actual change in heart rate induced by such infusions is the result of these two opposing effects.**

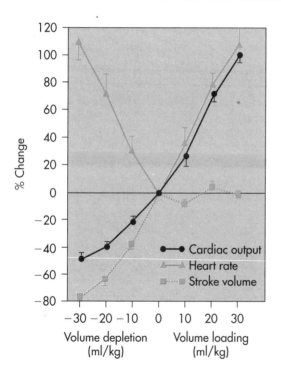

Figure 4-10 ■ **Effects of blood transfusion and of bleeding on cardiac output, heart rate, and stroke volume in unanesthetized dogs.** (From Vatner SF, Boettcher DH: *Circ Res* 42:557, 1978.)

tended by an increase of sympathetic activity to the peripheral arterioles.

Stimulation of the atrial receptors also increases the urine volume. Reduced activity in the renal sympathetic nerve fibers might be partially responsible for this diuresis. However, the principal mechanism appears to be a neurally mediated reduction in the secretion of **vasopressin (antidiuretic hormone)** by the posterior pituitary gland.

A peptide, called **atrial natriuretic peptide (ANP),** is released from atrial tissue in response to increases in blood volume, presumably because of the resulting stretch of the atrial walls. ANP consists of 28 amino acids. It has potent diuretic and natriuretic effects on the kidneys, and it has vasodilator effects on the resistance and capacitance blood vessels. Thus ANP is an important regulator of blood volume and blood pressure.

A Common Cardiac Dysrhythmia Is Induced by Respiration

Rhythmic variations in heart rate, occurring at the frequency of respiration, are detectable in most individuals and tend to be more pronounced in children. Typically, the cardiac rate

In **congestive heart failure,** sodium chloride (NaCl) and water are retained, mainly because of the increased release of aldosterone from the adrenal cortex, consequent to stimulation by the renin-angiotensin system. The plasma level of ANP is also increased in congestive heart failure. This peptide acts to enhance the renal excretion of NaCl and water and thereby attenuates the fluid retention and consequent elevations of central venous pressure and cardiac preload.

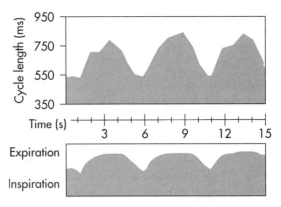

Figure 4-11 ■ **Respiratory sinus dysrhythmia in a resting, unanesthetized dog. Note that the cardiac cycle length increases during expiration and decreases during inspiration.** (Modified from Warner MR, de Tarnowsky JM, Whitson CC, et al: *Am J Physiol* 251:H1134, 1986.)

accelerates during inspiration and decelerates during expiration (Figure 4-11).

Recordings from the autonomic nerves to the heart reveal that the neural activity increases in the sympathetic fibers during inspiration, whereas the neural activity in the vagal fibers increases during expiration (Figure 4-12). The acetylcholine released at the vagal endings is removed so rapidly that the rhythmic changes in activity are able to elicit rhythmic variations in heart rate. Conversely, the norepinephrine released at the sympathetic endings is removed more slowly, thus damping out the effects of rhythmic variations in norepinephrine release on heart rate. Hence rhythmic changes in heart rate are ascribable almost entirely to the oscillations in vagal activity. Respiratory sinus dysrhythmia is exaggerated when vagal tone is enhanced.

Both reflex and central factors contribute to the genesis of the respiratory cardiac dysrhythmia (Figure 4-13). During inspiration, intrathoracic pressure decreases, and therefore venous return to the right side of the heart is accelerated (see also Chapter 9), which elicits the Bainbridge reflex (Figure 4-13). After the time delay required for the increased venous return to reach the left side of the heart, left ventricular output increases and raises arterial blood pres-

sure. This in turn reduces heart rate reflexly through baroreceptor stimulation (Figure 4-13).

Fluctuations in sympathetic activity to the arterioles cause peripheral resistance to vary at the respiratory frequency. Consequently, arterial blood pressure fluctuates rhythmically, which affects heart rate via the baroreceptor reflex. Stretch receptors in the lungs may also affect heart rate (Figure 4-13). Moderate pulmonary inflation may increase heart rate reflexly. The afferent and efferent limbs of this reflex are located in the vagus nerves.

Central factors are also responsible for respiratory cardiac dysrhythmia (Figure 4-13). The respiratory center in the medulla influences the cardiac autonomic centers. In heart-lung bypass experiments conducted on animals, the chest is open, the lungs are collapsed, venous return is diverted to a pump-oxygenator, and arterial blood pressure is maintained at a constant level. In such experiments, rhythmic movements of the rib cage attest to the activity of the medullary respiratory centers, and the movements of the rib cage are often accompanied by rhythmic

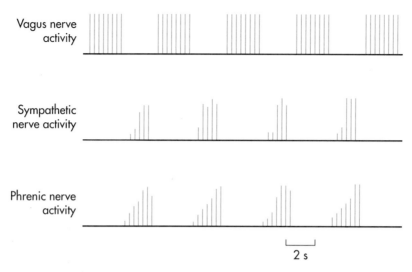

Figure 4-12 ■ Respiratory fluctuations in efferent neural activity in the cardiac nerves of an anesthetized dog. Note that the sympathetic nerve activity occurs synchronously with the phrenic nerve discharges (which initiate diaphragmatic contraction), whereas the vagus nerve activity occurs between the phrenic nerve discharges. (From Kollai M, Koizumi K: *J Auton Nerv Syst* 1:33, 1979.)

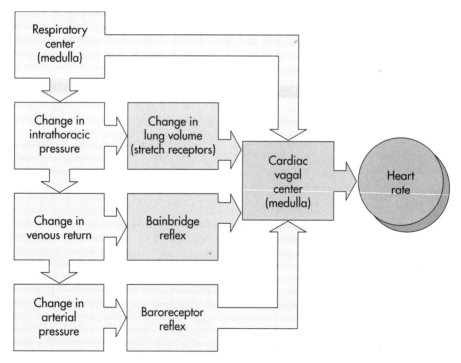

Figure 4-13 ■ Respiratory sinus dysrhythmia is generated by a direct interaction between the respiratory and cardiac centers in the medulla, as well as by reflexes originating from stretch receptors in the lungs, stretch receptors in the right atrium (Bainbridge reflex), and baroreceptors in the carotid sinuses and aortic arch.

changes in heart rate at the respiratory frequency. *This respiratory cardiac dysrhythmia is almost certainly induced by an interaction between the respiratory and cardiac centers in the medulla* (Figure 4-13).

Activation of the Chemoreceptor Reflex Affects Heart Rate

The cardiac response to peripheral (or arterial) chemoreceptor stimulation merits special consideration because it illustrates the complexity that may be introduced when one stimulus excites two organ systems simultaneously. In intact animals, stimulation of the arterial chemoreceptors consistently increases ventilatory rate and depth, but heart rate usually changes only slightly.

The directional change in heart rate is evoked by the peripheral chemoreceptors related to the enhancement of pulmonary ventilation, as shown in Figure 4-14. When respiratory stimulation is mild, heart rate usually diminishes; when the increase in pulmonary ventilation is more pronounced, heart rate usually accelerates.

The cardiac response to arterial chemoreceptor stimulation is the result of primary and secondary reflex mechanisms (Figure 4-15). The primary reflex effect of arterial chemoreceptor excitation is mainly to facilitate the medullary vagal center and thereby to decrease heart rate. Secondary effects are mediated by the respiratory system. Respiratory stimulation by the arterial chemoreceptors tends to inhibit the medullary vagal center. This inhibitory effect varies with concomitant stimulation of respiration.

An example of the primary inhibitory influence of arterial chemoreceptor stimulation is displayed in Figure 4-16. In this experiment on an anesthetized dog, the lungs were completely collapsed and blood oxygenation was accomplished by an artificial oxygenator. When the carotid chemoreceptors were stimulated, an intense bradycardia and some degree of AV block

ensued. Such effects are mediated primarily by efferent vagal fibers.

The pulmonary hyperventilation that is ordinarily evoked by carotid chemoreceptor stimulation influences heart rate secondarily, both by initiating more pronounced pulmonary inflation reflexes and by producing hypocapnia (Figure 4-15). Each of these influences tends to depress the primary cardiac response to chemoreceptor stimulation and thereby to accelerate the heart. Hence when pulmonary hyperventilation is not prevented, the primary and secondary effects tend to neutralize each other, and carotid chemoreceptor stimulation affects heart rate only minimally.

Box 4-2

The identical primary vagal inhibitory effect also operates in humans. The electrocardiogram shown in Figure 4-17 was recorded from a quadriplegic patient who could not breathe spontaneously but required tracheal intubation and artificial respiration. When the tracheal catheter was briefly disconnected to permit nursing care, the patient quickly developed a profound bradycardia. His heart rate was 65 beats per minute just before the tracheal catheter was disconnected. In fewer than 10 s after cessation of artificial respiration, his heart rate dropped to about 20 beats per minute. This bradycardia could be prevented by blocking the effects of efferent vagal activity with atropine, and its onset could be delayed considerably by hyperventilating the patient before disconnecting the tracheal catheter.

The Ventricular Receptor Reflexes Play a Minor Role in the Regulation of Heart Rate

Sensory receptors near the endocardial surfaces of the ventricular walls initiate reflex effects similar to those elicited by the arterial baroreceptors. Excitation of these endocardial recep-

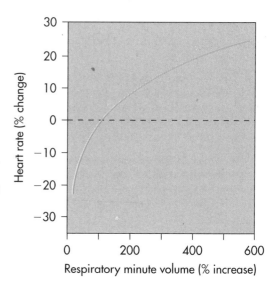

Figure 4-14 ■ Relationship between the change in heart rate and the change in respiratory minute volume during carotid chemoreceptor stimulation in spontaneously breathing cats and dogs. When respiratory stimulation was relatively slight, heart rate usually diminished; when respiratory stimulation was more pronounced, heart rate usually increased. (Modified from Daly MdeB, Scott MJ: *J Physiol* 144:148, 1958.)

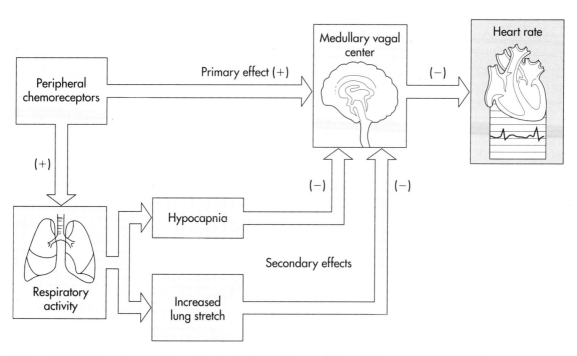

Figure 4-15 ■ The primary effect of stimulation of the peripheral chemoreceptors on heart rate is to excite the cardiac vagal center in the medulla and thus to decrease heart rate. Peripheral chemoreceptor stimulation also excites the respiratory center in the medulla. This effect produces hypocapnia and increases lung inflation, both of which secondarily inhibit the medullary vagal center. Thus these secondary influences attenuate the primary reflex effect of peripheral chemoreceptor stimulation of heart rate.

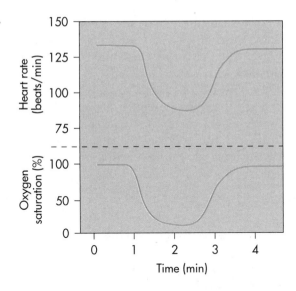

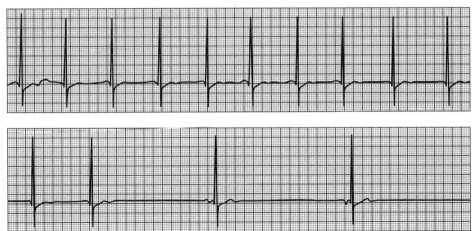

Figure 4-16 ■ Changes in heart rate during carotid chemoreceptor stimulation in an anesthetized dog on total heart bypass. The lungs remain deflated and respiratory gas exchange is accomplished by an artificial oxygenator. The lower tracing represents the oxygen saturation of the blood perfusing the carotid chemoreceptors. The blood perfusing the remainder of the animal, including the myocardium, was fully saturated with oxygen throughout the experiment. (Modified from Levy MN, DeGeest H, Zieske H: *Circ Res* 18:67, 1966.)

Figure 4-17 ■ Electrocardiogram of a 30-year-old quadriplegic man who could not breathe spontaneously and required tracheal intubation and artificial respiration. The two strips are continuous. The tracheal catheter was temporarily disconnected from the respirator at the beginning of the top strip. (Modified from Berk JL, Levy MN: *Eur Surg Res* 9:75, 1977.)

tors diminishes heart rate and peripheral resistance. Other sensory receptors have been identified in the epicardial regions of the ventricles. Ventricular receptors are excited by a variety of mechanical and chemical stimuli, but their physiological functions are not clear.

■ MYOCARDIAL PERFORMANCE IS REGULATED BY INTRINSIC MECHANISMS

Just as the heart can initiate its own beat in the absence of any nervous or hormonal control, so also can the myocardium adapt to changing hemodynamic conditions by mechanisms that are

Ventricular receptors are suspected of being involved in the initiation of **vasovagal syncope,** which is lightheadedness or brief loss of consciousness that may be triggered by psychological or orthostatic stress. The ventricular receptors are believed to be stimulated by a reduced ventricular filling volume combined with a vigorous ventricular contraction. In a person standing quietly, ventricular filling is diminished because blood tends to pool in the veins in the abdomen and legs, as explained in Chapter 9. Consequently, the reduction in cardiac output and arterial blood pressure leads to a generalized increase in sympathetic neural activity via the baroreceptor reflex (Figure 4-8). The enhanced sympathetic activity to the heart evokes a vigorous ventricular contraction, which thereby stimulates the ventricular receptors. Excitation of the ventricular receptors appears to initiate the autonomic neural changes that evoke vasovagal syncope, namely, a combination of a profound, vagally mediated bradycardia and a generalized arteriolar vasodilation mediated by a diminution in sympathetic neural activity.

intrinsic to cardiac muscle itself. Experiments on denervated hearts reveal that this organ adjusts remarkably well to stress. For example, racing greyhounds with denervated hearts perform almost as well as those with intact innervation. Their maximal running speed was found to be only 5% less after complete cardiac denervation. In these dogs the threefold to fourfold increase in cardiac output during exertion was achieved principally by an increase in stroke volume. In normal dogs the increase of cardiac output with exercise is accompanied by a proportionate increase of heart rate; stroke volume does not change much (see Chapter 12). It is unlikely that the cardiac adaptation in the denervated animals is achieved entirely by intrinsic mechanisms; cir-

culating catecholamines undoubtedly contribute. If the β-adrenergic receptors are blocked in greyhounds with denervated hearts, their racing performance is severely impaired.

The intrinsic cardiac adaptation that has received the greatest attention involves changes in the resting length of the myocardial fibers. This adaptation is designated **Starling's law of the heart** or the **Frank-Starling mechanism.** The mechanical, ultrastructural, and physiological bases for this mechanism have been explained in Chapter 3.

The Frank-Starling Mechanism Is an Important Regulator of Myocardial Contractility

Isolated Hearts In 1895 the German physiologist Otto Frank described the response of the isolated heart of the frog to alterations in the load on the myocardial fibers just before ventricular contraction. He observed that as the load was increased, the heart responded with a more forceful contraction.

In 1914 the English physiologist Ernest Starling described the intrinsic response of the heart to changes in right atrial and aortic pressure in the canine isolated heart-lung preparation. In this preparation the right ventricular filling pressure is varied by altering the height of a reservoir connected to the right atrium. The ventricular filling pressure just before ventricular contraction constitutes the **preload** for the myocardial fibers in the ventricular wall (see also Chapter 3). The right ventricle then pumps this blood through the pulmonary vessels to the left atrium. The lungs are artificially ventilated. Blood is pumped by the left ventricle into the aortic arch and then through some external tubing back to the right atrial reservoir. A resistance device in the external tubing allows the investigator to control the aortic pressure; this pressure constitutes the **afterload** for left ventricular ejection (see also Chapter 3).

When the blood reservoir is abruptly raised to increase the preload, the stroke volume and the end-diastolic ventricular volume increase progressively over the next several beats; heart rate and afterload remain constant. In the brief period during which the stroke volume and ventricular volume gradually increase, a disparity must exist between ventricular inflow during diastole and ventricular output during systole. Thus during this transient period before equilibrium is attained, the stroke volume must be less than the filling volume. The consequent accumulation of blood dilates the ventricles and lengthens the individual myocardial fibers that make up the walls of the ventricles.

The increased diastolic fiber length somehow facilitates ventricular contraction and enables the ventricles to pump a greater stroke volume, so that cardiac output exactly matches the augmented venous return at equilibrium. Increased fiber length alters cardiac performance in part by changing the number of myofilament cross-bridges that can interact, but mainly by changing the calcium sensitivity of the myofilaments (see also Chapter 3). An optimal fiber length apparently exists beyond which contraction is actually impaired. Therefore excessively high filling pressures may depress rather than enhance the pumping capacity of the ventricles by overstretching the myocardial fibers. Such excessive degrees of stretch are rarely encountered under normal conditions.

Changes in diastolic fiber length also permit the isolated heart to compensate for an increase in peripheral resistance. In a Starling preparation, when the arterial resistance is abruptly increased but ventricular filling rate is held constant, the stroke volume diminishes initially in response to the sudden increase in arterial resistance. However, after a brief period the stroke volume increases to equal the constant ventricular filling volume. Concomitantly, the arterial pressure and end-diastolic ventricular volume

are greater than the respective values that prevailed before the experimentally induced increase in afterload. Thus when the afterload is first increased, the stroke volume ejected by the ventricles during systole is less than the filling volume that enters the ventricles during diastole. The consequent excess of volume in the ventricles stretches the myocardial fibers in the ventricular walls. This increase in myocardial fiber length enables the ventricles to eject a given stroke volume against an increased afterload.

Changes in ventricular volume are also involved in the cardiac adaptation to alterations in heart rate. During bradycardia, for example, the increased duration of diastole permits greater ventricular filling. The consequent augmentation of myocardial fiber length increases stroke volume. Therefore the reduction in heart rate may be fully compensated by the increase in stroke volume, such that cardiac output may remain constant (see Figure 9-16).

When cardiac compensation involves ventricular dilation, the force required by each myocardial fiber to generate a given intraventricular systolic pressure must be appreciably greater than that developed by the fibers in a nondilated ventricle. The relationship between wall tension and cavity pressure resembles the Laplace relationship for cylindric tubes (see Chapter 7) in that for a constant internal pressure, wall tension varies directly with the radius. As a consequence, the dilated heart requires considerably more oxygen to perform a given amount of external work than does the normal heart.

The relatively rigid pericardium that encloses the heart determines the pressure-volume relationship at high levels of pressure and volume. The pericardium exerts this limitation of volume even under normal conditions—when an individual is at rest and the heart rate is slow (see also Chapter 3).

Intact Preparations The major problem of assessing the role of the Frank-Starling mecha-

In the cardiac dilation and hypertrophy that accompanies **chronic heart failure,** the pericardium is stretched considerably (Figure 4-18). The pericardial limitation of cardiac filling is exerted at pressures and volumes entirely different from those in normal individuals.

nism in intact animals and humans is the difficulty of measuring end-diastolic myocardial fiber length. The Frank-Starling mechanism has been represented graphically by plotting some index of ventricular performance along the ordinate and some index of fiber length along the abscissa. The most commonly used indexes of ventricular performance are cardiac output, stroke volume, and stroke work. The indexes of fiber length include ventricular end-diastolic volume, ventricular end-diastolic pressure, ventricular circumference, and mean atrial pressure.

The Frank-Starling mechanism is better represented by a family of so-called ventricular function curves than by a single curve. To construct a control ventricular function curve, the blood volume of an experimental animal is altered over a range of values, and stroke work and end-diastolic pressure are measured at each step. Similar observations are then made during the desired experimental intervention. For example, the ventricular function curve obtained during a norepinephrine infusion lies above and to the left of a control ventricular function curve (Figure 4-19). It is evident that, for a given level of left ventricular end-diastolic pressure, the left ventricle performs more work during a norepinephrine infusion than under control conditions. Hence a shift of the ventricular function curve to the left usually signifies an improvement of ventricular **contractility** (see Chapter 3); a shift to the right usually indicates an impairment of contractility and a consequent tendency toward **cardiac failure.** Contractility is a measure of cardiac performance at a given level of preload and afterload. The end-diastolic

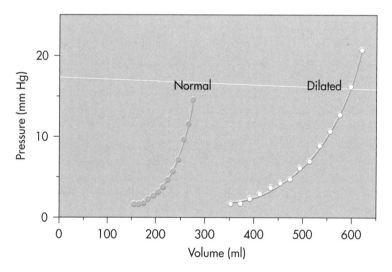

Figure 4-18 ■ Pericardial pressure-volume relations in a normal dog and in a dog with experimentally induced chronic cardiac hypertrophy. (Modified from Freeman GL, Le Winter MM: *Circ Res* 54:294, 1984.)

pressure is ordinarily a good index of preload, whereas the aortic systolic pressure is a good index of afterload.

The Frank-Starling mechanism is ideally suited for matching cardiac output to venous return. Any sudden, excessive output by one ventricle soon increases the venous return to the other ventricle. The consequent increase in diastolic fiber length in the second ventricle augments the output of that ventricle to correspond with the output of its mate. *Therefore it is the*

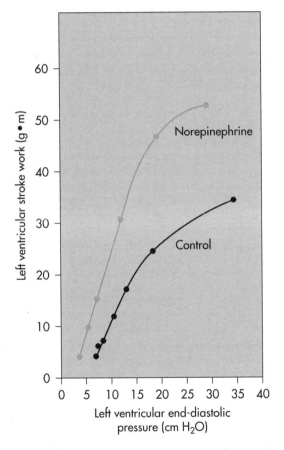

Figure 4-19 ■ **A constant infusion of norepinephrine in a dog shifts the ventricular function curve to the left. This shift signifies an enhancement of ventricular contractility.** (Redrawn from Sarnoff SJ, Brockman SK, Gilmore JP, et al: *Circ Res* 8:1108, 1960.)

Frank-Starling mechanism that maintains a precise balance between the outputs of the right and left ventricles. Because the two ventricles are arranged in series in a closed circuit, even a small, maintained imbalance in the outputs of the two ventricles would otherwise be catastrophic.

The curves that relate cardiac output to mean atrial pressure for the two ventricles are not coincident; the curve for the left ventricle usually lies below that for the right, as shown in Figure 4-20. At equal right and left atrial pressures (points *A* and *B*), right ventricular output would exceed left ventricular output. Hence venous return to the left ventricle (a function of right ventricular output) would exceed left ventricular output, and therefore left ventricular diastolic volume and pressure would rise. By the Frank-Starling mechanism, left ventricular output would increase (from *B* toward *C*). Only when the outputs of both ventricles are identical (points *A* and *C*) would the equilibrium be stable. Under such conditions, however, left atrial pressure *(C)* would exceed right atrial pressure *(A),* and this is precisely the relationship that ordinarily prevails in normal subjects.

Changes in Heart Rate Affect Contractile Force

The effects of the frequency of contraction on the force developed in an isometrically contracting cat papillary muscle are shown in Figure 4-21. Initially, the strip of cardiac muscle

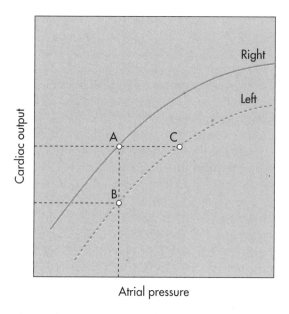

Figure 4-20 ■ Outputs of the right and left ventricles as functions of the mean right and left atrial pressure, respectively. At a given level of cardiac output, mean left atrial pressure (e.g., point *C*) exceeds mean right atrial pressure (point *A*).

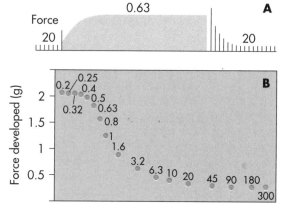

Figure 4-21 ■ Changes in force development in an isolated papillary muscle from a cat as the interval between contractions is varied. The numbers in both panels denote the interval (in seconds) between beats. (Redrawn from Koch-Weser J, Blinks JR: *Pharmacol Rev* 15:601, 1963.)

was stimulated to contract only once every 20 s (Figure 4-21, *A*). When the muscle was suddenly made to contract once every 0.63 s, the developed force increased progressively over the next several beats. This progressive increase in developed force induced by a change in contraction frequency is known as the **staircase,** or t**reppe, phenomenon.**

At the new steady state, the developed force was more than five times as great as it was during stimulation at the larger contraction interval. A return to the larger interval (20 s) had the opposite influence on developed force.

The effect of the interval between contractions on the steady-state level of developed force is shown in Figure 4-21, *B* for a wide range of intervals. As the interval is diminished from

300 s down to about 20 s, developed force changes only slightly. As the interval is reduced further, to a value of about 0.5 s, force increases sharply. Further reduction of the interval to 0.2 s has little additional effect on developed force.

The initial progressive rise in developed force when the interval between beats is suddenly decreased (e.g., from 20 to 0.63 s in Figure 4-21, *B*) is achieved by a gradual increase in intracellular Ca^{++} content. Two mechanisms contribute to the rise in Ca^{++} content: (1) an increase in the number of depolarizations per minute and (2) an increase in the inward Ca^{++} current per depolarization.

With respect to the first mechanism, Ca^{++} enters the myocardial cell during each action potential plateau (see Figure 2-21). As the inter-

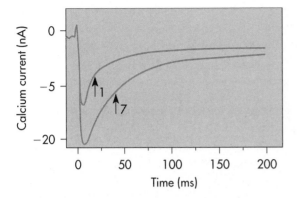

Figure 4-22 ▪ Calcium currents induced in a guinea pig myocyte during the first and seventh depolarizations in a sequence of depolarizations. *Arrows* indicate the half-times of inactivation. Note that during the seventh depolarization, the maximal inward Ca^{++} current and the half-time of inactivation were greater than the respective values for the first depolarization. (Modified from Lee KS: *Proc Natl Acad Sci USA* 84:3941, 1987.)

val between beats is diminished, the number of plateaus per minute increases. Even though the duration of each action potential (and of each plateau) decreases as the interval between beats is reduced (see Figure 2-21), the overriding effect of the increased number of plateaus per minute on the influx of Ca^{++} would increase the intracellular content of Ca^{++}.

With respect to the second mechanism, as the interval between beats is suddenly diminished, the inward Ca^{++} current (i_{Ca}) progressively increases with each successive beat until a new steady state is attained at the new basic cycle length. Figure 4-22 shows that in an isolated ventricular myocyte that was subjected to repetitive depolarizations, the Ca^{++} current into the myocyte increased on successive beats. For example, the maximal i_{Ca} was considerably greater during the seventh depolarization than it was during the first depolarization. Furthermore, the decay of that current (i.e., its inactiva-

tion) was substantially slower during the seventh depolarization than during the first depolarization. Both of these characteristics of the i_{Ca} would result in a greater influx of Ca^{++} into the myocyte during the seventh depolarization than during the first depolarization. The greater influx of Ca^{++} would strengthen the contraction.

Transient changes in the intervals between beats also affect the strength of contraction. When a premature ventricular systole (Figure 4-23, beat *A*) occurs, the premature contraction (extrasystole) itself is feeble, whereas the beat *(B)* after the subsequent pause is very strong. In intact animals, this response depends partly on the Frank-Starling mechanism. Inadequate ventricular filling just before the premature beat accounts partly for the weak premature contraction. The exaggerated degree of filling associated with the subsequent pause explains in part the vigorous postextrasystolic contraction.

Although the Frank-Starling mechanism is certainly involved in the usual ventricular adaptation to a premature beat, it is not the exclusive mechanism. Directionally similar results are obtained even from isovolumically contracting ventricles. In the experiment shown in Figure 4-23, an anesthetized animal was subjected to total heart-lung bypass. The coronary circulation was perfused with oxygenated blood, a balloon was inserted into the left ventricle, and it was filled with enough saline to fill the entire ventricle. In this preparation the left ventricle contracts against an incompressible fluid; that is, the ventricle contracts isovolumically. Figure 4-23 shows the changes in pressure that were recorded from this balloon during a series of contraction. Note that the premature beat *(A)* was much weaker than the preceding beat, and that the postextrasystolic beat *(B)* that immediately followed the premature beat was very strong. Such enhanced contractility in contraction B is an example of **postextrasystolic po-**

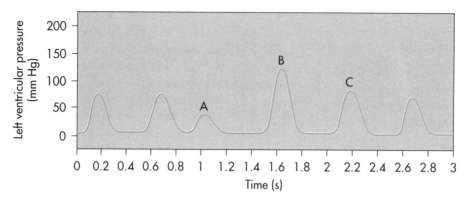

Figure 4-23 ▪ In an isovolumic canine left ventricle preparation, a premature ventricular systole (beat *A*) is typically feeble, whereas the postextrasystolic contraction (beat *B*) is characteristically strong, and the enhanced contractility may persist to a diminishing degree over a few beats (e.g., contraction *C*). In this preparation the animal is placed on total heart-lung bypass, and a balloon filled with saline is positioned in the left ventricle. (From Levy MN: Unpublished tracing.)

tentiation, and it may persist for one or more additional beats (e.g., contraction *C*).

The weakness of the premature beat is directly related to the degree of prematurity. Conversely, as the time **(coupling interval)** between the premature beat and the preceding beat is increased, the more nearly normal will be the strength of the premature beat. The curve that relates the strength of contraction of a premature beat to the coupling interval is called a **mechanical restitution curve.** Figure 4-24 shows the restitution curve obtained by varying the coupling intervals of test beats in an isolated ventricular muscle preparation from a guinea pig.

The restitution of contractile strength probably depends on the time course of the intracellular circulation of Ca^{++} during the contraction and relaxation process (see Figure 3-5). During relaxation, the Ca^{++} that dissociates from the contractile proteins is taken up by the sarcoplasmic reticulum for subsequent release. However, about 500 to 800 ms are required before the Ca^{++} that had been taken up becomes

available for release in response to the next depolarization.

The premature beat itself (Figure 4-23, beat *A*) is feeble probably because not enough time has elapsed to allow much of the Ca^{++} taken up by the sarcoplasmic reticulum during the preceding relaxation to become available for release in response to the premature depolarization. Conversely, the postextrasystolic beat (Figure 4-23, beat *B*) is considerably stronger than normal. The reason is that after the pause between beats *A* and *B*, the sarcoplasmic reticulum had available for release the Ca^{++} that had been taken up during two heartbeats: the extrasystole (beat *A*) and the preceding normal beat.

▪ MYOCARDIAL PERFORMANCE IS REGULATED BY NERVOUS AND HUMORAL FACTORS

Although the completely isolated heart can adapt well to changes in preload and afterload, various extrinsic factors also influence the heart in the intact animal. Under many normal conditions these extrinsic regulatory mechanisms

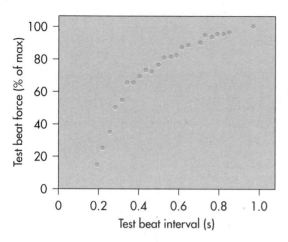

Figure 4-24 ■ **Force generated during premature contractions in a guinea pig isolated ventricular muscle preparation. The muscle was driven to contract once per second. Periodically, the muscle was stimulated to contract prematurely. The scale along the abscissa denotes the time between the driven and premature beat. The ordinate denotes the ratio of the contractile force of the premature beat to that of the driven beat.** (Modified from Seed WA, Walker JM: *Cardiovasc Res* 22:303, 1988.)

may overwhelm the intrinsic mechanisms. These extrinsic regulatory factors may be subdivided into nervous and chemical components.

Nervous Control

Sympathetic Influences Sympathetic nervous activity enhances atrial and ventricular contractility. The effects of increased cardiac sympathetic activity on the ventricular myocardium are asymmetric. The cardiac sympathetic nerves on the left side of the body usually have a much greater effect on left ventricular contraction than do those on the right side (see Figure 4-6).

The alterations in left ventricular contraction, evoked by electrical stimulation of the left stellate ganglion in a canine isovolumic left ventricle preparation, are shown in Figure 4-25. The peak pressure and the maximal rate of pressure

rise (dP/dt) during systole are markedly increased. Also, the duration of systole is reduced and the rate of ventricular relaxation is increased during the early phases of diastole. The shortening of systole and more rapid ventricular relaxation would enhance ventricular filling in the intact circulatory system. For a given cardiac cycle length, the abbreviation of systole allows more time for diastole and hence for ventricular filling. In the experiment shown in Figure 4-26, for example, the animal's heart was paced at a constant rapid rate. Sympathetic stimulation *(right panel)* shortened systole, which allowed substantially more time for ventricular filling.

Sympathetic nervous activity enhances myocardial performance. Neurally released norepinephrine or circulating catecholamines interact with β-adrenergic receptors on the cardiac cell membranes (see Figure 4-5). This reaction activates adenylyl cyclase, which raises the intracellular levels of cAMP. As a consequence, protein kinases are activated that promote the phosphorylation of various proteins within the myocardial cells. Phosphorylation of specific sarcolemmal proteins activates the calcium channels in the myocardial cell membranes. Phosphorylation of another specific protein, **phospholamban,** facilitates the reuptake of systolic Ca^{++} by the sarcoplasmic reticulum, and thus it accelerates the relaxation of myocardial cells (see also Chapter 3).

Activation of the calcium channels increases the influx of Ca^{++} during the action potential plateau, and more Ca^{++} is released from the sarcoplasmic reticulum in response to each cardiac excitation. The contractile strength of the heart is thereby increased. Figure 4-27 shows the correlation between the contractile force developed by a thin strip of ventricular muscle and the Ca^{++} concentration (as reflected by the aequorin light signal) in the myocytes as the concentration of isoproterenol (a β-adrenergic agonist) was increased in the tissue bath.

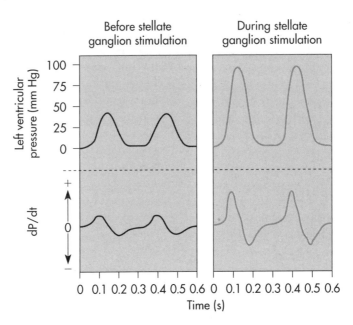

Figure 4-25 ■ **In an isovolumic left ventricle preparation, stimulation of cardiac sympathetic nerves evokes a substantial rise in peak left ventricular pressure and in the maximal rates of intraventricular pressure rise and fall *(dP/dt)*.** (From Levy MN: Unpublished tracing.)

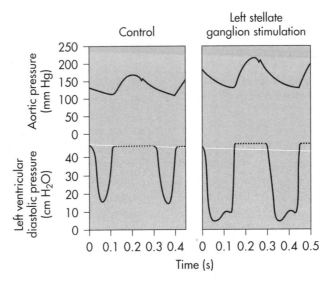

Figure 4-26 ■ **Stimulation of the left stellate ganglion of a dog increases arterial pressure, stroke volume, and stroke work despite a concomitant reduction in ventricular end-diastolic pressure. Note also the abridgment of systole, thereby allowing more time for ventricular filling; the heart was paced at a constant rate. In the ventricular pressure tracings, the pen excursion is limited at 45 mm Hg; actual ventricular pressures during systole can be estimated from the aortic pressure tracings.** (Redrawn from Mitchell JH, Linden RJ, Sarnoff SJ: *Circ Res* 8:1100, 1960.)

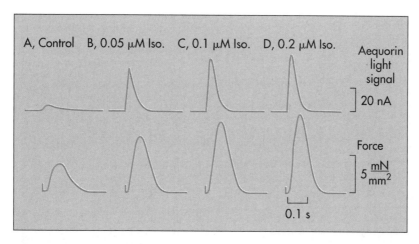

Figure 4-27 ■ **Effects of various concentrations of isoproterenol *(Iso)* on the aequorin light signal (in nA) and contractile force (in mN/mm²) in a rat ventricular muscle injected with aequorin. The aequorin light signal reflects the instantaneous changes in intracellular Ca⁺⁺ concentration.** (Modified from Kurihara S, Konishi M: *Pflugers Arch* 409:427, 1987.)

The overall effect of increased cardiac sympathetic activity in intact animals can best be appreciated in terms of families of ventricular function curves. When stepwise increases in the frequency of electrical stimulation are applied to the left stellate ganglion, the ventricular function curves shift progressively to the left. The changes parallel those produced by catecholamine infusions (Figure 4-19). Hence for any given left ventricular end-diastolic pressure, the ventricle is capable of performing more work as the level of sympathetic nervous activity is raised.

During cardiac sympathetic stimulation the enhanced cardiac response is usually accompanied by a reduction in left ventricular end-diastolic pressure (see Figure 4-26). This reduction in end-diastolic pressure represents a decrease in the preload. The reason for the reduction in ventricular preload is explained in Chapter 9.

Parasympathetic Influences The vagus nerves inhibit the cardiac pacemaker, atrial myocardium, and AV conduction tissue. The vagus nerves also depress the ventricular myocardium, but the ventricular effects are less pronounced. In the isovolumic left ventricle preparation, vagal stimulation decreases the peak left ventricular pressure, maximal rate of pressure development (dP/dt), and maximal rate of pressure decline during diastole (Figure 4-28). In pumping heart preparations, vagal stimulation affects the relation between ventricular performance and preload such that the ventricular function curve shifts to the right.

The vagal effects on the ventricular myocardium are achieved by at least two mechanisms, as shown in Figure 4-5. The acetylcholine (ACh) released from the vagal endings can interact with muscarinic (M) receptors in the cardiac cell membrane. This interaction inhibits adenylyl cyclase. The consequent diminution in the intracellular concentration of cAMP diminishes the Ca⁺⁺ conductance of the cardiac cell membrane and hence decreases myocardial contractility.

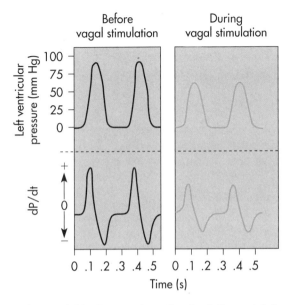

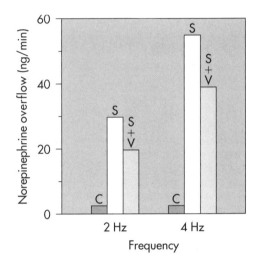

Figure 4-28 ■ In an isovolumic left ventricle preparation, when the ventricle is paced at a constant frequency, vagal stimulation decreases the peak left ventricular pressure and diminishes the maximal rates of pressure rise and fall *(dP/dt)*. (From Levy MN: Unpublished tracing.)

Figure 4-29 ■ Mean rates of overflow of norepinephrine into the coronary sinus blood in a group of seven dogs under control conditions *(C)*, during cardiac sympathetic stimulation *(S)* at 2 or 4 Hz and during combined sympathetic and vagal stimulation *(S + V)*. The combined stimulus consisted of sympathetic stimulation at 2 or 4 Hz, and vagal stimulation at 15 Hz. (Redrawn from Levy MN, Blattberg B: *Circ Res* 38:81, 1976.)

The ACh released from the vagal endings can also inhibit the release of norepinephrine from neighboring sympathetic nerve endings (see Figure 4-5). The experiment illustrated in Figure 4-29 demonstrates that stimulation of the cardiac sympathetic nerves *(S)* results in the overflow of substantial amounts of norepinephrine into the coronary sinus blood. Concomitant vagal stimulation *(S + V)* reduces the overflow of norepinephrine by about 30%. The amount of norepinephrine that overflows into the coronary sinus blood probably parallels the amount of norepinephrine released at the cardiac sympathetic terminals. Thus vagal activity can decrease ventricular contractility partly by antagonizing the facilitatory effects of any concomitant sympathetic activity. The tendency for vagal activity to diminish the release of norepinephrine from neighboring sympathetic nerve endings also accounts for the preponderance of vagal influence over the sympathetic influence on heart rate, as reflected by the experimental results shown in Figure 4-4. Similarly, sympathetic nerves release norepinephrine and certain neuropeptides, including **neuropeptide Y (NPY)**; norepinephrine and NPY both inhibit the release of acetylcholine from neighboring vagal fibers (see Figure 4-5).

Baroreceptor Reflex Not only does stimulation of the carotid sinus and aortic arch baroreceptors change heart rate (see Figure 4-7), but also stimulation of these receptors alters myocar-

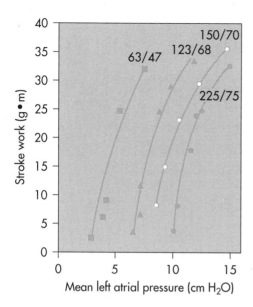

Figure 4-30 ■ **As the pressure in the isolated carotid sinus is progressively raised, the ventricular function curves shift to the right. The numbers at the tops of each curve represent the systolic/diastolic perfusion pressures (in millimeters of mercury) in the carotid sinus regions of the dog.** (Redrawn from Sarnoff SJ, Gilmore JP, Brockman SK, et al: *Circ Res* 8:1123, 1960.)

dial performance. Evidence of reflex alterations of ventricular contractility is presented in Figure 4-30. Ventricular function curves were obtained at four levels of carotid sinus pressure. With each successive rise in pressure, the ventricular function curves were displaced farther and farther to the right, denoting a progressively greater reflex depression of ventricular performance.

Cardiac Performance Is Also Regulated by Hormonal Substances

Hormones

Adrenomedullary Hormones The adrenal medulla is essentially a component of the autonomic nervous system. The principal hormone secreted by the adrenal medulla is epinephrine, although some norepinephrine is also released.

The rate of secretion of catecholamines by the adrenal medulla is largely regulated by the same mechanisms that control sympathetic nervous activity. The concentrations of catecholamines in the blood rise under the same conditions that activate the sympathoadrenal system. However, the cardiovascular effects of circulating catecholamines are probably minimal under normal resting conditions.

The changes in myocardial contractility induced by norepinephrine infusions have been tested in resting, unanesthetized dogs. The maximal rate of rise of left ventricular pressure (dP/dt), an index of myocardial contractility, was found to be proportional to the norepinephrine concentration in the blood (Figure 4-31). In these same animals, moderate exercise increased the maximal dP/dt by almost 100%, but it raised the circulating catecholamines by only 500 pg/ml. Such a rise in blood norepinephrine concentration, by itself, would have had only a negligible effect on left ventricular dP/dt (Figure 4-31). Hence the pronounced change in dP/dt observed during exercise must have been achieved mainly by the norepinephrine released from the cardiac sympathetic nerve fibers rather than by the catecholamines released from the adrenal medulla.

Adrenocortical Hormones The influence of adrenocortical steroids on the myocardium is controversial. Cardiac muscle removed from adrenalectomized animals and placed in a tissue bath is more likely to fatigue than that obtained from normal animals. In some species the adrenocortical hormones enhance contractility. Furthermore, hydrocortisone potentiates the cardiotonic effects of the catecholamines. This potentiation may be mediated in part by an inhibition of the uptake mechanisms for the catecholamines by the adrenocortical steroids.

Thyroid Hormones Numerous studies on intact animals and humans have demonstrated that thyroid hormones enhance myocardial con-

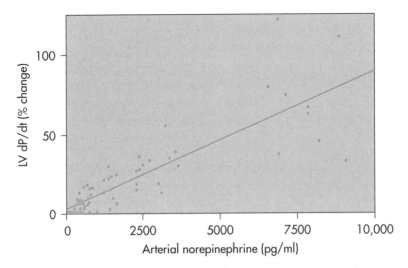

Figure 4-31 ▪ **Effect of norepinephrine infusions on ventricular contractility in a group of resting, unanesthetized dogs.** The plasma concentrations of norepinephrine *(pg/ml)* plotted along the abscissa are the increments above the control values. The maximal rate of rise of left ventricular pressure *(LV dP/dt)* is plotted along the ordinate as percentage change from the control value; it is an index of contractility. (Redrawn from Young MA, Hintze TH, Vatner SF: *Am J Physiol* 248:H82, 1985.)

Box 4-6

Cardiovascular problems are common in adrenocortical insufficiency **(Addison's disease).** The blood volume tends to fall, which may lead to severe hypotension and cardiovascular collapse, the so-called **addisonian crisis.**

tractility. The rates of Ca^{++} uptake and of ATP hydrolysis by the sarcoplasmic reticulum are increased in response to excess thyroid hormones, and the opposite effects occur when thyroid hormones are inadequate. Thyroid hormones increase protein synthesis in the heart, which leads to cardiac hypertrophy. These hormones also affect the composition of myosin isoenzymes in cardiac muscle. They increase principally those isoenzymes with the greatest ATPase activity, and thereby enhance myocardial contractility.

Box 4-7

The cardiovascular changes in thyroid dysfunction also depend on indirect mechanisms. Thyroid hyperactivity increases the body's metabolic rate, and this in turn results in arteriolar vasodilation. The consequent reduction in total peripheral resistance increases cardiac output (see Chapter 9). Substantial evidence indicates that hyperthyroidism increases the density of β-adrenergic receptors in cardiac tissue and it increases the responsiveness of the heart to sympathetic neural activity. Cardiac activity is sluggish in patients with inadequate thyroid function **(hypothyroidism);** that is, the heart rate is slow and cardiac output is diminished. The converse is true in patients with overactive thyroid glands **(hyperthyroidism).** Characteristically, hyperthyroid patients exhibit tachycardia, high cardiac output, palpitations, and dysrhythmias (such as atrial fibrillation).

Insulin Insulin has a prominent, direct, positive inotropic effect on the heart. The effect of insulin is evident even when hypoglycemia is prevented by glucose infusions and when the β-adrenergic receptors are blocked. In fact, the positive inotropic effect of insulin is potentiated by β-adrenergic receptor blockade.

Glucagon Glucagon has potent positive inotropic and chronotropic effects on the heart. The endogenous hormone probably plays no significant role in the normal regulation of the cardiovascular system, but it has been used to treat various cardiac conditions. The effects of glucagon on the heart closely resemble those of the catecholamines, and certain of their metabolic effects are similar. Both glucagon and catecholamines activate adenylyl cyclase to increase the myocardial tissue levels of cAMP. The catecholamines activate adenylyl cyclase by interacting with β-adrenergic receptors, but glucagon activates this enzyme through a different mechanism.

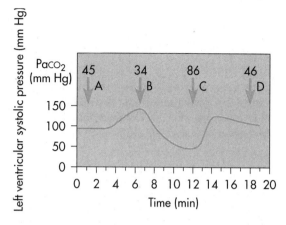

Figure 4-32 ▪ Decrease in PaCO$_2$ increases left ventricular systolic pressure (arrow *B*) in an isovolumic left ventricle preparation; a rise in PaCO$_2$ (arrow *C*) has the reverse effect. When PaCO$_2$ is returned to the control level (arrow *D*), left ventricular systolic pressure returns to its original value (arrow *A*). (Levy MN: Unpublished tracing.)

Blood Gases

Oxygen Changes in oxygen tension (PaO$_2$) of the blood perfusing the brain and the peripheral chemoreceptors affect the heart through nervous mechanisms, as described earlier in this chapter. These indirect cardiac effects of hypoxia are usually prepotent. Moderate degrees of systemic hypoxia characteristically increase heart rate, cardiac output, and myocardial contractility. These changes are largely mediated by the sympathetic nervous system, and they are effectively abolished by β-adrenergic receptor blockade.

The PaO$_2$ of the blood perfusing the myocardium also influences myocardial performance directly. Moderate-to-severe degrees of hypoxia depress myocardial contractility. The principal mechanism for the diminished contractility has not been established. Certain studies indicate that the sensitivity of the contractile proteins to Ca^{++} is reduced; other studies show that the impaired contractility is produced by increased intracellular concentrations of inorganic phosphate and of hydrogen ions.

Carbon Dioxide and Acidosis Changes in PaCO$_2$ may also affect the myocardium directly and indirectly. The indirect, neurally mediated effects produced by increased PaCO$_2$ are similar to those evoked by a decrease in PaO$_2$.

With respect to the direct effects on the heart, alterations in myocardial performance elicited by changes of PaCO$_2$ in the coronary arterial blood are illustrated in Figure 4-32. In this experiment on an isolated left ventricle preparation, the control PaCO$_2$ was 45 mm Hg (arrow *A*). Decreasing the PaCO$_2$ to 34 mm Hg (arrow *B*) was stimulatory, whereas increasing PaCO$_2$ to 86 mm Hg (arrow *C*) was depressant. In intact animals, systemic hypercapnia activates the sympatho-adrenal system, which tends to compensate for the direct depressant effect of the increased PaCO$_2$ on the heart.

Figure 4-33 ■ Effect of pH on the relationship between relative force and pCa in a "skinned" ventricular fiber from a rat. Relative force is the force developed by the preparation under the various experimental conditions, expressed as a percentage of the maximal force developed by the preparation when intracellular pH was normal (i.e., 7.1) and pCa was less than 4.6. The "skinned" fiber was prepared by treating the preparation with a detergent to solubilize the cell membranes, thus exposing the contractile proteins in the fiber to the concentrations of H^+ and of Ca^{++} that prevailed in the bathing solution. (Modified from Mayoux E, Coutry N, Lechêne P, et al: *Am J Physiol* 266:H2051, 1994.)

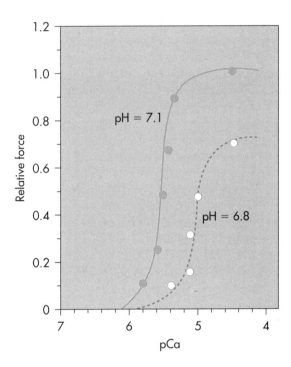

Neither the $PaCO_2$ nor the blood pH are primary determinants of myocardial behavior. The associated change in intracellular pH is the critical factor. The reduced intracellular pH diminishes the amount of Ca^{++} released from the sarcoplasmic reticulum in response to excitation. The diminished pH also decreases the sensitivity of the myofilaments to Ca^{++}. This effect of acidosis on sensitivity to Ca^{++} is reflected by a shift in the relationship between developed force and pCa (the negative logarithm of the intracellular Ca^{++} concentration). Figure 4-33 illustrates such a shift in an experiment on isolated ventricular fibers immersed in a tissue bath. When the pH of the bath was changed from 7.1 to 6.8, the curve of contractile force as a function of pCa was shifted substantially to the right (normal intracellular pH is about 7.1). Furthermore, in this same preparation, at high intracellular Ca^{++} concentrations (i.e., at values of pCa below about 4.6), a reduction in pH diminishes the maximal developed force. This reduction in maximal force suggests that the low pH depresses the actomyosin interactions.

Summary

- Cardiac function is regulated by intrinsic and extrinsic mechanisms.
- Sympathetic nervous activity increases heart rate, whereas parasympathetic (vagal) activity decreases heart rate. When both systems are active, the vagal effects usually dominate.
- The baroreceptor, chemoreceptor, pulmonary inflation, atrial receptor (Bainbridge), and ven-

tricular receptor reflexes regulate heart rate.

- A change in the resting length of the muscle influences the subsequent contraction in part by altering the affinity of the myofilaments for calcium; this is called the Frank-Starling mechanism.

- A sustained change in contraction frequency affects the strength of contraction by altering the influx of Ca^{++} into the cell per minute. A transient change in contraction frequency alters contractile strength because an appreciable delay exists between the time that Ca^{++} is taken up by the sarcoplasmic reticulum and the time that it becomes available again for release.

- The autonomic nervous system regulates myocardial performance mainly by varying the Ca^{++} conductance of the cell membrane via the adenylyl cyclase system.

- Various hormones, including epinephrine, adrenocortical steroids, thyroid hormones, insulin, glucagon, and anterior pituitary hormones, regulate myocardial performance.

- Changes in the blood concentrations of O_2, CO_2, and H^+ alter cardiac function directly (by interacting with the contractile proteins), and reflexly (via the central and peripheral chemoreceptors).

■ **BIBLIOGRAPHY**

1. Armour JA, Ardell JL, editors: *Neurocardiology,* New York, 1994, Oxford University Press.
2. Cechetto E, Hachinski V, editors: *Neurocardiology,* London, 1997, Baillière Tindall.
3. Dampney RAL: Functional organization of central pathways regulating the cardiovascular system. *Physiol Rev* 74:323, 1994.
4. Fuchs F: Mechanical modulation of the Ca^{2+} regulatory protein complex in cardiac muscle. *News Physiol Sci* 10:6, 1995.
5. Hainsworth R: Reflexes from the heart. *Physiol Rev* 71:617, 1991.
6. Levy MN, Schwartz PJ, editors: *Vagal control of the heart: experimental basis and clinical implications,* Armonk, NY, 1994, Futura.
7. Löffelholz K, Pappano AJ: The parasympathetic neuroeffector junction of the heart. *Pharmacol Rev* 37:1, 1985.
8. Marshall JM: Peripheral chemoreceptors and cardiovascular regulation. *Physiol Rev* 74:543, 1994.
9. Morgan JP: Abnormal intracellular modulation of calcium as a major cause of cardiac contractile dysfunction. *N Engl J Med* 325:625, 1991.
10. Rea RF, Thames MD: Neural control mechanisms and vasovagal syncope. *J Cardiovasc Electrophysiol* 4:587, 1993.
11. Rowell LB: *Human cardiovascular control,* New York, 1993, Oxford University Press.
12. Share L, editor: *Hormones and the heart in health and disease,* Totowa, NJ, 1999, Human Press.
13. Shepherd JT, Vatner SF, editors: *Nervous control of the heart,* Amsterdam, 1996, Harwood Academic Press.
14. Sperelakis N, editor: *Physiology and pathophysiology of the heart,* ed 3, Boston, 1995, Kluwer Academic.
15. Spyer KM: Central nervous mechanisms contributing to cardiovascular control. *J Physiol (Lond)* 474:1, 1994.

■ CASE 4

HISTORY

A 48-year-old woman was susceptible to occasional, usually brief, episodes of lightheadedness. She noticed that her heart rate was very rapid during these episodes and that the lightheadedness disappeared when the heart rate returned to normal. Her doctor noted no significant abnormalities on physical examination. Review of a 24-hour recording of the patient's electrocardiogram revealed a 7-minute period during which the patient's heart rate increased abruptly from a resting value of about 75 beats per minute to a steady level of about 145 beats per minute. At the end of the 7-minute period of tachycardia, the heart rate decreased within 1 minute to the resting value of about 75 beats per minute. The patient's problem was diagnosed as paroxysmal supraventricular tachycardia, which is a sudden, pronounced increase in heart rate; this problem is mediated usually by a reentry circuit in the atrioventricular junction.

During a subsequent visit to her doctor, the paroxysmal tachycardia appeared spontaneously. The doctor was able to terminate the tachycardia promptly by carotid sinus massage (i.e., massaging the patient's neck just below the angles of the jaw, in the region of the bifurcations of the common carotid arteries). The physician noted that the patient's arterial blood pressure during tachycardia was 95/75 mm Hg and that it returned to a value of 130/85 mm Hg (the patient's usual resting blood pressure) soon after the termination of the tachycardia.

QUESTIONS

1. A reduction in the patient's mean arterial pressure during the paroxysmal tachycardia would cause a reflex
   a. Decrease in myocardial contractility
   b. Increase in cardiac cycle duration
   c. Decrease in AV conduction velocity
   d. Increase in norepinephrine release from the cardiac sympathetic nerves
   e. Decrease in calcium conductance of myocytes during the action potential plateau

2. A sudden, substantial increase in efferent vagal activity (induced by carotid sinus massage, for example) would
   a. Strengthen the contraction of atrial myocytes
   b. Strengthen the stimulatory action of any concurrent sympathetic activity
   c. Increase the speed of impulse conduction in the ventricular Purkinje fibers
   d. Decrease the heart rate within one or two cardiac cycles
   e. Shorten the AV conduction time

3. When the subject was in a normal sinus rhythm, administration of a drug that antagonizes the muscarinic cholinergic receptors would
   a. Dampen any changes in heart rate that occur at the subject's respiratory frequency
   b. Weaken the contractions of the atrial myocytes
   c. Delay AV conduction
   d. Decrease the action potential duration in atrial myocytes
   e. Hyperpolarize the atrial myocytes during the resting phase (phase 4) of the action potential

4. If the patient had a prominent respiratory sinus dysrhythmia when she was not afflicted by the paroxysmal tachycardia, the following functional change would take place
   a. Efferent vagal activity would decrease during inspiration.
   b. Efferent cardiac sympathetic activity would decrease during inspiration.
   c. The slope of the slow diastolic depolarization of the sinoatrial cells would decrease during inspiration.
   d. The respiratory sinus dysrhythmia would become more pronounced in response to hemorrhage.
   e. Propranolol would abolish the respiratory sinus dysrhythmia.

5. When neural activity in the vagus nerves suddenly ceases, the heart rate response to that vagal activity disappears rapidly because
   a. The cardiac cells gradually become more responsive to acetylcholine.
   b. The vagus nerve endings rapidly take up the released acetylcholine.
   c. The cardiac myocytes rapidly take up the released acetylcholine.
   d. The acetylcholine in the nerve endings is rapidly depleted.
   e. The abundant acetylcholinesterase rapidly degrades the released acetylcholine.

CHAPTER 5

Hemodynamics

Objectives

1. Define the relation between the velocity of blood flow and vascular cross-sectional area.

2. Describe the factors that govern the relationship between blood flow and pressure gradient.

3. Distinguish between resistances in series and resistances in parallel.

4. Distinguish between laminar and turbulent flow.

5. Describe the influence of the particulates in blood on blood flow.

THE PRECISE MATHEMATICAL EXPRES-sion of the pulsatile flow of blood through the cardiovascular system is insuperable. The heart is a complicated pump, and its behavior is affected by a variety of physical and chemical factors. The blood vessels are multibranched, elastic conduits of continuously varying dimensions. The blood itself is not a simple, homogeneous solution but is instead a complex suspension of red and white corpuscles, platelets, and lipid globules dispersed in a colloidal solution of proteins.

Despite these complex factors, considerable insight may be gained from an understanding of the elementary principles of fluid mechanics as they pertain to simple physical systems. Such principles are expounded in this chapter to explain the interrelationships among the blood flow, the blood pressure, and the dimensions of the various components of the systemic circulation.

■ VELOCITY OF THE BLOODSTREAM DEPENDS ON BLOOD FLOW AND VASCULAR AREA

In describing the variations in blood flow in different vessels, one must first distinguish between the terms **velocity** and **flow.** The former term, sometimes designated as **linear velocity,** refers to the rate of displacement with respect to time and it has the dimensions of distance per unit time, for example, cm/s. The flow is frequently designated as **volume flow** and it has the dimensions of volume per unit time,

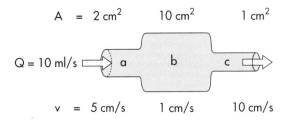

Figure 5-1 ■ As fluid flows through a tube of variable cross-sectional area, _A,_ the linear velocity, _v,_ varies inversely as the cross-sectional area.

for example, cm³/s. In a conduit of varying cross-sectional dimensions, velocity, v, flow, Q, and cross-sectional area, A, are related by the equation:

$$v = Q/A \qquad (1)$$

The interrelationships among velocity, flow, and area are portrayed in Figure 5-1. The flow of an incompressible fluid past successive cross-sections of a rigid tube must be constant. For a given constant flow, the velocity varies inversely as the cross-sectional area (see Figure 1-3). Thus for the same volume of fluid per second passing from section _a_ into section _b,_ where the cross-sectional area is five times greater, the velocity diminishes to one fifth of its previous value. Conversely, when the fluid proceeds from section _b_ to section _c,_ where the cross-sectional area is one tenth as great, the velocity of each particle of fluid must increase tenfold.

The velocity at any point in the system depends not only on the cross-sectional area, but also on the flow, Q. This in turn depends on the pressure gradient, properties of the fluid, and dimensions of the entire hydraulic system, as discussed in the next section. For any given flow, however, the ratio of the velocity past one cross-section relative to that past a second cross-section depends only on the inverse ratio of the respective area; that is,

$$v_1/v_2 = A_2/A_1 \qquad (2)$$

This rule pertains regardless of whether a given cross-sectional area applies to a system that consists of a single large tube or to a system made up of several smaller tubes in parallel.

As shown in Figure 1-3, velocity decreases progressively as the blood traverses the aorta, its larger primary branches, the smaller secondary branches, and the arterioles. Finally, a minimal value is reached in the capillaries. As the blood then passes through the venules and continues centrally toward the venae cavae, the velocity progressively increases again. The relative velocities in the various components of the circulatory system are related only to the respective cross-sectional areas. Thus each point on the cross-sectional area curve is inversely proportional to the corresponding point on the velocity curve (see Figure 1-3).

■ BLOOD FLOW DEPENDS ON THE PRESSURE GRADIENT

In that portion of a hydraulic system in which the total energy remains virtually constant, changes in velocity may be accompanied by appreciable alterations in the measured pressure. Consider three sections (**A, B,** and **C**) of the hydraulic system depicted in Figure 5-2. Six pressure probes, or **Pitot tubes,** have been inserted. The openings of three of these (**2, 4,** and **6**) are tangential to the direction of flow and hence measure the **lateral,** or **static,** pressure within the tube. The openings of the remaining three Pitot tubes (**1, 3,** and **5**) face upstream. Therefore they detect the **total pressure,** which is the lateral pressure plus a dynamic pressure component that reflects the kinetic energy of the flowing fluid. This dynamic component, P_d, of the total pressure may be calculated from the following equation:

$$P_d = \rho v^2/2 \qquad (3)$$

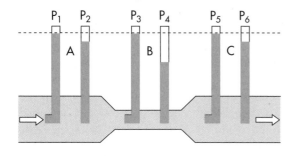

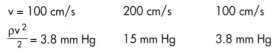

Figure 5-2 ■ In a narrow section, B, of a tube, the linear velocity, v, and hence the dynamic component of pressure, $\dfrac{\rho v^2}{2}$, are greater than in the wide sections, A and C, of the same tube. If the total energy is virtually constant throughout the tube (i.e., if the energy loss because of viscosity is negligible), the total pressures (P_1, P_3, and P_5) will not be detectably different, but the lateral pressure, P_4, in the narrow section will be less than the lateral pressures (P_2 and P_6) in the wide sections of the tube.

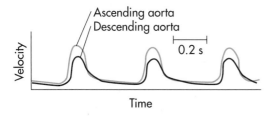

Figure 5-3 ■ Velocity of the blood in the ascending and descending aorta of a dog. (Redrawn from Falsetti HL, Kiser KM, Francis GP, et al: *Circ Res* 31:328, 1972.)

where ρ is the density of the fluid and v is the velocity. If the midpoints of segments *A, B,* and *C* are at the same hydrostatic level, the corresponding total pressure, P_1, P_3, and P_5, will be equal, provided that the energy loss from viscosity in these segments is negligible. However, because of the changes in cross-sectional area, the concomitant velocity changes alter the dynamic component.

In sections *A* and *C*, let $\rho = 1$ g/cm^3 and $v = 100$ cm/s. From equation 3

$$P_d = 5000 \text{ dynes/cm}^2$$

$$= 3.8 \text{ mm Hg}$$

because 1330 dynes/cm^2 = 1 mm Hg. In the narrow section, *B,* let the velocity be twice as great as in sections *A* and *C.* Therefore

$$P_d = 20,000 \text{ dynes/cm}^2$$

$$= 15 \text{ mm Hg}$$

Hence in the wide sections of the conduit, the lateral pressures (P_2 and P_6) will be only 3.8 mm Hg less than the respective total pressures (P_1 and P_5), whereas in the narrow section the lateral pressure (P_4) is 15 mm Hg less than the total pressure (P_3).

The peak velocity of flow in the ascending aorta of normal dogs is about 150 cm/s. Therefore the measured pressure at this site may vary significantly, depending on the orientation of the pressure probe. In the descending thoracic aorta the peak velocity is substantially less than that in the ascending aorta (Figure 5-3), and lesser velocities have been recorded in still more distal arterial sites. In most arterial locations the dynamic component is a negligible fraction of the total pressure, and the orientation of the pressure probe does not materially influence the pressure recorded. At the site of a constriction, however, the dynamic pressure component may attain substantial values. In **aortic stenosis,** for example, the entire output of the left ventricle is ejected through a narrow aortic valve orifice. The high flow velocity is associated with a large kinetic energy, and therefore the lateral pressure is correspondingly reduced.

The reduction of lateral pressure in the region of the stenotic valve orifice influences

The pressure tracings shown in Figure 5-4 were obtained from two pressure transducers inserted into the left ventricle of a patient with aortic stenosis. The transducers were located on the same catheter and were 5 cm apart. When both transducers were well within the left ventricular cavity (Figure 5-4, *A*), they both recorded the same pressures. However, when the proximal transducer was positioned in the aortic valve orifice (Figure 5-4, *B*), the lateral pressure recorded during ejection was much less than that recorded by the transducer in the ventricular cavity. This pressure difference was associated almost entirely with the much greater velocity of flow in the narrowed valve orifice than in the ventricular cavity. The pressure difference reflects mainly the conversion of some potential energy to kinetic energy. When the catheter was withdrawn still farther, so that the proximal transducer was in the aorta (Figure 5-4, *C*), the pressure difference was even more pronounced, because substantial energy was lost through friction (viscosity) as blood flowed rapidly through the narrow aortic valve.

coronary blood flow in patients with aortic stenosis. The orifices of the right and left coronary arteries are located in the sinuses of Valsalva, just behind the valve leaflets. The initial segments of these vessels are oriented at right angles to the direction of blood flow through the aortic valves. Therefore the lateral pressure is that component of total pressure that propels the blood through the two major coronary arteries. During the ejection phase of the cardiac cycle, the lateral pressure is diminished by the conversion of potential energy to kinetic energy. This process is grossly exaggerated in aortic stenosis because of the high flow velocities.

■ RELATIONSHIP BETWEEN PRESSURE AND FLOW DEPENDS ON THE CHARACTERISTICS OF THE CONDUITS

The most fundamental law that governs the flow of fluids through cylindrical tubes was derived empirically by the French physiologist Poiseuille. He was primarily interested in the physical determinants of blood flow, but he substituted simpler liquids for blood in his measurements of flow through glass capillary tubes. His work was so precise and important that his observations have been designated **Poiseuille's law.** Subsequently, this same law has been derived theoretically.

Poiseuille's law is applicable to the flow of fluids through cylindrical tubes only under special conditions. It applies to the case of steady, laminar flow of newtonian fluids. The term **steady flow** signifies the absence of variations of flow in time, that is, a nonpulsatile flow. **Laminar flow** is the type of motion in which the fluid moves as a series of individual layers, with each stratum moving at a different velocity from its neighboring layers (Figure 5-5). In the case of flow through a tube, the fluid consists of a series of infinitesimally thin concentric tubes sliding past one another. Laminar flow is described in greater detail below, where it is distinguished from turbulent flow. Also, a **newtonian fluid** is defined more precisely. For the present discussion, it may be considered to be a homogeneous fluid, such as water, in contradistinction to a suspension, such as blood.

Pressure is one of the principal determinants of the rate of flow. The pressure, P, in dynes/cm^2, at a distance h centimeters below the surface of a liquid is

$$P = h\rho g \qquad (4)$$

where ρ is the density of the liquid in g/cm^3 and g is the acceleration of gravity in cm/s^2. For convenience, however, pressure is frequently expressed simply in terms of height, h, of the col-

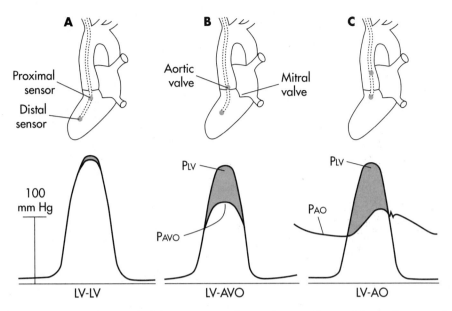

Figure 5-4 ■ Pressures *(P)* recorded by two transducers in a patient with aortic stenosis. A, Both transducers were in the left ventricle *(LV-LV)*. B, One transducer was in the left ventricle and the other was in the aortic valve orifice *(LV-AVO)*. C, One transducer was in the left ventricle and the other was in the ascending aorta *(LV-AO)*. (Redrawn from Pasipoularides A, Murgo JP, Bird JJ, et al: *Am J Physiol* 246:H542, 1984.)

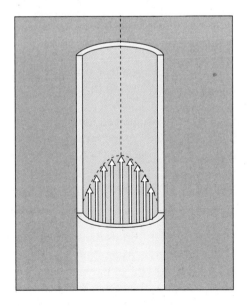

Figure 5-5 ■ In laminar flow, all elements of the fluid move in streamlines that are parallel to the axis of the tube; movement does not occur in a radial or circumferential direction. The layer of fluid in contact with the wall is motionless; the fluid that moves along the axis of the tube has the maximal velocity.

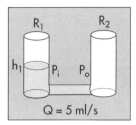

A, When R_2 is empty, fluid flows from R_1 to R_2 at a rate proportional to the pressure in R_1.

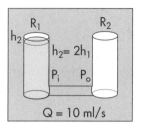

B, When the fluid level in R_1 is increased twofold, the flow increases proportionately.

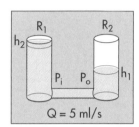

C, Flow from R_1 to R_2 is proportional to the difference between the pressures in R_1 and R_2.

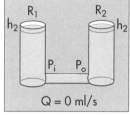

D, When pressure in R_2 rises to equal the pressure in R_1, flow ceases in the connecting tube.

Figure 5-6 ■ The flow, Q, of fluid through a tube connecting two reservoirs, R_1 and R_2, is proportional to the difference between the pressure at the inflow end (P_i) and the pressure at the outflow end (P_o) of the tube.

umn of liquid above some arbitrary reference point.

Consider the tube connecting reservoirs R_1 and R_2 in Figure 5-6, A. Let reservoir R_1 be filled with liquid to height h_1, and let reservoir R_2 be empty, as in panel A of Figure 5-6. The outflow pressure, P_o, is therefore equal to the atmospheric pressure, which shall be designated as the zero, or reference, level. The inflow pressure, P_i, is then equal to the same reference level plus the height, h_1, of the column of liquid in reservoir R_1. Under these conditions, let the flow, Q, through the tube be 5 ml/s.

If reservoir R_1 is filled to height h_2, which is twice h_1, and reservoir R_2 is again empty (as in panel B), the flow will be twice as great, that is,

10 ml/s. Thus with reservoir R_2 empty, the flow will be directly proportional to the inflow pressure, P_i.

If reservoir R_2 is now allowed to fill to height h_1, and the fluid level in R_1 is maintained at h_2 (as in panel C), the flow will again become 5 ml/s. Thus flow is directly proportional to the difference between inflow and outflow pressures:

$$Q \propto P_i - P_o \qquad (5)$$

If the fluid level in R_2 attains the same height as in R_1, flow will cease (panel D).

For any given pressure difference between the two ends of a tube, the flow will depend on the dimensions of the tube. Consider the tube connected to the reservoir in Figure 5-7, A. With

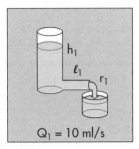

A, Reference condition: for a given pressure, length, radius, and viscosity, let the flow (V_1) equal 10 ml/s.

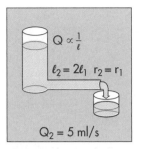

B, If tube length doubles, flow decreases by 50%.

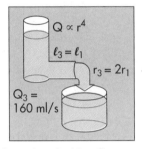

C, If tube radius doubles, flow increases 16-fold.

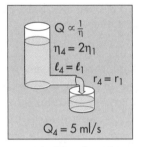

D, If viscosity doubles, flow decreases by 50%.

Figure 5-7 ■ The flow, Q, of fluid through a tube is inversely proportional to the length, ℓ, and the viscosity, η, and is directly proportional to the fourth power of the radius, r.

length ℓ_1 and radius r_1, the flow Q_1 is observed to be 10 ml/s.

The tube connected to the reservoir in panel *B* has the same radius but is twice as long. Under those conditions the flow Q_2 is found to be 5 ml/s, or only half as great as Q_1. Conversely, for a tube half as long as ℓ_1, the flow would be twice as great as Q_1. In other words, flow is inversely proportional to the length of the tube:

$$Q \propto 1/\ell \qquad (6)$$

The tube connected to the reservoir in Figure 5-7, *C* is the same length as ℓ_1, but the radius is twice as great. Under these conditions, the flow

Q_3 is found to increase to a value of 160 ml/s, which is 16 times greater than Q_1. The precise measurements of Poiseuille revealed that flow varies directly as the fourth power of the radius:

$$Q \propto r^4 \qquad (7)$$

Because $r_3 = 2r_1$ in the example above (Figure 5-7, *C*), Q_3 will be proportional to $(2r_1)^4$, or $16r_1^4$; therefore Q_3 will equal $16Q_1$.

Finally, for a given pressure difference and for a cylindrical tube of given dimensions, the flow will vary as a function of the nature of the fluid itself. This flow-determining property of fluids is termed **viscosity,** η, which has been

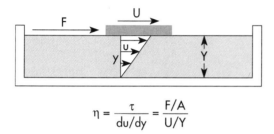

$$\eta = \frac{\tau}{du/dy} = \frac{F/A}{U/Y}$$

Figure 5-8 ■ **For a newtonian fluid, the viscosity, η, is defined as the ratio of shear stress, τ, to shear rate, *du/dy*. For a plate of contact area, *A*, moving across the surface of a liquid, τ equals the ratio of the force, *F*, applied in the direction of motion to the contact area, *A*, and *du/dy* equals the ratio of the velocity of the plate, *U*, to the depth of the liquid, *Y*.**

defined by Newton as the ratio of **shear stress** to the **shear rate** of the fluid. Those fluids for which the shear rate is proportional to the shear stress are known as **newtonian fluids.** If the shear rate is not proportional to the shear stress, the fluid is **nonnewtonian.**

These terms may be comprehended most clearly by considering the flow of a homogeneous fluid between parallel plates. In Figure 5-8, let the bottom plate (the bottom of a large basin) be stationary, and let the upper plate move at a constant velocity along the upper surface of the fluid. The **shear stress,** τ, is defined as the ratio of F:A, where F is the force applied to the upper plate in the direction of its motion along the upper surface of the fluid, and A is the area of the upper plate in contact with the fluid. The **shear rate** is du/dy, where u is the velocity of a minute element of the fluid in the direction parallel to the motion of the upper plate, and y is the distance of that fluid element above the bottom, stationary plate.

For a movable plate traveling with constant velocity across the surface of a homogeneous fluid, the velocity profile of the fluid will be lin-

ear. The fluid layer in contact with the upper plate will adhere to it and therefore will move at the same velocity, U, as the plate. Each minute element of fluid between the plates will move at a velocity, u, proportional to its distance, y, from the lower plate. Therefore the shear rate will be U/Y, where Y is the total distance between the two plates. Because viscosity, η, is defined as the ratio of shear stress, τ, to the shear rate, du/dy, in the example illustrated in Figure 5-8,

$$\eta = (F/A)/(U/Y) \qquad (8)$$

Thus the dimensions of viscosity are dynes/cm^2 divided by (cm/s)/cm, or dynes/cm^2. In honor of Poiseuille, 1 dyne/cm^2 has been termed a poise. The viscosity of water at 20° C is approximately 0.01 poise, or 1 centipoise.

With regard to the flow of newtonian fluids through cylindrical tubes, the flow varies inversely as the viscosity. Thus in the example of flow from the reservoir in Figure 5-7, *D*, if the viscosity of the fluid in the reservoir were doubled, the flow would be halved (5 ml/s instead of 10 ml/s).

In summary, for the steady, laminar flow of a newtonian fluid through a cylindrical tube, the flow, Q, varies directly as the pressure difference, $P_i - P_o$, and the fourth power of the radius, r, of the tube, and it varies inversely as the length, ℓ, of the tube and the viscosity, η, of the fluid. The full statement of Poiseuille's law is

$$Q = \frac{\pi(P_i - P_o)r^4}{8\eta\ell} \qquad (9)$$

where $\pi/8$ is the constant of proportionality.

■ RESISTANCE TO FLOW

In electrical theory the resistance, R, is defined as the ratio of voltage drop, E, to current flow, I. Similarly, in fluid mechanics the hydraulic resistance, R, may be defined as the ratio of pressure drop, $P_i - P_o$, to flow, Q; P_i and P_o are the pressures at the inflow and outflow ends, respectively, of the hydraulic system. For the steady, laminar flow of a newtonian fluid through a cylindrical tube, the physical components of hydraulic resistance may be appreciated by rearranging Poiseuille's law to give the **hydraulic resistance equation**

$$R = \frac{P_i - P_o}{Q} = \frac{8\eta\ell}{\pi r^4} \qquad (10)$$

Thus when Poiseuille's law applies, the resistance to flow depends only on the dimensions of the tube and on the characteristics of the fluid.

The principal determinant of the resistance to blood flow through any individual vessel within the circulatory system is its caliber; this is because resistance varies with the fourth power of the tube radius. The resistance to flow through small blood vessels in cat mesentery has been measured, and the resistance per unit length of vessel (R/ℓ) is plotted against the vessel diameter in Figure 5-9. The resistance is highest in the capillaries (diameter 7 μm), and it diminishes as the vessels increase in diameter on the arterial and venous sides of the capillaries. The values of R/ℓ were found to be virtually proportional to the fourth power of the diameter (or radius) for the larger vessels on both sides of the capillaries.

Figures 1-2 and 1-3 show that the greatest upstream to downstream drop in internal pressure occurs in the arterioles and small arteries. Because the total flow is the same through the various series components of the circulatory system, it follows that the greatest resistance to flow resides in the arterioles. For example, if R_a represents the resistance of the arterioles, and R_x represents the resistance of any other component of the vascular system in series with the arterioles, then by the definition of hydraulic resistance (equation 10),

$$R_a = (P_i - P_o)_a / Q_a \qquad (11)$$

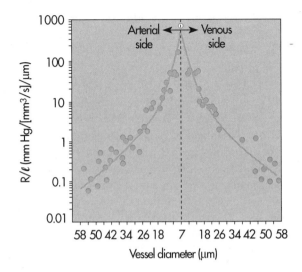

Figure 5-9 ■ **The resistance per unit length (R/ℓ) for individual small blood vessels in the cat mesentery. The capillaries, diameter 7 μm, are denoted by the vertical dashed line. Resistances of the arterioles are plotted to the left and resistances of the venules are plotted to the right of the vertical dashed line. The solid circles represent the actual data. The two curves through the data represent the following regression equations for the arteriole and venule data, respectively: (a) arterioles, $R/\ell = 1.02 \times 10^6 D^{-4.04}$, and (b) venules, $R/\ell = 1.07 \times 10^6 D^{-3.94}$. Note that for both types of vessels, the resistance per unit length is inversely proportional to the fourth power (within 1%) of the vessel diameter (D).** (Redrawn from Lipowsky HH, Kovalcheck S, Zweifach BW: *Circ Res* 43:738, 1978.)

for the arterioles, and

$$R_x = (P_i - P_o)_x / Q_x \qquad (12)$$

for the other vascular component.

However, the two components are in series, $Q_a = Q_x$, as stated above. Therefore

$$R_a / R_x = (P_i - P_o)_a / (P_i - P_o)_x \qquad (13)$$

That is, the ratio of the pressure drop across the length of the arterioles to the pressure drop across the length of any other series component of the vascular system is equal to the ratio of the hydraulic resistances of these two vascular components.

The reason why the highest resistance does not reside in the capillaries (as might otherwise be suspected from Figure 5-9) is related to the relative numbers of parallel capillaries and parallel arterioles, as explained below (see Figure 5-11). The arterioles are vested with a thick coat of circularly arranged smooth muscle fibers, by means of which the lumen radius may be varied. From the hydraulic resistance equation, wherein R varies inversely as r^4, it is clear that small changes in radius will alter resistance greatly.

Resistances in Series and in Parallel

In the cardiovascular system the various types of vessels listed along the horizontal axis in Figures 1-2 and 1-3 lie in series with one another. For two vessels arranged in series, a red blood cell that flows through the upstream vessel will also flow through the downstream vessel. Furthermore, the individual members of a given category of vessels are ordinarily arranged in parallel with one another (see Figure 1-4). For two vessels arranged in parallel, a red cell will pass through one of these vessels but not through the other during one circuit around the body. For example, the capillaries throughout the body are in most instances parallel elements. However, notable exceptions are the renal vasculature (wherein the peritubular capillaries are in series with the glomerular capillaries) and the splanchnic vasculature (wherein the intestinal and hepatic capillaries are aligned in series). Formulas for the total hydraulic resistance of tubes arranged in series and in parallel have been derived in the same manner as those for similar combinations of electrical resistances.

Three hydraulic resistances, R_1, R_2, and R_3, are arranged in series in the schema depicted in Figure 5-10. The pressure drop across the entire

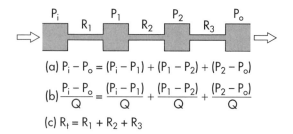

(a) $P_i - P_o = (P_i - P_1) + (P_1 - P_2) + (P_2 - P_o)$

(b) $\dfrac{P_i - P_o}{Q} = \dfrac{(P_i - P_1)}{Q} + \dfrac{(P_1 - P_2)}{Q} + \dfrac{(P_2 - P_o)}{Q}$

(c) $R_t = R_1 + R_2 + R_3$

Figure 5-10 ■ For resistances (R_1, R_2, and R_3) arranged in series, the total resistance, R_t, equals the sum of the individual resistances.

system—that is, the difference between inflow pressure, P_i, and outflow pressure, P_o—consists of the sum of the pressure drops across each of the individual resistances (equation *a*). Under steady-state conditions, the flow, Q, through any given cross-section must equal the flow through any other cross-section. By dividing each component in equation *a* by Q (equation *b*), it becomes evident from the definition of resistance (equation *c*) that *the total resistance, R_t, of the entire system of tubes in series equals the sum of the individual resistances,* that is,

$$R_t = R_1 + R_2 + R_3 \qquad (14)$$

For resistances in parallel, as illustrated in Figure 5-11, the inflow and outflow pressures are the same for all tubes. Under steady-state conditions, the total flow, Q_t, through the system equals the sum of the flows through the individual parallel elements (equation *a*). Because the pressure gradient ($P_i - P_o$) is identical for all parallel elements, each term in equation *a* may be divided by that pressure gradient to yield equation *b*. From the definition of resistance, equation *c* may be derived. This states that *the reciprocal of the total resistance, R_t, of tubes in parallel equals the sum of the reciprocals of the individual resistances,* that is,

$$\frac{1}{R_t} = \frac{1}{R_1} + \frac{1}{R_2} + \frac{1}{R_3} \qquad (15)$$

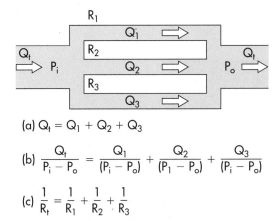

(a) $Q_t = Q_1 + Q_2 + Q_3$

(b) $\dfrac{Q_t}{P_i - P_o} = \dfrac{Q_1}{(P_i - P_o)} + \dfrac{Q_2}{(P_1 - P_o)} + \dfrac{Q_3}{(P_i - P_o)}$

(c) $\dfrac{1}{R_t} = \dfrac{1}{R_1} + \dfrac{1}{R_2} + \dfrac{1}{R_3}$

Figure 5-11 ■ **For resistances (R_1, R_2, and R_3) arranged in parallel, the reciprocal of the total resistance, R_t, equals the sum of the reciprocals of the individual resistances.**

Stated in another way, if we define hydraulic **conductance** as the reciprocal of resistance, it becomes evident that, *for tubes in parallel, the total conductance is the sum of the individual conductances.*

By considering a few simple illustrations, some of the fundamental properties of parallel hydraulic systems become apparent. For example, if the resistance of the three parallel elements in Figure 5-11 were all equal, then

$$R_1 = R_2 = R_3 \qquad (16)$$

Therefore

$$1/R_t = 3/R_1 \qquad (17)$$

and

$$R_t = R_1/3 \qquad (18)$$

Thus the total resistance is less than any of the individual resistances. After further consideration, it becomes evident that for any parallel arrangement, the total resistance must be less than that of any individual component. For example, consider a system in which a very high-resistance tube is added in parallel to a low-resistance tube. The total resistance must be less than that of the low-resistance component by itself, because the high-resistance component affords an additional pathway, or conductance, for fluid flow.

■ FLOW MAY BE LAMINAR OR TURBULENT

Under certain conditions, the flow of a fluid in a cylindrical tube is **laminar** (sometimes called **streamlined**), as illustrated in Figure 5-5. The thin layer of fluid in contact with the wall of the tube adheres to the wall and thus is motionless. The layer of fluid just central to this external lamina must shear against this motionless layer and therefore moves slowly, but with a finite velocity. Similarly, the adjacent, more central layer travels still more rapidly. The longitudinal velocity profile is that of a paraboloid (see Figure 5-5). The velocity of the fluid adjacent to the wall is zero, whereas the velocity at the center of the stream is maximum and equal to twice the mean velocity of flow across the entire cross-section of the tube. In laminar flow, fluid elements remain in one lamina, or streamline, as the fluid progresses longitudinally along the tube.

Irregular motions of the fluid elements may develop in the flow of fluid through a tube; this flow is called **turbulent.** Under such conditions, fluid elements do not remain confined to definite laminae, but rapid, radial mixing occurs (Figure 5-12). A considerably greater pressure is required to force a given flow of fluid through the same tube when the flow is turbulent than when it is laminar. In turbulent flow the pressure drop is approximately proportional to the square of the flow rate, whereas in laminar flow the pressure drop is proportional to the first power of the flow rate. Hence to produce a given flow, a pump such as the heart must do considerably more work to generate a given flow if turbulence develops.

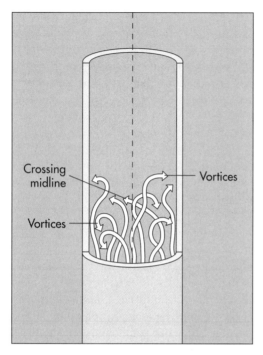

Figure 5-12 ■ **In turbulent flow the elements of the fluid move irregularly in axial, radial, and circumferential directions. Vortices frequently develop.**

Whether turbulent or laminar flow will exist in a tube under given conditions may be predicted on the basis of a dimensionless number called **Reynold's number,** N_R. This number represents the ratio of inertial to viscous forces. For a fluid flowing through a cylindric tube,

$$N_R = \rho D \bar{v}/\eta \qquad (19)$$

where D is the tube diameter, $\bar{v}$ is the mean velocity, ρ is the density, and η is the viscosity. For $N_R < 2000$, the flow is usually laminar; for $N_R > 3000$, the flow is turbulent. Various possible conditions may develop in the transition range of N_R between 2000 and 3000. Because flow tends to be laminar at low N_R and turbulent at high N_R, the definition of N_R indicates that

large diameters, high velocities, and low viscosities predispose to turbulence.

Turbulence is usually accompanied by audible vibrations. When turbulent flow exists within the cardiovascular system, it is usually detected as a **murmur.** The factors listed above that predispose to turbulence may account for murmurs heard clinically. In severe anemia, **functional cardiac murmurs** (murmurs not caused by structural abnormalities) are frequently detectable. The physical basis for such murmurs resides in (1) the reduced viscosity of blood in anemia and (2) the high flow velocities associated with the high cardiac output that usually prevails in anemic patients. Turbulence also occurs when the cross-secional area of the bloodstream suddenly changes, as when the blood passes through a narrowed (stenotic) cardiac valve or when it passes through an abnormal widening (aneurysm) of a large artery. Such abrupt changes in dimensions of the bloodstream cause audible murmurs.

Blood clots, or **thrombi,** are much more likely to develop in turbulent than in laminar flow. One of the problems with the use of artificial valves in the surgical treatment of valvular heart disease is that thrombi may occur in association with the prosthetic valve. The thrombi may be dislodged and occlude a crucial artery. It is thus important to design such valves to avert turbulence.

■ SHEAR STRESS ON THE VESSEL WALL

In Figure 5-8 an external force is applied to a plate floating on the surface of a liquid in a large basin. This force, exerted parallel to the surface, causes a shearing stress on the liquid below and thereby produces a differential motion of each layer of liquid relative to the adjacent layers. At the bottom of the basin, the flowing liquid exerts a shearing stress on the surface of the basin in contact with the liquid. By rearranging the equation for viscosity stated in Figure 5-8, it is apparent that the shear stress, τ, equals η (du/dy); that is, the shear stress equals the product of the viscosity and the shear rate. Hence *the greater the rate of flow, the greater the shear stress that the liquid exerts on the walls of the container in which it flows.*

For precisely the same reasons, the rapidly flowing blood in a large artery tends to pull the endothelial lining of the artery along with it. This force **(viscous drag)** is proportional to the shear rate (du/dy) of the layers of blood very close to the wall. For a flow regimen that obeys Poiseuille's law,

$$\tau = 4\eta Q/\pi r^3 \qquad (20)$$

The greater the rate of blood flow (Q) in the artery, the greater will be du/dy near the arterial wall, and the greater will be the viscous drag (τ).

Box 5-3

In certain types of arterial disease, particularly in patients with hypertension, the subendothelial layers tend to degenerate locally, and small regions of the endothelium may lose their normal support. The viscous drag on the arterial wall may cause a tear between a normally supported and an unsupported region of the endothelial lining. Blood may then flow from the vessel lumen through the rift in the lining and dissect between the various layers of the artery. Such a lesion is called a **dissecting aneurysm.** It occurs most commonly in the proximal portions of the aorta and is extremely serious. One reason for its predilection for this site is the high velocity of blood flow, with the associated large values of du/dy at the endothelial wall. The shear stress at the vessel wall also influences many other vascular functions, such as the permeability of the vascular walls to large molecules, the biosynthetic activity of the endothelial cells, the integrity of the formed elements in the blood, and the coagulation of the blood.

■ RHEOLOGIC PROPERTIES OF BLOOD

The viscosity of a newtonian fluid, such as water, may be determined by measuring the rate of flow of the fluid at a given pressure gradient through a cylindrical tube of known length and radius. As long as the fluid flow is laminar, the viscosity may be computed by substituting these values into Poiseuille's equation. The viscosity of a given newtonian fluid at a specified temperature will be constant over a wide range of tube dimensions and flows. However, for a non-newtonian fluid, the viscosity calculated by substituting into Poiseuille's equation may vary considerably as a function of tube dimensions and flows. Therefore in considering the rheologic properties of a suspension such as blood, the term **viscosity** does not have a unique meaning. The terms **anomalous viscosity** and **apparent viscosity** are frequently applied to the value of viscosity obtained for blood under the particular conditions of measurement.

Rheologically, blood is a suspension of formed elements, principally erythrocytes, in a relatively homogeneous liquid, the blood plasma. For this reason, the apparent viscosity of blood varies as a function of the **hematocrit ratio** (ratio of volume of red blood cells to volume of whole blood). In Figure 5-13 the upper curve represents the ratio of the apparent viscosity of whole blood to that of plasma over a range of hematocrit ratios from 0% to 80%, measured in a tube 1 mm in diameter. The viscosity of plasma is 1.2 to 1.3 times that of water. Figure 5-13 *(upper curve)* shows that blood, with a normal hematocrit ratio of 45%, has an apparent viscosity 2.4 times that of plasma.

For any given hematocrit ratio, the apparent viscosity of blood depends on the dimensions of the tube employed in estimating the viscosity. Figure 5-14 demonstrates that the apparent viscosity of blood diminishes progressively as tube diameter decreases below a value of about 0.3 mm. The diameters of the highest-resistance blood vessels, the arterioles, are considerably less than this critical value. This phenomenon therefore reduces the resistance to flow in the blood vessels that possess the greatest resistance.

The apparent viscosity of blood, when measured in living tissues, is considerably less than when it is measured in a conventional capillary tube viscometer with a diameter greater than 0.3 mm. In the lower curve of Figure 5-13, the apparent viscosity of blood was assessed by using the hind leg of an anesthetized dog as a biological viscometer. Over the entire range of hematocrit ratios, the apparent viscosity was less when measured in the living tissue than in the capillary tube viscometer *(upper curve),* and the disparity was greater the higher the hematocrit ratio.

The influence of tube diameter on apparent viscosity depends in part on the change in actual composition of the blood as it flows through small tubes. The composition changes because the red blood cells tend to accumulate in the faster axial stream in the blood vessels, whereas the blood component that flows in the slower marginal layers is mainly plasma.

To illustrate this phenomenon, a reservoir such as R_1 in Figure 5-6, *C* has been filled with blood possessing a given hematocrit ratio. The blood in R_1 was constantly agitated to prevent settling and was permitted to flow through a narrow capillary tube into reservoir R_2. As long as the tube diameter was substantially greater than the diameter of the red blood cells, the hematocrit ratio of the blood in R_2 was not detectably different from that in R_1. Surprisingly, however, the hematocrit ratio of the blood contained within the tube was found to be considerably

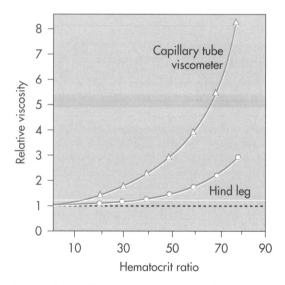

Figure 5-13 ■ **The viscosity of whole blood, relative to that of plasma, increases at a progressively greater rate as the hematocrit ratio increases. For any given hematocrit ratio, the apparent viscosity of blood is less when measured in a biological viscometer (such as the hind leg of a dog) than in a conventional capillary tube viscometer.** (Redrawn from Levy MN, Share L: *Circ Res* 1:247, 1953.)

lower than the hematocrit ratio of the blood in either reservoir.

In Figure 5-15, the relative hematocrit is the ratio of the hematocrit in the tube to that in the reservoir at either end of the tube. For tubes of 300 μm diameter or greater, the relative hematocrit ratio was close to 1. However, as the tube diameter was reduced below 300 μm, the relative hematocrit ratio progressively diminished;

for a tube diameter of 30 μm, the relative hematocrit ratio was only 0.65.

The fact that this phenomenon results from a disparity in the relative velocities of the red cells and plasma can be appreciated on the basis of the following analogy. Consider the flow of automobile traffic across a bridge that is 3 miles long. Let the cars move in one lane at a speed of 60 miles per hour and the trucks in another lane at 20 miles per hour, as illustrated in Figure 5-16. If one car and one truck start out across the bridge each minute, then except for the initial few minutes of traffic flow across the bridge, one car and one truck will arrive at the other end each minute. Yet, if one counts the actual number of cars and trucks on the bridge at any moment, there will be three times more of the slower trucks than of the faster cars.

Because the axial portions of the bloodstream contain a greater proportion of red cells and move with a greater velocity, the red cells tend to traverse the tube in less time than does the plasma. Therefore the red cells correspond to the fast cars in the analogy, and the plasma corresponds to the slow trucks. Measurement of transit times through various organs has shown that red cells do travel faster than the plasma. Furthermore, the hematocrit ratios of the blood

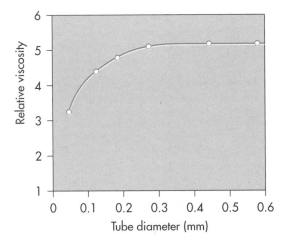

Figure 5-14 ■ **The viscosity of blood, relative to that of water, increases as a function of tube diameter up to a diameter of about 0.3 mm.** (Redrawn from Fåhraeus R, Lindqvist T: *Am J Physiol* 96:562, 1931.)

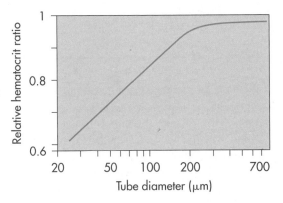

Figure 5-15 ■ **The relative hematocrit ratio of blood flowing from a feed reservoir through capillary tubes of various calibers, as a function of the tube diameter. The relative hematocrit is the ratio of the hematocrit of the blood in the tubes to that of the blood in the feed reservoir.** (Redrawn from Barbee JH, Cokelet GR: *Microvasc Res* 3:6, 1971.)

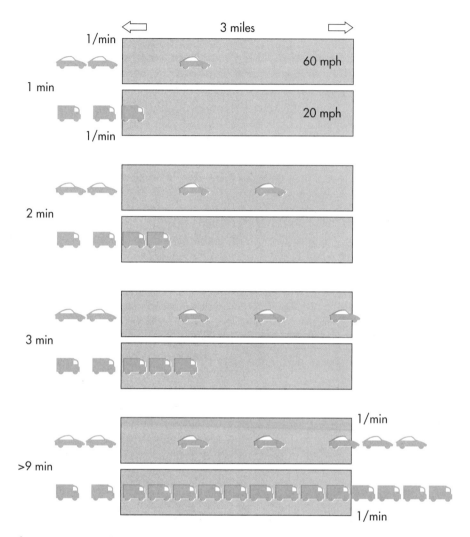

Figure 5-16 ■ **When the car velocity is three times as great as the truck velocity, the ratio of the number of cars to trucks on a bridge will be 1:3, even though one of each type of vehicle enters and leaves the bridge each minute.**

contained in the smallest vessels in various tissues are lower than those in blood samples withdrawn from large arteries or veins in the same animal (Figure 5-17).

The physical forces responsible for the drift of the erythrocytes toward the axial stream and away from the vessel walls are not fully understood. One factor is the great flexibility of the red blood cells. At low flow (or shear) rates, comparable with those in the microcirculation, rigid particles do not migrate toward the axis of a tube, whereas flexible particles do migrate. The concentration of flexible particles near the tube axis is enhanced by increasing the shear rate.

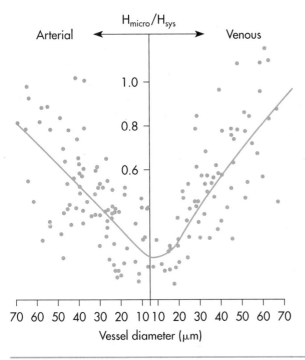

Figure 5-17 ■ The hematocrit ratio (*H$_{micro}$*) of the blood in various-sized arterial and venous microvessels in the cat mesentery, relative to the hematocrit ratio (*H$_{sys}$*) in the large systemic vessels. The hematocrit ratio is least in the capillaries and tiny venules. (Modified from Lipowsky HH, Usami S, Chien S: *Microvasc Res* 19:297, 1980.)

The apparent viscosity of blood diminishes as the shear rate is increased (Figure 5-18), a phenomenon called **shear thinning.** The greater tendency of the erythrocytes to accumulate in the axial laminae at higher flow rates is partly responsible for this nonnewtonian behavior. However, a more important factor is that at very slow rates of shear, the suspended cells tend to form aggregates, which would increase viscosity. As the flow is increased, this aggregation would decrease and so would the apparent viscosity (Figure 5-18).

The tendency for the erythrocytes to aggregate at low flows depends on the concentration in the plasma of the larger protein molecules, especially fibrinogen. For this reason, the changes in blood viscosity with shear rate are much more pronounced when the concentration of fibrinogen is high. Also, at low flow rates, the leukocytes tend to adhere to the endothelial cells of

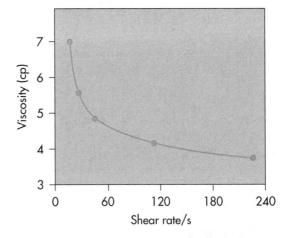

Figure 5-18 ■ Decrease in the viscosity of blood (centipoise) at increasing rates of shear. The shear rate refers to the velocity of one layer of fluid relative to that of the adjacent layers and is directionally related to the rate of flow. (Redrawn from Amin TM, Sirs JA: *Q J Exp Physiol* 70:37, 1985.)

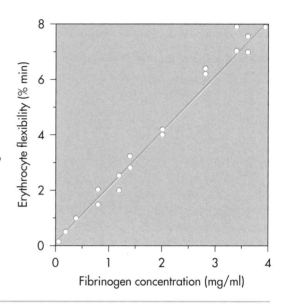

Figure 5-19 ■ **The effect of the plasma fibrinogen concentration on the flexibility of human erythrocytes.** (Redrawn from Amin TM, Sirs JA: *Q J Exp Physiol* 70:37, 1985.)

the microvessels and thereby increase the apparent viscosity.

The deformability of the erythrocytes is also a factor in shear thinning, especially at high hematocrit ratios. The mean diameter of human red blood cells is about 8 μm, yet they are able to pass through openings with a diameter of only 3 μm. As blood that is densely packed with erythrocytes is caused to flow at progressively greater rates, the erythrocytes become more and more deformed, which diminishes the apparent viscosity of the blood. The flexibility of human erythrocytes is enhanced as the concentration of fibrinogen in the plasma increases (Figure 5-19).

Box 5-5

If the red blood cells become hardened, as they are in certain **spherocytic anemias,** shear thinning may become much less prominent. When erythrocytes are extremely deformed, especially in **sickle cell anemia,** they tend to aggregate and completely block flow in small vessels; the tissues supplied by those vessels frequently become infarcted.

Summary

- The vascular system is composed of two major subdivisions in series with one another—the systemic circulation and the pulmonary circulation.

- Each subdivision consists of several types of vessels (e.g., arteries, arterioles, capillaries) aligned in series with one another. In general, the vessels of a given type are arranged in parallel with each other.

- The mean velocity (v) of blood flow in a given type of vessel is directly proportional to the total blood flow (Q_t) being pumped by the heart, and it is inversely proportional to the cross-sectional area (A) of all the parallel vessels of that type; i.e., $v = Q_t/A$.

- The laterally directed pressure in the bloodstream decreases as the flow velocity increases; the decrement in lateral pressure is proportional to the square of the velocity.

- When blood flow is steady and laminar in vessels larger than arterioles, the flow (Q) is proportional to the pressure drop down the vessel ($P_i - P_o$) and to the fourth power of the radius (r), and it is inversely proportional to the length (ℓ) of the vessel and to the viscosity (η) of the fluid; i.e., $Q = \pi(P_i - P_o)r^4/8\eta\ell$ (Poiseuille's law).

- For resistances aligned in series, the total resistance equals the sum of the individual resistances.

- For resistances aligned in parallel, the reciprocal of the total resistance equals the sum of the reciprocals of the individual resistances.

- Flow tends to become turbulent when flow velocity is high, when fluid viscosity is low, when tube diameter is large, or when the wall of the vessel is very irregular.

- Blood flow is nonnewtonian in very small vessels; i.e., Poiseuille's law is not applicable. The apparent viscosity of blood diminishes as shear rate (flow) increases and as the tube dimensions decrease.

■ BIBLIOGRAPHY

1. Alonso C, Pries AR, Kiesslich O, et al: Transient rheological behavior of blood in low-shear tube flow: velocity profiles and effective viscosity. *Am J Physiol* 268:H25, 1995.
2. Badeer HS, Hicks JW: Hemodynamics of vascular "waterfall": is the analogy justified? *Resp Physiol* 87:205, 1992.
3. Cokelet GR, Goldsmith HI: Decreased hydrodynamic resistance in the two-phase flow of blood through small vertical tubes at low flow rates. *Circ Res* 68:1, 1991.
4. Hoeks APG, Samijo SK, Brands PJ, et al: Noninvasive determination of shear-rate distribution across the arterial wall. *Hypertension* 26:26, 1995.
5. Jonsson V, et al: Significance of plasma skimming and plasma volume expansion. *J Appl Physiol* 72:2047, 1992.
6. Klanchar M, Tarbell JM, Wang D-M: In vitro study of the influence of radial wall motion on wall shear stress in an elastic tube model of the aorta. *Circ Res* 66:1624, 1990.
7. Lee RT, Kamm RD: Vascular mechanics for the cardiologist. *J Am Coll Cardiol* 23:1289, 1994.
8. Lowe GDO: *Clinical blood rheology*, vol I, Boca Raton, FL, 1988, CRC Press.
9. Maeda N, Shiga T: Velocity of oxygen transfer and erythrocyte rheology. *News Physiol Sci* 9:22, 1994.
10. Melkumyants AM, Balashov SA, Khayutin VM: Control of arterial lumen by shear stress on endothelium. *News Physiol Sci* 10:204, 1995.
11. Morita T, Kurihara H, Maemura K, et al: Role of Ca^{2+} and protein kinase C in shear stress–induced actin depolymerization and endothelin 1 gene expression. *Circ Res* 75:630, 1994.
12. Pries AR, Secomb TW, Gaetgens P: Design principles of vascular beds *Circ Res* 77:1017, 1995.
13. Pries AR, Secomb TW, Gessner T, et al: Resistance to blood flow in microvessels in vivo. *Circ Res* 75:904, 1994.
14. Reinhart WH, Boulanger CM, Lüscher TF, et al: Influence of endothelial surface on flow velocity in vitro. *Am J Physiol* 265:H523, 1993.
15. White KC, Kavanaugh JF, Wang D-M, et al: Hemodynamics and wall shear rate in the abdominal aorta of dogs: effects of vasoactive agents. *Circ Res* 75:637, 1994.

■ CASE 5

HISTORY

A 70-year-old man complained of severe pain in his right leg whenever he walked briskly; the pain disappeared soon after he stopped walking. His doctor referred him to a vascular surgeon, who carried out several hemodynamic tests. Angiography showed partial obstruction by large arteriosclerotic plaques about 3 cm distal to the origin of the right femoral artery. The left femoral artery appeared to be normal. The mean arterial pressure in the left femoral artery with the patient at rest was 100 mm Hg, and the blood flow in this artery was 500 ml/min. The mean arterial pressure in the right femoral artery proximal to the obstruction was 100 mm Hg, and just distal to the obstruction, it was 80 mm Hg. The blood flow in this artery was 300 mm Hg/ml/min. The mean venous pressure was 10 mm Hg in the left and right femoral veins.

QUESTIONS

1. The resistance to blood flow in the vascular bed perfused by the right femoral artery was
   a. 0.03 mm Hg/ml/min
   b. 0.30 mm Hg/ml/min
   c. 3.00 mm Hg/ml/min
   d. 3.33 mm Hg/ml/min
   e. 33.3 mm Hg/ml/min

2. The resistance to blood flow (R_t) in the combined vascular beds perfused by both femoral arteries was
   a. 0.48 mm Hg/ml/min
   b. 0.84 mm Hg/ml/min
   c. 1.10 mm Hg/ml/min
   d. 0.11 mm Hg/ml/min
   e. 11.1 mm Hg/ml/min

3. The resistance to flow imposed by the arteriosclerotic obstruction in the right femoral artery amounted to
   a. 0.066 mm Hg/ml/min
   b. 0.660 mm Hg/ml/min
   c. 0.15 mm Hg/ml/min
   d. 1.50 mm Hg/ml/min
   e. 15.0 mm Hg/ml/min

CHAPTER 6

The Arterial System

Objectives

1. Explain how the pulsatile blood flow in the large arteries is converted into a steady flow in the capillaries.

2. Explain the factors that determine the mean, systolic, and diastolic arterial pressures and the arterial pulse pressure.

3. Describe the common procedure for measuring the arterial blood pressure in humans.

■ THE HYDRAULIC FILTER CONVERTS PULSATILE FLOW TO STEADY FLOW

The principal function of the systemic and pulmonary arterial systems is to distribute blood to the capillary beds throughout the body. The arterioles, which are the terminal components of the arterial system, regulate the distribution of flow to the various capillary beds. Between the heart and the arterioles, the aorta and pulmonary artery and their major branches constitute a system of conduits of considerable volume and distensibility. An arterial system composed of elastic conduits and high-resistance terminals constitutes a **hydraulic filter** analogous to the resistance-capacitance filters of electrical circuits.

Hydraulic filtering converts the intermittent output of the heart to a steady flow through the capillaries. This important function of the large elastic arteries has been likened to the **Windkessels** of antique fire engines. The Windkessel contained a large volume of trapped air. The compressibility of the trapped air converted the intermittent inflow of water to a steady outflow at the nozzle of the fire hose.

The analogous function of the large elastic arteries is illustrated in Figure 6-1. The heart is an intermittent pump. The entire stroke volume is discharged into the arterial system during systole, which usually occupies approximately one third of the duration of the cardiac cycle. In fact, as shown in Figure 3-11, most of the stroke volume is pumped during the rapid ejection phase, which constitutes about half of systole. Part of the energy of cardiac contraction is dissipated as forward capillary flow during systole; the remainder is stored in the arteries as potential en-

135

Compliant arteries

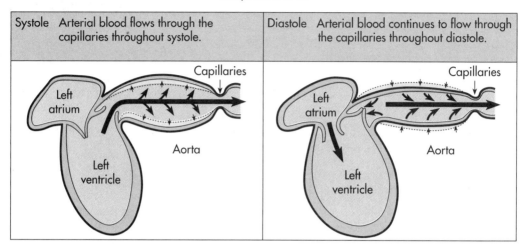

A, When the arteries are normally compliant, a substantial fraction of the stroke volume is stored in the arteries during ventricular systole. The arterial walls are stretched.

B, During ventricular diastole the previously stretched arteries recoil. The volume of blood that is displaced by the recoil furnishes continuous capillary flow throughout diastole.

Rigid arteries

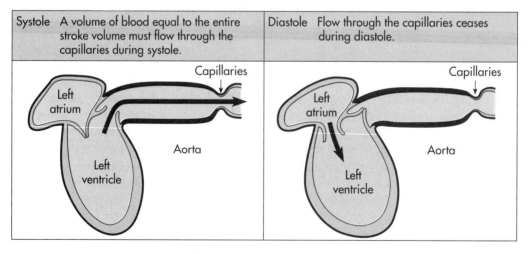

C, When the arteries are rigid, virtually none of the stroke volume can be stored in the arteries.

D, Rigid arteries cannot recoil appreciably during diastole.

Figure 6-1 ■ **When the arteries are normally compliant, blood flows through the capillaries throughout the cardiac cycle. When the arteries are rigid, blood flows through the capillaries during systole, but flow ceases during diastole.**

ergy, in that much of the stroke volume is retained by stretching the distensible arteries (Figure 6-1, *A-B*). During diastole the elastic recoil of the arterial walls converts this potential energy into capillary blood flow. If the arterial walls were rigid, capillary flow would cease during diastole (Figure 6-1, *C-D*).

Hydraulic filtering minimizes the workload of the heart. More work is required to pump a given flow intermittently than steadily; the more effective the filtering, the less is the excess work. A simple example will illustrate this point.

Consider first the steady flow of a fluid at a rate of 100 ml/s through a hydraulic system with a resistance of 1 mm Hg/ml/s. This combination of flow and resistance would result in a constant pressure of 100 mm Hg, as shown in Figure 6-2, *A*. Neglecting any inertial effect, hydraulic work, W, may be defined as

$$W = \int_{t_1}^{t_2} PdV \qquad (1)$$

that is, each small increment of volume, dV, pumped is multiplied by the pressure, P, existing at the time, and the products are integrated over the time interval of interest, $t_2 - t_1$, to give the total work, W. For steady flow,

$$W = PV \qquad (2)$$

In the example in Figure 6-2, *A,* the work done in pumping the fluid for 1 s would be 10,000 mm Hg · ml (or 1.33×10^7 dyne-cm).

Next, consider an intermittent pump that puts out the same volume per second but pumps the entire volume at a steady rate over 0.5 s and then pumps nothing during the next 0.5 s. Hence it pumps at the rate of 200 ml/s for 0.5 s, as shown in Figure 6-2, *B* and *C*. In *B* the conduit is rigid and the fluid is incompressible, but the system has the same resistance as in *A*. During the pumping phase of the cycle (systole) the flow of 200 ml/s through a resistance of 1 mm Hg/ml/s would produce a pressure of 200 mm Hg. During

the filling phase of the pump (diastole) the pressure would be 0 mm Hg in this rigid system. The work done during systole would be 20,000 mm Hg · ml, which is twice that required in the example shown in Figure 6-2, *A*.

If the system were very distensible, hydraulic filtering would be very effective and the pressure would remain virtually constant throughout the entire cycle (Figure 6-2, *C*). Of the 100 ml of fluid pumped during the 0.5 s of systole, only 50 ml would be emitted through the high-resistance outflow end of the system during systole. The remaining 50 ml would be stored by the distensible conduit during systole and would flow out during diastole. Hence the pressure would be virtually constant at 100 mm Hg throughout the cycle. The fluid pumped during systole would be ejected at only half the pressure that prevailed in Figure 6-2, *B*, and therefore the work would be only half as great. With nearly perfect filtering, as in Figure 6-2, *C,* the work would be identical to that for steady flow (Figure 6-2, *A*).

Naturally, the filtering accomplished by the systemic and pulmonic arterial systems is intermediate between the examples in Figure 6-2, *B* and *C*. Ordinarily, the additional work imposed by intermittency of pumping, in excess of that for steady flow, is about 35% for the right ventricle and about 10% for the left ventricle. These fractions change, however, with variations in heart rate, peripheral resistance, and arterial distensibility.

The increased cardiac energy requirement imposed by a rigid arterial system is illustrated by the experimental results shown in Figure 6-3. In a group of anesthetized dogs, the cardiac output pumped by the left ventricle could be allowed to flow through the natural route (the aorta), or it could be diverted through a stiff plastic tube to the peripheral arteries. The total peripheral resistance (TPR) readings were virtually identical regardless of which pathway was selected. The

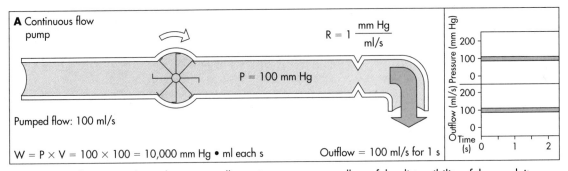

A, The pump flow is steady, and pressure will remain constant regardless of the distensibility of the conduit.

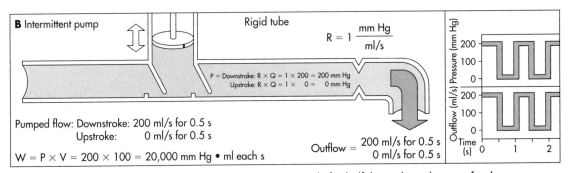

B, The flow (Q) produced by the pump is intermittent; it is steady for half the cycle and ceases for the remainder of the cycle. The conduit is rigid, and therefore the flow produced by the pump during its downstroke must exit through the resistance during the same 0.5 second that elapses during the downstroke. The pump must do twice as much work as the pump in **A.**

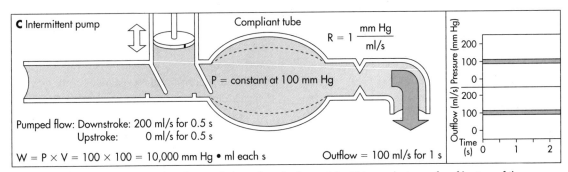

C, The pump operates as in **B,** but the conduit is infinitely distensible. This results in perfect filtering of the pressure; that is, the pressure is steady, and the outflow through the resistance is also steady. The work equals that in **A.**

Figure 6-2 ■ **The relationships between pressure and flow for three hydraulic systems. In each the overall flow is 100 ml/s and the resistance is 1 mm Hg/ml/s.**

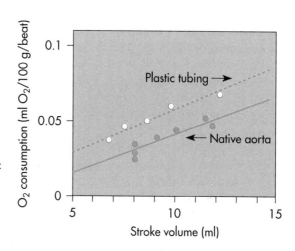

Figure 6-3 ■ The relationship between myocardial oxygen consumption (ml/100 g/beat) and stroke volume (ml) in an anesthetized dog whose cardiac output could be pumped by the left ventricle either through the aorta or through a stiff plastic tube to the peripheral arteries. (Modified from Kelly RP, Tunin R, Kass DA: *Circ Res* 71:490, 1992.)

data (Figure 6-3) from a representative animal show that for any given stroke volume, the myocardial oxygen consumption (MVO$_2$) was substantially greater when the blood was diverted through the plastic tubing than when it flowed through the aorta. This increase in MVO$_2$ indicates that the left ventricle had to expend more energy to pump blood through a less compliant conduit than through a more compliant conduit.

■ ARTERIAL ELASTICITY COMPENSATES FOR THE INTERMITTENT FLOW DELIVERED BY THE HEART

The elastic properties of the arterial wall may be appreciated by considering first the **static pressure-volume relationship** for the aorta. To obtain the curves shown in Figure 6-4, aortas were obtained at autopsy from individuals in different age groups. All branches of the aorta were ligated and successive volumes of liquid were injected into this closed elastic system. After each increment of volume, the internal pressure was measured. In Figure 6-4 the curve that relates pressure to volume for the youngest age group (curve *a*) is sigmoidal. Although the curve is nearly linear over most of its extent, the slope decreases at the upper and lower ends. At

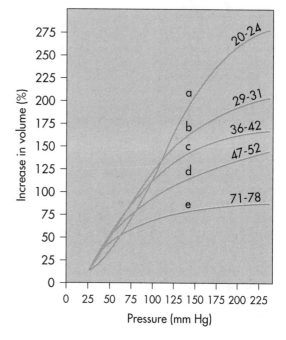

Figure 6-4 ■ Pressure-volume relationships for aortas obtained at autopsy from humans in different age groups (denoted by the numbers at the right end of each of the curves). (Redrawn from Hallock P, Benson IC: *J Clin Invest* 16:595, 1937.)

any point, the slope (dV/dP) represents the aortic **compliance.** Thus in young individuals the aortic compliance is least at very high and low pressures and greatest over the usual range of pressure variations. This sequence of compliance changes resembles the familiar compliance changes encountered in inflating a balloon. The greatest difficulty in introducing air into the balloon is experienced at the beginning of inflation and again at near-maximal volume, just before rupture of the balloon. At intermediate volumes, the balloon is relatively easy to inflate; that is, it is more compliant.

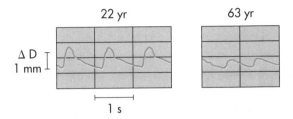

Figure 6-5 ▪ **The pulsatile changes in diameter, measured ultrasonically, in a 22-year-old and in a 63-year-old man.** (Modified from Imura T, Yamamoto K, Kanamori K, et al: *Cardiovasc Res* 20:208, 1986.)

> ### BOX 6-1
>
> It is also apparent from Figure 6-4 that the curves become displaced downward and the slopes diminish as a function of advancing age. Thus for any pressure above about 80 mm Hg, the compliance decreases with age, a manifestation of increased rigidity **(atherosclerosis)** caused by progressive changes in the collagen and elastin contents of the arterial walls.

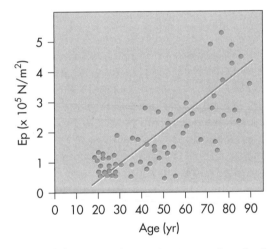

Figure 6-6 ▪ **The effects of age on the elastic modulus *(Ep)* of the abdominal aorta in a group of 61 human subjects.** (Modified from Imura T, Yamamoto K, Kanamori K, et al: *Cardiovasc Res* 20:208, 1986.)

The above effects of the subject's age on the elastic characteristics of the arterial system were derived from aortas removed at autopsy (see Figure 6-4). Such age-related changes have been confirmed in living subjects by ultrasound imaging techniques. These studies disclosed that the increase in the diameter of the aorta produced by each cardiac contraction is much less in elderly persons than in young persons (Figure 6-5). The effects of aging on the elastic modulus of the aorta in healthy subjects are shown in Figure 6-6. The elastic modulus, Ep, is defined as

$$E_p = \Delta P/(\Delta D/D) \qquad (3)$$

where ΔP is the aortic pulse pressure (Figure 6-7), D is the mean aortic diameter during the cardiac cycle, and ΔD is the maximal change in aortic diameter during the cardiac cycle.

The fractional change in diameter ($\Delta D/D$) of the aorta during the cardiac cycle reflects its change in volume as the left ventricle ejects its stroke volume into the aorta each systole. Thus E_p is **inversely** related to compliance, which is the ratio of ΔV to ΔP. Consequently, the **increase** in elastic modulus with aging (Figure 6-6) and the **decrease** in compliance with aging (Fig-

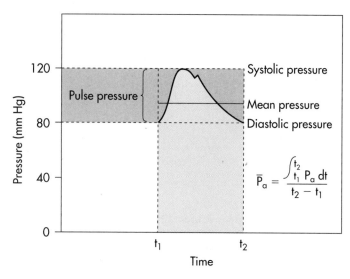

Figure 6-7 ■ **Arterial systolic, diastolic, pulse, and mean pressures. The mean arterial pressure ($\overline{P}_a$) represents the area under the arterial pressure curve (*colored area*) divided by the cardiac cycle duration ($t_2 - t_1$).**

ure 6-4) both reflect the stiffening of the arterial walls **(atherosclerosis)** as individuals age.

■ THE ARTERIAL BLOOD PRESSURE IS DETERMINED BY PHYSICAL AND PHYSIOLOGICAL FACTORS

The determinants of the pressure within the arterial system of intact subjects cannot be evaluated precisely. Nevertheless, arterial blood pressure is routinely measured in patients and provides a useful clue to the cardiovascular status. We therefore take a simplified approach to explain the principal determinants of arterial blood pressure. To accomplish this, the determinants of **mean arterial pressure** (defined in the next section) are first analyzed. **Systolic** and **diastolic arterial pressures** are then considered as the upper and lower limits of periodic oscillations about this mean pressure. Finally, the changes in arterial pressure as the pulse wave progresses from the origin of the aorta toward the capillaries is discussed.

The determinants of arterial blood pressure may be arbitrarily subdivided into "physical" and "physiological" factors (Figure 6-8). The arterial system is assumed to be a static, elastic system, and the only two "physical" factors considered are the **blood volume** within the arterial system and the **elastic characteristics** (compliance) of the system. Certain "physiological" factors will be considered: cardiac output, which equals **heart rate × stroke volume,** and **peripheral resistance.** *Such physiological factors will be shown to operate through one or both of the physical factors.*

Mean Arterial Pressure

Mean arterial pressure is the pressure in the large arteries, averaged over time. It may be obtained from an arterial pressure tracing by measuring the area under the pressure curve and dividing this area by the time interval involved, as shown in Figure 6-7. The mean arterial pressure, $\overline{P}_a$, can usually be approximated satisfactorily

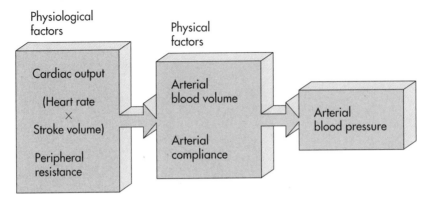

Figure 6-8 ■ **Arterial blood pressure is determined directly by two major physical factors, the arterial blood volume and the arterial compliance. These physical factors are affected in turn by certain physiological factors, primarily the heart rate, stroke volume, cardiac output (heart rate × stroke volume), and peripheral resistance.**

from the measured values of the systolic (P_s) and diastolic (P_d) pressures by means of the following empirical formula:

$$\overline{P}_a \cong P_d + \tfrac{1}{3} (P_s - P_d) \qquad (4)$$

The mean pressure will be considered to depend only on the mean blood volume in the arterial system and on the arterial compliance (Figure 6-8). The arterial volume, V_a, in turn depends on the rate of inflow, Q_h, from the heart into the arteries **(cardiac output)** and the rate of outflow, Q_r, from the arteries through the resistance vessels **(peripheral runoff)**; expressed mathematically,

$$dV_a/dt = Q_h - Q_r \qquad (5)$$

This equation is an expression of the law of conservation of mass. It states that the change in arterial blood volume per unit time (dV_a/dt) represents the difference between the rate at which blood is pumped into the arterial system by the heart (Q_h) and the rate at which it leaves the arterial system through the resistance vessels (Q_r).

If arterial inflow exceeds outflow, arterial volume increases, the arterial walls are stretched more, and pressure rises. The converse happens when arterial outflow exceeds inflow. When inflow equals outflow, arterial pressure remains constant.

Cardiac Output

The change in pressure in response to an alteration of cardiac output can be better appreciated by considering some simple examples. Under control conditions, let cardiac output be 5 L/min and mean arterial pressure ($\overline{P}_a$) be 100 mm Hg (Figure 6-9, *A*). From the definition of total peripheral resistance,

$$R = (\overline{P}_a - \overline{P}_{ra})/Q_r \qquad (6)$$

If $\overline{P}_{ra}$ (mean right atrial pressure) is negligible compared with $\overline{P}_a$,

$$R \cong \overline{P}_a/Q_r \qquad (7)$$

Therefore in the example, R is 100/5, or 20 mm Hg/L/min.

Now let cardiac output, Q_h, suddenly increase to 10 L/min (Figure 6-9, *B*). Instantaneously, $\overline{P}_a$ will be unchanged. Because the outflow, Q_r, from the arteries depends on $\overline{P}_a$ and R,

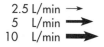

2.5 L/min →
5 L/min →
10 L/min →

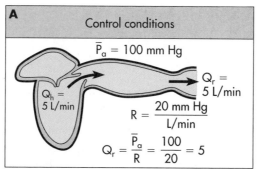

A, Under control conditions Q_h = 5 L/min, $\bar{P}_a$ = 100 mm Hg, and R = 20 mm Hg/L/min. Q_r must equal Q_h, and therefore the mean blood volume $(\bar{V}_a)$ in the arteries will remain constant from heartbeat to heartbeat.

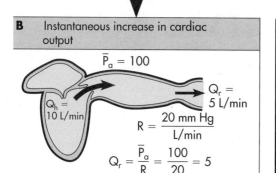

B, If Q_h suddenly increases to 10 L/min, Q_h will initially exceed Q_r, and therefore $\bar{P}_a$ will begin to rise rapidly.

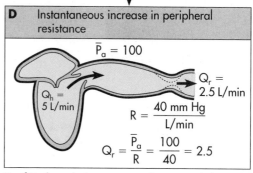

D, If R abruptly increases to 40 mm Hg/L/min, Q_r suddenly decreases and therefore Q_h exceeds Q_r. Thus $\bar{P}_a$ will rise progressively.

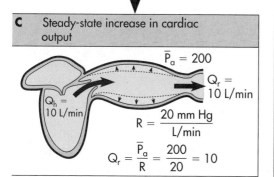

C, The disparity between Q_h and Q_r progressively increases arterial blood volume. The volume continues to increase until $\bar{P}_a$ reaches a level of 200 mm Hg.

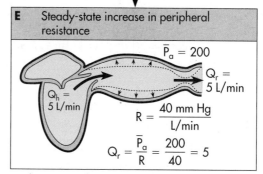

E, The excess of Q_h over Q_r accumulates blood in the arteries. Blood continues to accumulate until $\bar{P}_a$ rises to a level of 200 mm Hg.

Figure 6-9 ■ The relationship of mean arterial blood pressure $(\bar{P}_a)$ to cardiac output (Q_h), peripheral runoff (Q_r), and peripheral resistance (R) under control conditions (A), in response to an increase in cardiac output (B and C), and in response to an increase in peripheral resistance (D and E).

Q_r will also remain unchanged at first. Therefore Q_h, now 10 L/min, will exceed Q_r, still only 5 L/min. This will increase the mean arterial blood volume ($\overline{V}_a$). From equation 5, when $Q_h > Q_r$, $d\overline{V}_a/dt > 0$; that is, volume is increasing.

Because $\overline{P}_a$ depends on the mean arterial blood volume, $\overline{V}_a$, and the arterial compliance, C_a, an increase in $\overline{V}_a$ will raise the $\overline{P}_a$. By definition,

$$C_a = d\overline{V}_a/d\overline{P}_a \qquad (8)$$

Therefore

$$d\overline{V}_a = C_a d\overline{P}_a \qquad (9)$$

and

$$\frac{d\overline{V}_a}{dt} = C_a \frac{d\overline{P}_t}{dt} \qquad (10)$$

From equation 5,

$$\frac{d\overline{P}_a}{dt} = \frac{Q_h - Q_r}{C_a} \qquad (11)$$

Hence $\overline{P}_a$ will rise when $Q_h > Q_r$, will fall when $Q_h < Q_r$, and will remain constant when $Q_h = Q_r$.

In this example, in which Q_h is suddenly increased to 10 L/min, $\overline{P}_a$ will continue to rise as long as Q_h exceeds Q_r. It is evident from equation 7 that Q_r will not attain a value of 10 L/min until $\overline{P}_a$ reaches a level of 200 mm Hg, as long as R remains constant at 20 mm Hg/L/min. Hence as $\overline{P}_a$ approaches 200, Q_r will almost equal Q_h, and $\overline{P}_a$ will rise very slowly. When Q_h is first raised, however, Q_h is greatly in excess of Q_r, and therefore $\overline{P}_a$ will rise sharply. The pressure-time tracing in Figure 6-10 indicates that, regardless of the value of C_a, the slope gradually diminishes as pressure rises, to approach a final value asymptotically.

Furthermore, the **height** to which $\overline{P}_a$ will rise is independent of the elastic characteristics of the arterial walls. $\overline{P}_a$ must rise to a level such that peripheral runoff will equal cardiac output;

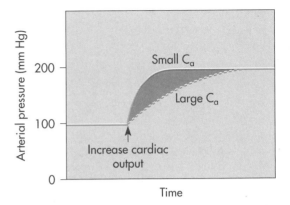

Figure 6-10 ■ When cardiac output is suddenly increased, the arterial compliance *(C$_a$)* determines the rate at which the mean arterial pressure will attain its new, elevated value but will not determine the magnitude of the new pressure.

that is, $Q_r = Q_h$. It is apparent from equation 6 that Q_r depends only on the pressure gradient and the resistance to flow. Hence C_a determines only the rate at which the new equilibrium value of $\overline{P}_a$ will be approached, as illustrated in Figure 6-10. When C_a is small (rigid vessels), a relatively slight increment in $\overline{V}_a$ (caused by a transient excess of Q_h over Q_r) increases $\overline{P}_a$ greatly. Hence $\overline{P}_a$ attains its new equilibrium level quickly. Conversely, when C_a is large, considerable volumes can be accommodated with relatively small pressure changes. Therefore the new equilibrium value of $\overline{P}_a$ is reached at a slower rate.

Peripheral Resistance

Similar reasoning may now be applied to explain the changes in $\overline{P}_a$ that accompany alterations in peripheral resistance. Let the control conditions be identical with those of the preceding example, that is, $Q_h = 5$, $\overline{P}_a = 100$, and R = 20 (Figure 6-9, *A*). Then, let R suddenly be increased to 40 (Figure 6-9, *D*). Instantaneously, $\overline{P}_a$ will be unchanged. With $\overline{P}_a = 100$ and R =

40, $Q_r = \overline{P}_a/R = 2.5$ L/min. Thus the peripheral runoff will momentarily be only 2.5 L/min, even though cardiac output equals 5 L/min. If Q_h remains constant at 5 L/min, $Q_h \geq Q_r$ and $\overline{V}_a$ will increase; hence $\overline{P}_a$ will rise. $\overline{P}_a$ will continue to rise until it reaches 200 mm Hg (Figure 6-9, *E*). At this level, $Q_r = 200/40 = 5$ L/min, which equals Q_h. $\overline{P}_a$ will then remain at this new elevated equilibrium level as long as Q_h and R do not change.

Therefore it is clear that *the level of the mean arterial pressure depends on cardiac output and peripheral resistance.* It is immaterial whether any change in cardiac output is accomplished by an alteration of heart rate, of stroke volume, or of both. Any change in heart rate that is balanced by a concomitant, oppositely directed change in stroke volume will not alter Q_h. Hence $\overline{P}_a$ will not be affected.

Pulse Pressure

If we assume (Figure 6-8) that the arterial pressure, P_a, at any moment depends on the two physical factors arterial blood volume, V_a, and arterial capacitance, C_a, it then follows that the arterial **pulse pressure** (difference between systolic and diastolic pressures) is principally a function of **stroke volume** and **arterial compliance.**

Stroke Volume

The effect of a change in stroke volume on pulse pressure may be analyzed under conditions in which C_a remains virtually constant over a substantial range of pressures. C_a is constant over any linear region of the pressure-volume curve (Figure 6-11). Volume is plotted along the vertical axis, and pressure is plotted along the horizontal axis; the slope, dV/dP, equals the compliance, C_a.

In an individual with such a linear $P_a:V_a$ curve, the arterial pressure would oscillate about some mean value ($\overline{P}_A$ in Figure 6-11) that

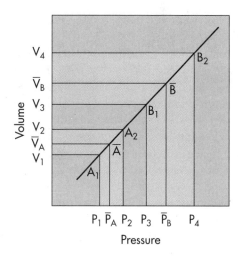

Figure 6-11 ■ **Effect of a change in stroke volume on pulse pressure in a system in which arterial compliance is constant over the range of pressures and volumes involved. A larger volume increment ($V_4 - V_3$ as compared with $V_2 - V_1$) results in a greater mean pressure ($\overline{P}_B$ as compared with $\overline{P}_A$) and a greater pulse pressure ($P_4 - P_3$ as compared with $P_2 - P_1$).**

depends entirely on cardiac output and peripheral resistance, as explained previously. This mean pressure corresponds to some mean arterial blood volume, $\overline{V}_A$. The coordinates $\overline{P}_A, \overline{V}_A$ define point $\overline{A}$ on the graph. During diastole, peripheral runoff from the arterial system occurs in the absence of ventricular ejection of blood, and P_a and V_a diminish to minimal values, P_1 and V_1, just before the next ventricular ejection. P_1 is then, by definition, the diastolic pressure.

During the rapid ejection phase of systole, the volume of blood introduced into the arterial system exceeds the volume that exits through the arterioles. Arterial pressure and volume therefore rise from point A_1 toward point A_2 in Figure 6-11. The maximal arterial volume, V_2, is reached at the end of the rapid ejection phase (see Figure 3-11), and this volume corresponds to a peak pressure, P_2, which is the **systolic pressure.**

The pulse pressure is the difference between systolic and diastolic pressures ($P_2 - P_1$ in Figure 6-11), and it corresponds to some arterial volume increment, $V_2 - V_1$. *This increment equals the volume of blood discharged by the left ventricle during the rapid ejection phase minus the volume that has run off to the periphery during this same phase of the cardiac cycle.* When a normal heart beats at a normal frequency, the volume increment during the rapid ejection phase is a large fraction of the stroke volume (about 80%). It is this increment that will raise arterial volume rapidly from V_1 to V_2 and hence will cause the arterial pressure to rise from the diastolic to the systolic level (P_1 to P_2 in Figure 6-11). During the remainder of the cardiac cycle, peripheral runoff will exceed cardiac ejection. During diastole, of course, cardiac ejection equals zero. The resulting arterial blood volume decrement will cause volumes and pressures to fall from point A_2 back to point A_1.

If stroke volume is now doubled, while heart rate and peripheral resistance remain constant, the mean arterial pressure will be doubled, to $\overline{B}$ in Figure 6-11. Thus the arterial pressure will now oscillate each heartbeat about this new value of the mean arterial pressure. A normal, vigorous heart will eject this greater stroke volume during a fraction of the cardiac cycle. This fraction is approximately equal to the fraction that prevailed at the lower stroke volume. Therefore the arterial volume increment, $V_4 - V_3$, will be a large fraction of the new stroke volume, and hence it will be approximately *twice as great* as the previous volume increment ($V_2 - V_1$). If the P_a:V_a curve is linear, the greater volume increment will be reflected by a pulse pressure ($P_4 - P_3$) approximately twice as great as the original pulse pressure ($P_2 - P_1$). Inspection of Figure 6-11 reveals that with a rise in both mean and pulse pressures, the rise in systolic pressure (from P_2 to P_4) exceeds the rise in diastolic pressure (from P_1 to P_3). Thus an increase in stroke volume raises systolic pressure more than it raises diastolic pressure.

Arterial Compliance

To assess how arterial compliance affects pulse pressure, the relative effects of a given volume increment ($V_2 - V_1$ in Figure 6-12) in a young person (curve A) and in an elderly person (curve B) will be compared. Let cardiac output and TPR be the same in both people; therefore $\overline{P}_a$ will be the same. It is apparent from Figure 6-12 that the same volume increment ($V_2 - V_1$) will cause a greater pulse pressure ($P_4 - P_1$) in the less distensible arteries of the elderly individual than in the more compliant arteries of the young person ($P_3 - P_2$). For the reasons enunciated on page 137, this will impose a greater workload on the left ventricle of the elderly person than on that of the young person, even if the stroke volumes, TPR, and mean arterial pressures are equivalent.

Figure 6-13 displays the effects of changes in arterial compliance and in peripheral resistance, R_p, on arterial pressure in an isolated cat heart preparation. As the compliance was reduced

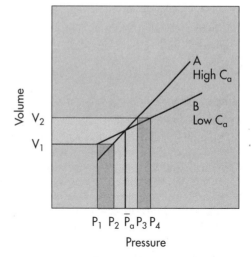

Figure 6-12 ■ **For a given volume increment (V$_2$ − V$_1$), a reduced arterial compliance (curve *B* as compared with curve *A*) results in an increased pulse pressure (P$_4$ − P$_1$ as compared with P$_3$ − P$_2$).**

from 43 to 14 to 3.6 units, the pulse pressure increased significantly. In this preparation, the stroke volume decreased as the arterial compliance was diminished. This accounts for the failure of the mean arterial pressure to remain constant at the different levels of arterial compliance. The effects of changes in peripheral resistance in this same preparation are described in the next section.

Total Peripheral Resistance and Arterial Diastolic Pressure

It is often asserted that increased TPR affects the diastolic more than the systolic arterial pressure. The validity of such an assertion deserves close scrutiny. First, let TPR be increased in an individual with a linear P$_a$:V$_a$ curve, as depicted in Figure 6-14, *A*. If the person's heart rate and stroke volume remain constant, an increase in TPR will increase $\overline{P}_a$ proportionately (from P$_2$ to P$_5$). If the volume increments (V$_2$ − V$_1$ and V$_4$ − V$_3$) are equal at both levels of TPR, the pulse pressures (P$_3$ − P$_1$ and P$_6$ − P$_4$) will also be equal. Hence systolic (P$_6$) and diastolic (P$_4$) pressures will have been elevated by exactly the same amounts from their respective control levels (P$_3$ and P$_1$).

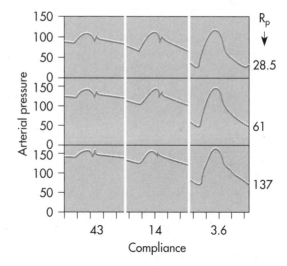

Figure 6-13 ■ **The changes in aortic pressure induced by changes in arterial compliance and peripheral resistance (R$_p$) in an isolated cat heart preparation.** (Modified from Elizinga G, Westerhof N: *Circ Res* 32:178, 1973.)

The combination of an increased resistance and diminished arterial compliance on arterial blood pressure would be represented in Figure 6-13 by a shift in direction from the top left panel to the bottom right panel; that is, both the mean pressure and the pulse pressure would be increased significantly. These results also coincide with the changes predicted by Figure 6-14, *B*.

BOX 6-3

Chronic **hypertension,** a condition characterized by a persistent elevation of TPR, occurs more commonly in older persons than in younger persons. The P_a:V_a curve for a hypertensive patient would therefore resemble that shown in Figure 6-14, *B*, which is like the curves in Figure 6-4 for older individuals. In Figure 6-14, *B*, the slope of the P_a:V_a curve diminishes as pressure and volume are increased. Hence C_a is less at higher than at lower pressures. As before, if cardiac output remains constant, an increase in TPR would increase $\overline{P}_a$ proportionately (from P_2 to P_5). For equivalent increases in TPR, the elevation of pressure from P_2 to P_5 will be the same in panel *A* as in panel *B*, for reasons discussed in relation to Figure 6-10. If the volume increment ($V_4 - V_3$ in Figure 6-14, *B*) at elevated TPR were equal to the control increment ($V_2 - V_1$), the pulse pressure ($P_6 - P_4$) in the hypertensive range would greatly exceed that ($P_3 - P_1$) at normal pressure levels. In other words, a given volume increment produces a greater pressure increment (i.e., pulse pressure) when the arteries are more rigid than when they are more compliant. Hence the rise in systolic pressure ($P_6 - P_3$) will exceed the increase in diastolic pressure ($P_4 - P_1$).

These hypothetical changes in arterial pressure closely resemble those actually seen in patients with **hypertension.** Diastolic pressure is indeed elevated in such individuals, but ordinarily not more than 10 to 40 mm Hg above the average normal level of 80 mm Hg. Conversely, it is not uncommon for systolic pressures to be elevated by 50 to 150 mm Hg above the average normal level of 120 mm Hg. *Thus an increase in peripheral resistance will usually raise systolic pressure more than it will raise diastolic pressure.*

■ THE PRESSURE CURVES CHANGE IN ARTERIES AT DIFFERENT DISTANCES FROM THE HEART

The radial stretch of the ascending aorta brought about by left ventricular ejection initiates a pressure wave that is propagated down the aorta and its branches. *The pressure wave travels much faster than does the blood itself.* It is this pressure wave that one perceives by palpating a peripheral artery.

The velocity of the pressure wave varies inversely with the vascular compliance. Accurate measurement of the transmission velocity has provided valuable information about the elastic characteristics of the arterial tree. In general, transmission velocity increases with age. This finding confirms the observation that the arteries become less compliant with advancing age (Figures 6-4 and 6-6). Also, pulse wave velocity increases progressively as the pulse wave travels from the ascending aorta toward the periphery. This indicates that vascular compliance is less in the more distal than in the more proximal portions of the arterial system.

The arterial pressure contour becomes distorted as the wave is transmitted down the arterial system; the changes in configuration of the pulse with distance are shown in Figure 6-15. Aside from the increasing delay in the onset of the initial pressure rise, three major changes occur in the arterial pulse contour as the pressure wave travels distally. First, the high-frequency components of the pulse, such as the **incisura** (the notch that appears at the end of ventricular ejection), are damped out and soon disappear. Second, the systolic portions of the pressure wave become narrowed and elevated. In the curves shown in Figure 6-15, the systolic pressure at the level of the knee was 39 mm Hg greater than that recorded in the aortic arch. Third, a hump may appear on the diastolic portion of the pressure wave. These changes in contour are pronounced in young individuals but diminish with age. In elderly patients the pulse

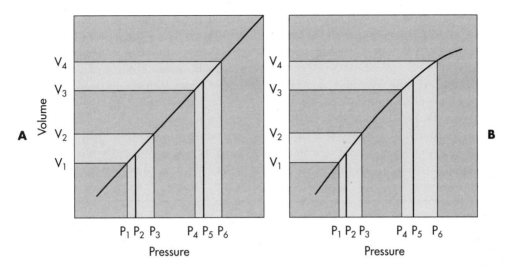

Figure 6-14 ■ **Effect of a change in total peripheral resistance (volume increment remaining constant) on pulse pressure when the pressure-volume curve for the arterial system is rectilinear (A) or curvilinear** (B).

wave may be transmitted virtually unchanged from the ascending aorta to the periphery.

The damping of the high-frequency components of the arterial pulse is caused largely by the viscoelastic properties of the arterial walls. The precise mechanism for the peaking of the pressure wave is controversial. Probably several factors contribute, including reflection, tapering of the arteries, resonance, and changes in transmission velocity with pressure level.

■ BLOOD PRESSURE IS MEASURED BY A SPHYGMOMANOMETER IN HUMAN PATIENTS

In hospital intensive care units, arterial blood pressure can be measured **directly** by introducing a needle or catheter into a peripheral artery. Ordinarily, however, the blood pressure is estimated **indirectly** by means of a **sphygmomanometer.** This instrument consists of an inextensible cuff containing an inflatable bag. The cuff is wrapped around the extremity (usually the arm, occasionally the thigh) so that the in-

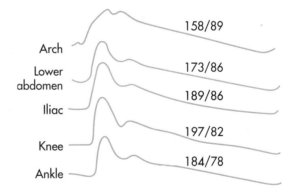

Figure 6-15 ■ **Arterial pressure curves recorded from various sites in an anesthetized dog.** (From Remington JW, O'Brien LJ: *Am J Physiol* 218:437, 1970.)

flatable bag lies between the cuff and the skin, directly over the artery to be compressed. The artery is occluded by inflating the bag, by means of a rubber squeeze bulb, to a pressure in excess of arterial systolic pressure. The pressure in the bag is measured by means of a mercury or an aneroid manometer. Pressure is released from the bag at a rate of 2 or 3 mm Hg per heartbeat by means of a needle valve in the inflating bulb (Figure 6-16).

When blood pressure readings are taken from the arm, the systolic pressure may be estimated by palpating the radial artery at the wrist **(palpatory method).** When pressure in the bag exceeds the systolic level, no pulse will be perceived. As the pressure falls just below the

systolic level (Figure 6-16, *A*), a spurt of blood will pass through the brachial artery under the cuff during the peak of systole, and a slight pulse will be felt at the wrist.

The **auscultatory method** is a more sensitive and therefore a more precise method for measuring systolic pressure, and it also permits estimation of diastolic pressure. The practitioner listens with a stethoscope applied to the skin of the antecubital space over the brachial

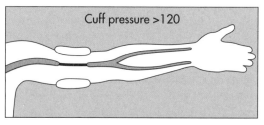

B, When the cuff pressure exceeds the systolic arterial pressure (120 mm Hg), no blood progresses through the arterial segment under the cuff, and no sounds can be detected by a stethoscope bell placed on the arm distal to the cuff.

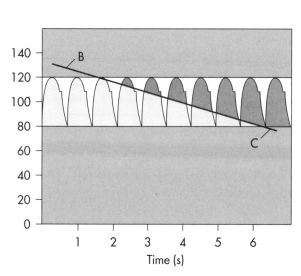

A, Consider that the arterial blood pressure is being measured in a patient whose blood pressure is 120/80 mm Hg. The pressure (represented by the *oblique line*) in a cuff around the patient's arm is allowed to fall from greater than 120 mm Hg (point *B*) to below 80 mm Hg (point *C*) in about 6 seconds.

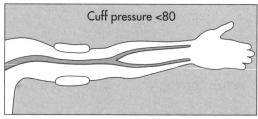

C, When the cuff pressure falls below the diastolic arterial pressure, arterial flow past the region of the cuff is continuous, and no sounds are audible. When the cuff pressure is between 120 and 80 mm Hg, spurts of blood traverse the artery segment under the cuff with each heartbeat, and the Korotkoff sounds are heard through the stethoscope.

Figure 6-16 ■ **Measurement of arterial blood pressure with a sphygmomanometer.**

artery. While the pressure in the bag exceeds the systolic pressure, the brachial artery is occluded and no sounds are heard (Figure 6-16, *B*). When the inflation pressure falls just below the systolic level (120 mm Hg in Figure 6-16, *A*), small spurts of blood escape through the cuff and slight tapping sounds (called **Korotkoff sounds**) are heard with each heartbeat. The pressure at which the first sound is detected represents the **systolic pressure.** It usually corresponds closely with the directly measured systolic pressure.

As inflation pressure continues to fall, more blood escapes under the cuff per beat and the sounds become louder thuds. As the inflation pressure approaches the diastolic level, the Korotkoff sounds become muffled. As they fall just below the diastolic level (80 mm Hg in Figure 6-16, *A*), the sounds disappear; this indicates the **diastolic pressure.** The origin of the Korotkoff sounds is related to the spurt of blood passing under the cuff and meeting a static column of blood; the impact and turbulence generate audible vibrations. Once the inflation pressure is less than the diastolic pressure, flow is continuous in the brachial artery and sounds are no longer heard (Figure 6-16, *C*).

SUMMARY

- The arteries serve not only to conduct blood from the heart to the capillaries, but they also store some of the ejected blood during each cardiac systole. Therefore blood can continue to flow through the capillaries during cardiac diastole.
- The aging process diminishes the compliance of the arteries.
- The less compliant the arteries, the more work the heart must do to pump a given cardiac output.
- The mean arterial pressure varies directly with the cardiac output and total peripheral resistance.
- The arterial pulse pressure varies directly with the stroke volume, but inversely with the arterial compliance.
- The contour of the systemic arterial pressure wave is distorted as it travels from the ascending aorta to the periphery. The high-frequency components of the wave are damped, the systolic components are narrowed and elevated, and a hump may appear in the diastolic component of the wave.
- When blood pressure is measured by a sphygmomanometer in humans, systolic pressure is manifested by the occurrence of a tapping sound that originates in the artery distal to the cuff as the cuff pressure falls below peak arterial pressure. The diminished cuff pressure permits spurts of blood to pass through the compressed artery. Diastolic pressure is manifested by the disappearance of the sound as the cuff pressure falls below the minimal arterial pressure, which permits flow through the artery to become continuous.

■ BIBLIOGRAPHY

1. Armentano RL, Barra JG, Levenson J, et al: Arterial wall mechanics in conscious dogs: assessment of viscous, inertial, and elastic moduli to characterize aortic wall behavior. *Circ Res* 76:468, 1995.

2. Burattini R, Campbell KB: Effective distributed compliance of the canine descending aorta estimated by modified T-tube model. *Am J Physiol* 264:H1977, 1993.

3. Cernadas MR, Sanchez de Miguel L, Garcia-Duran M, et al: Expression of constitutive and inducible nitric oxide synthases in the vascular wall of young and aging rats. *Circ Res* 83:279, 1998.

4. Folkow B, Svanborg A: Physiology of cardiovascular aging. *Physiol Rev* 73:725, 1993.

5. Kelly RP, Ting C-T, Yang T-M, et al: Effective arterial elastance as index of arterial vascular load in humans. *Circulation* 86:513, 1992.

6. Kelly RP, Tunin R, Kass DA: Effects of reduced aortic compliance on cardiac efficiency and contractile function of in situ canine left ventricle. *Circ Res* 71:490, 1992.

7. Kingwell BA, Cameron JD, Gillies KJ, et al: Arterial compliance may influence baroreflex function in athletes and hypertensives. *Am J Physiol* 268:H411, 1995.

8. Lee RT, Kamm RD: Vascular mechanics for the cardiologist. *J Am Coll Cardiol* 23:1289, 1994.

9. Mulvany MJ, Aalkjaer C: Structure and function of small arteries. *Physiol Rev* 70:921, 1990.

10. O'Rourke M: Mechanical principles in arterial disease. *Hypertension* 26:2, 1995.

11. O'Rourke M, Kelly R, Avolio A: *Arterial pulse,* Baltimore, 1992, Williams & Wilkins.

12. Perloff D, Grim C, Flack J, et al: Human blood pressure determination by sphygmomanometry. *Circulation* 88:2460, 1993.

13. Piene H: Pulmonary arterial impedance and right ventricular function. *Physiol Rev* 66:606, 1986.

14. Rabbany SY, Drzewiecke GM, Noordergraaf A: Peripheral vascular effects on auscultatory blood pressure measurement. *J Clin Monit* 9:9, 1993.

15. Stergiopulos N, Meister JJ, Westerhof N: Evaluation of methods for estimation of total arterial compliance. *Am J Physiol* 268:H1540, 1995.

16. Westerhof N, Gross DR: *Vascular dynamics,* New York, 1989, Plenum Press.

■ CASE 6

HISTORY

A 33-year-old man complained about chest pain on exertion. He was referred to a cardiologist, who carried out a number of studies, including right- and left-sided cardiac catheterization (for hemodynamic information) and coronary angiography (to image the status of the coronary arteries). Among the data that were obtained during these studies were the findings that the patient's pulmonary artery and aortic pressures, in mm Hg, were as follows:

	Pulmonary artery	Aorta
Systolic	30	120
Diastolic	15	80
Pulse	15	40
Mean	20	93

The hemodynamic and angiographic studies disclosed no serious abnormalities. The patient's physicians recommended certain changes in lifestyle and diet, and the patient continued to do well for about 20 years. At this time, the physician found that the patient's systemic arterial blood pressure was 190/100 mm Hg, and his mean arterial pressure was estimated to be 130 mm Hg. These and other findings led his physicians to the diagnosis of essential hypertension.

QUESTIONS

1. At the time of the initial examination, the patient's mean aortic pressure (93 mm Hg) was so much higher than his mean pulmonary arterial pressure (20 mm Hg) because

   a. His systemic vascular resistance was much greater than his pulmonary vascular resistance.

   b. His aortic compliance was much greater than his pulmonary arterial compliance.

   c. His left ventricular stroke volume was much greater than his right ventricular stroke volume.

   d. The total cross-sectional area of his pulmonary capillary bed was much greater than the total cross-sectional area of his systemic capillary bed.

   e. The duration of the rapid ejection phase of the left ventricle exceeded the duration of the rapid ejection phase of the right ventricle.

2. When the patient became hypertensive, his arterial pulse pressure (90 mm Hg) became

much greater than his prehypertension pulse pressure (40 mm Hg) because

a. His systemic vascular resistance is much less than it was before he became hypertensive.
b. The duration of the reduced ejection phase of the left ventricle decreases as the arterial blood pressure rises.
c. His arterial compliance was diminished in part by virtue of the hypertension per se, and in part because of the effects of aging.
d. The total cross-sectional area of the systemic capillary bed increases substantially in hypertensive subjects.
e. His aortic compliance becomes greater than his pulmonary arterial compliance.

CHAPTER 7

The Microcirculation and Lymphatics

Objectives

1. Describe the regulation of regional blood flow by the arterioles.

2. Enumerate the physical and chemical factors that affect the microvessels.

3. Explain the roles of diffusion, filtration, and pinocytosis in transcapillary exchange.

4. Describe the balance between hydrostatic and osmotic forces under normal and abnormal conditions.

5. Describe the lymphatic circulation.

THE ENTIRE CIRCULATORY SYSTEM IS geared to supply the body tissues with blood in amounts commensurate with their requirements for oxygen and nutrients and to remove carbon dioxide and other waste products for excretion by the lungs and kidneys. The exchange of gases, water, and solutes between the vascular and interstitial fluid compartments occurs mainly across the capillaries, which consist of a single layer of endothelial cells. The arterioles, capillaries, and venules constitute the microcirculation, and blood flow through the microcirculation is regulated by the arterioles, also known as the **resistance vessels** (see Chapter 8). The large arteries serve solely as blood conduits whereas the veins serve as storage or **capacitance vessels** as well as blood conduits.

■ FUNCTIONAL ANATOMY

Arterioles Are the Stopcocks of the Circulation

The arterioles, which range in diameter from about 5 to 100 μm, have a thick smooth muscle layer, a thin adventitial layer, and an endothelial lining (see Figure 1-1). The arterioles give rise directly to the capillaries (5 to 10 μm in diameter) or in some tissues to metarterioles (10 to 20 μm in diameter), which then give rise to capillaries (Figure 7-1). The **metarterioles** can serve either as thoroughfare channels to the venules, bypassing the capillary bed, or as conduits to supply the capillary bed. There are often cross connections between arterioles and between venules, as well as in the capillary network. Arterioles that give rise directly to capillaries regulate flow through

155

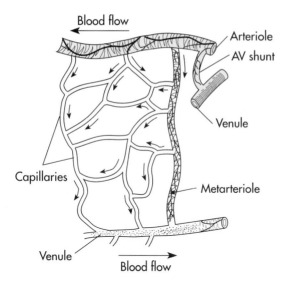

Figure 7-1 ▪ Composite schematic drawing of the microcirculation. The circular structures on the arteriole and venule represent smooth muscle fibers, and the branching solid lines represent sympathetic nerve fibers. The arrows indicate the direction of blood flow.

their cognate capillaries by constriction or dilation. The capillaries form an interconnecting network of tubes of different lengths with an average length of 0.5 to 1 mm.

Capillaries Permit the Exchange of Water, Solutes, and Gases

Capillary distribution varies from tissue to tissue. In metabolically active tissues, such as cardiac and skeletal muscle and glandular structures, capillaries are numerous, whereas in less active tissues, such as subcutaneous tissue or cartilage, **capillary density** is low. Also, all capillaries are not of the same diameter, and because some capillaries have diameters less than that of the erythrocytes, it is necessary for the cells to become temporarily deformed in their passage through these capillaries. Fortunately, the normal red cells are quite flexible

and readily change their shape to conform with that of the small capillaries.

Blood flow in the capillaries is not uniform and depends chiefly on the contractile state of the arterioles. The average velocity of blood flow in the capillaries is approximately 1 mm/s; however, it can vary from zero to several millimeters per second in the same vessel within a brief period. These changes in capillary blood flow may be of random type or may show rhythmical oscillatory behavior of different frequencies that are caused by contraction and relaxation (**vasomotion**) of the precapillary vessels. This vasomotion is to some extent an intrinsic contractile behavior of the vascular smooth muscle and is independent of external input. Furthermore, changes in **transmural pressure** (intravascular minus extravascular pressure) influence the contractile state of the precapillary vessels. An increase in transmural pressure, whether produced by an increase in venous pressure or by dilation of arterioles, results in contraction of the terminal arterioles at the points of origin of the capillaries, whereas a decrease in transmural pressure elicits precapillary vessel relaxation (see myogenic response, Chapter 8).

Although reduction of transmural pressure induces relaxation of the terminal arterioles, blood flow through the capillaries obviously cannot increase if the reduction in intravascular pressure is caused by severe constriction of the parent arterioles, metarterioles, or small arteries. Large arterioles and metarterioles also exhibit vasomotion, but in the contraction phase they usually do not completely occlude the lumen of the vessel and arrest blood flow, as may occur with contraction of the terminal arterioles (Figure 7-2). Thus *flow rate may be altered by contraction and relaxation of small arteries, arterioles, and metarterioles.*

Because blood flow through the capillaries provides for exchange of gases and solutes between blood and tissue, it has been termed **nu-**

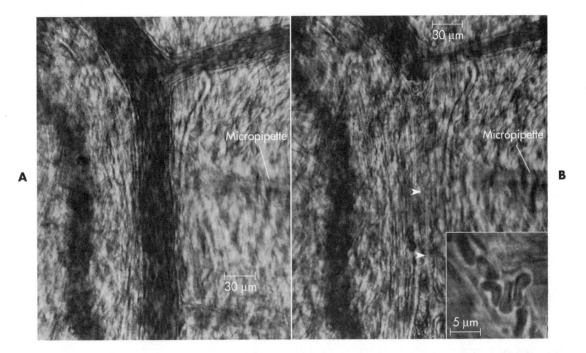

Figure 7-2 ■ A, **Arterioles of a hamster cheek pouch before microinjection of norepinephrine. B, After injection of norepinephrine. Note the complete closure of the arteriole between the arrows, and the narrowing of a branch arteriole at the upper right.** *Inset:* **Capillary with red cells during a period of complete closure of the feeding arteriole. Scale in A and B, 30 μm; in inset, 5 μm.** (Courtesy David N. Damon.)

tritional flow, whereas blood flow that bypasses the capillaries in traveling from the arterial to the venous side of the circulation has been termed **nonnutritional,** or **shunt, flow** (Figure 7-1). In some areas of the body (e.g., fingertips, ears), true **arteriovenous shunts** exist (see Figure 11-1). However, in many tissues, such as muscle, evidence of anatomical shunts is lacking. Nevertheless, nonnutritional flow can occur and has been termed **physiological shunting of blood flow.** It is the result of a greater flow of blood through previously open capillaries with either no change or an increase in the number of closed capillaries. In tissues that have metarterioles, shunt flow may be con-

tinuous from arteriole to venule during low metabolic activity when many precapillary vessels are closed. When metabolic activity increases in such tissues and more precapillary vessels open, blood passing through the metarterioles is readily available for capillary perfusion.

The true capillaries are devoid of smooth muscle and are therefore incapable of active constriction. Nevertheless, the endothelial cells that form the capillary wall contain actin and myosin and can alter their shape in response to certain chemical stimuli. There is no evidence, however, that changes in endothelial cell shape regulate blood flow through the capillaries. Hence *changes in capillary diameter are pas-*

TABLE 7-1		
Vessel wall tension in the aorta and a capillary		
	Aorta	Capillary
Radius (r)	1.5 cm	5×10^{-4} cm
Height of Hg column (h)	10 cm Hg	2.5 cm Hg
ρ	13.6 g/cm^3	13.6 g/cm^3
g	980 cm/s^2	980 cm/s^2
P	$10 \times 13.6 \times 980 = 1.33 \times 10^5$ dyne/cm^2	$2.5 \times 13.6 \times 980 = 3.33 \times 10^4$ dyne/cm^2
w	0.2 cm	1×10^{-4} cm
T = Pr	$(1.33 \times 10^5)(1.5) = 2 \times 10^5$ dyne/cm	$(3.33 \times 10^4)(5 \times 10^{-4}) = 16.7$ dyne/cm
$\sigma = \dfrac{Pr}{w}$	$\dfrac{2 \times 10^5}{0.2} = 1 \times 10^6$ dyne/cm^2	$\dfrac{16.7}{1 \times 10^{-4}} = 1.67 \times 10^5$ dyne/cm^2

sive and are caused by alterations in precapillary and postcapillary resistance.

The Law of Laplace Explains Why Capillaries Can Withstand High Intravascular Pressures

The law of Laplace is illustrated in the following comparison of wall tension of a capillary with that of the aorta (Table 7-1). The Laplace equation is

$$T = Pr$$

where T = Tension in the vessel wall
      P = Transmural pressure
      r = Radius of the vessel

Wall tension is the force per unit length tangential to the vessel wall that opposes the distending force (Pr) that tends to pull apart a theoretical longitudinal slit in the vessel (Figure 7-3). Transmural pressure is essentially equal to intraluminal pressure, because extravascular pressure is usually negligible. The Laplace equation applies to very thin-walled vessels, such as capillaries. Wall thickness must be taken into consideration when the equation is applied to thick-

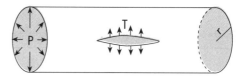

Figure 7-3 ■ Diagram of a small blood vessel to illustrate the law of Laplace—*T = Pr*, where *P* = intraluminal pressure, *r* = radius of the vessel, and *T* = wall tension as the force per unit length tangential to the vessel wall, tending to pull apart a theoretical longitudinal slit in the vessel.

walled vessels, such as the aorta. This is done by dividing Pr (pressure × radius) by wall thickness (w). The equation now becomes

$$\sigma \text{ (wall stress)} = Pr/w$$

Pressure in mm Hg (height of Hg column) is converted to dynes per square centimeter according to the equation P = hρg, where h = the height of a Hg column in centimeters, ρ = the density of Hg in g/cm^3, g = gravitational acceleration in cm/s^2, and wall stress (σ) = force per unit area.

Thus at normal aortic and capillary pressures the wall tension of the aorta is about 12,000 times greater than that of the capillary (Table 7-1). In a person standing quietly, capillary pressure in the feet may reach 100 mm Hg. Under such conditions, capillary wall tension increases to 66.5 dynes/cm, a value that is still only one three-thousandth that of the wall tension in the aorta at the same internal pressure. However, σ (wall stress), which takes wall thickness into consideration, is only about tenfold greater in the aorta than in the capillary.

In addition to providing an explanation for the ability of capillaries to withstand large internal pressures, the above calculations also point out that in dilated vessels, wall stress increases even when internal pressure remains constant.

The diameter of the resistance vessels is determined by the balance between the contractile force of the vascular smooth muscle and the distending force produced by the intraluminal pressure. The greater the contractile activity of the vascular smooth muscle of an arteriole, the smaller is its diameter, until a point is reached, in the case of small arterioles, when complete occlusion of the vessel occurs. This is caused by infolding of the endothelium and by trapping of the cells in the vessel. With progressive reduction in the intravascular pressure, vessel diameter decreases (as does tension in the vessel wall—law of Laplace).

THE ENDOTHELIUM PLAYS AN ACTIVE ROLE IN REGULATING THE MICROCIRCULATION

For many years, it was thought that the endothelium was an inert single layer of cells that served solely as a passive filter to permit passage of water and small molecules across the blood vessel wall and to retain blood cells and large molecules (proteins) within the vascular compartment. However, it is now recognized that the

BOX 7-1

Syphilitic aortic aneurysm (rare because syphilis is now less common) and abdominal aneurysm (caused by atherosclerotic degeneration of the aortic wall) are associated with murmurs caused by the turbulence in the dilated segment of the aorta. The diseased part of the aorta is also under severe stress, because of its increased radius and thinner wall. Unless treated, the aneurysm can rupture and cause immediate death. Treatment consists of resection of the aneurysm and replacement with a Dacron graft.

endothelium is a source of substances that elicit contraction or relaxation of the vascular smooth muscle.

As shown in Figure 7-4, prostacyclin can relax vascular smooth muscle via an increase in the cyclic adenosine monophosphate (cAMP) concentration. **Prostacyclin** is formed in the endothelium from arachidonic acid and may be released by shear stress caused by the pulsatile blood flow. The formation of prostacyclin is catalyzed by the enzyme prostacyclin synthase. The primary function of prostacyclin is to inhibit platelet adherence to the endothelium and platelet aggregation, thus preventing intravascular clot formation.

Of far greater importance in endothelial-mediated vascular dilation is the formation and release of the **endothelium-derived relaxing factor (EDRF)** (Figure 7-4), which has been identified as **nitric oxide (NO).** The discoverers of the role of NO were awarded the Nobel Prize for Medicine and Physiology in 1998. Stimulation of the endothelial cells in vivo, in isolated arteries, or in culture by acetylcholine or several other agents (adenosine triphosphate [ATP], bradykinin, serotonin, substance P, histamine) causes the production and release of NO.

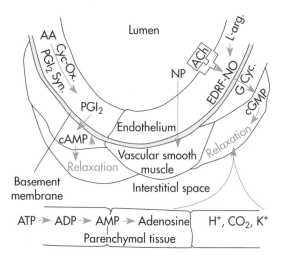

Figure 7-4 ■ **Endothelial- and nonendothelial-mediated vasodilation. Prostacyclin** *(PGI₂)* **is formed from arachidonic acid** *(AA)* **by the action of cyclooxygenase** *(Cyc-Ox)* **and prostacyclin synthase** *(PGI₂ Syn)* **in the endothelium, and elicits relaxation of the adjacent vascular smooth muscle via increases in cyclic adenosine monophosphate** *(cAMP)*. **Stimulation of the endothelial cells with acetylcholine** *(ACh)* **or other agents (see text) results in the formation and release of an endothelium-derived relaxing factor** *(EDRF)*, **identified as nitric oxide** *(NO)*. **The NO stimulates guanylyl cyclase** *(G Cyc)* **to increase cyclic guanosine monophosphate** *(cGMP)* **in the vascular smooth muscle to produce relaxation. The vasodilator agent nitroprusside** *(NP)* **acts directly on the vascular smooth muscle. Substances such as adenosine, hydrogen ions** *(H⁺)*, CO_2, **and potassium ions** *(K⁺)* **can arise in the parenchymal tissue and elicit vasodilation by direct action on the vascular smooth muscle (see p 184).**

In blood vessels from which the endothelium has been mechanically removed, these agents do not elicit vasodilation. The NO (synthesized from L-arginine) activates guanylyl cyclase in the vascular smooth muscle to increase the cyclic

guanosine monophosphate (cGMP) concentration, which produces relaxation by decreasing cytosolic free Ca^{++}. NO release can be stimulated by the shear stress of blood flow on the endothelium, but the physiologic role of NO in the local regulation of blood flow remains to be elucidated. The drug nitroprusside also increases cGMP, which produces vasodilation, but it acts directly on the vascular smooth muscle and is not endothelial-mediated (Figure 7-4). Vasodilator agents such as adenosine, hydrogen ions, CO_2, and potassium may be released from parenchymal tissue and act locally on the resistance vessels (Figure 7-4).

The endothelium can also synthesize **endothelin,** a very potent vasoconstrictor peptide. Endothelin can affect vascular tone and blood pressure in humans and may be involved in pathological states such as atherosclerosis, pulmonary hypertension, congestive heart failure, and renal failure.

■ THE ENDOTHELIUM PLAYS A PASSIVE ROLE IN TRANSCAPILLARY EXCHANGE

Solvent and solute move across the capillary endothelial wall by three processes: diffusion, filtration, and endothelial vesicles (pinocytosis).

The permeability of the capillary endothelial membrane is not the same in all body tissues. For example, the liver capillaries are quite permeable, and albumin escapes at a rate several times greater than that from the less permeable muscle capillaries. Also, there is not uniform permeability along the whole capillary; the venous ends are more permeable than the arterial ends, and permeability is greatest in the venules. The greater permeability at the venous end of the capillaries and in the venules is attributed to the greater number of pores in these regions of the microvessels.

The sites where filtration occurs have been a controversial subject for a number of years. Wa-

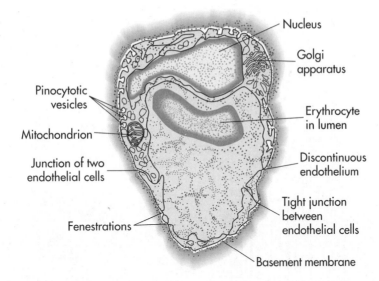

Figure 7-5 ■ Diagrammatic sketch of an electron micrograph of a composite capillary in cross section.

ter flows through the capillary endothelial cell membranes through water-selective channels, called **aquaporins,** a family of proteins that function as water channels. Water also flows through apertures (pores) in the endothelial wall of the capillaries (Figures 7-5 and 7-6). Calculations based on the transcapillary movement of solutes of small molecular size led to the prediction of capillary pores with diameters of about 4 nm in skeletal and cardiac muscle. In agreement with this prediction, electron microscopy revealed clefts between adjacent endothelial cells with a gap at the narrowest point of about 4 nm (Figures 7-5 and 7-6). The clefts (pores) are sparse and represent only about 0.02% of the capillary surface area. In cerebral capillaries, where a blood-brain barrier to many small molecules exists, pores are absent.

In addition to clefts, some of the more po-

rous capillaries (e.g., in kidney, intestine) contain **fenestrations** (Figure 7-5) 20 to 100 nm wide, whereas others (e.g., in the liver) have a **discontinuous endothelium** (Figure 7-5). Fenestrations and discontinuous endothelium permit passage of molecules that are too large to pass through the intercellular clefts of the endothelium.

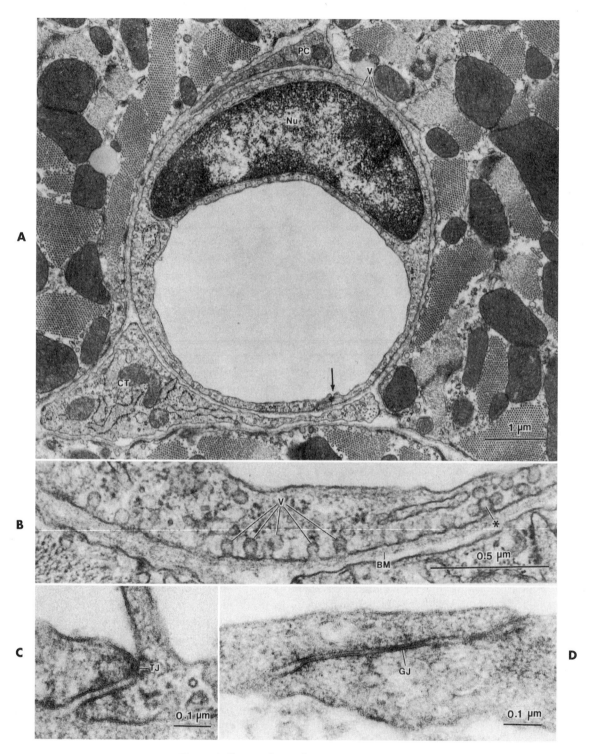

Figure 7-6 ■ For legend see opposite page.

Figure 7-6 ■ A, **Cross-sectioned capillary in a mouse ventricular wall. The luminal diameter is approximately 4 mm. In this thin section, the capillary wall is formed by a single endothelial cell (*Nu,* endothelial nucleus), which forms a functional complex *(arrow)* with itself. The thin pericapillary space is occupied by a pericyte *(PC)* and a connective tissue *(CT)* cell ("fibroblast"). Note the numerous endothelial vesicles *(V).* B, Detail of the endothelial cell in panel A, showing plasmalemmal vesicles *(V)* attached to the endothelial cell surface. These vesicles are especially prominent in vascular endothelium and are involved in transport of substances across the blood vessel wall. Note the complex alveolar vesicle (*). *BM,* Basement membrane. C, Junctional complex in a capillary of mouse heart. "Tight" junctions *(TJ)* typically form in these small blood vessels and appear to consist of fusions between apposed endothelial cell surface membranes. D, Interendothelial junction in a muscular artery of monkey papillary muscle. Although tight junctions similar to those of capillaries are found in these large blood vessels, extensive junctions that resemble gap junctions in the intercalated disks between myocardial cells often appear in arterial endothelium (example shown at *GJ).***

Diffusion Is the Most Important Means for Water and Solute Transfer Across the Endothelium

Under normal conditions, only about 0.06 ml of water per minute moves back and forth across the capillary wall per 100 g of tissue as a result of filtration and absorption, whereas 300 ml of water per minute per 100 g of tissue does so by diffusion, a 5000-fold difference.

When filtration and diffusion are related to blood flow, about 2% of the plasma passing through the capillaries is filtered. In contrast, the diffusion of water is 40 times greater than the rate by which it is brought to the capillaries by blood flow. The transcapillary exchange of solutes is also primarily governed by diffusion. Thus *diffusion is the key factor in providing exchange of gases, substrates, and waste products between the capillaries and the tissue cells.* However, *net* transfer of fluid across the capillary and venule endothelium is mainly attributable to filtration and absorption.

The process of diffusion is described by Fick's law:

$$J = -DA\frac{dc}{dx} \tag{1}$$

where J = Quantity of a substance moved per unit time (t)

D = Free diffusion coefficient for a particular molecule (the value is inversely related to the square root of the molecular weight)

A = Cross-sectional area of the diffusion pathway

$\dfrac{dc}{dx}$ = Concentration gradient of the solute

Fick's law is also expressed as

$$J = -PS(C_o - C_i) \tag{2}$$

where P = Capillary permeability of the substance

S = Capillary surface area

C_i = Concentration of the substance inside the capillary

C_o = Concentration of the substance outside the capillary

Hence the PS product provides a convenient expression of available capillary surface, because permeability is rarely altered under physiological conditions.

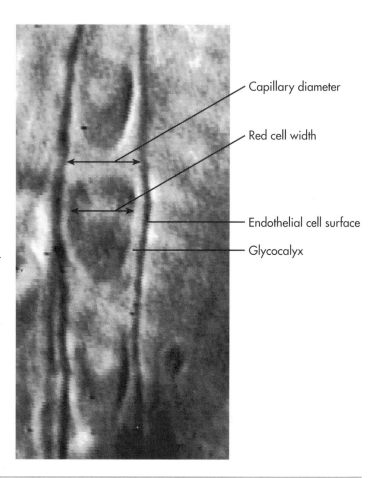

Capillary diameter

Red cell width

Endothelial cell surface

Glycocalyx

Figure 7-7 ■ A single capillary in a hamster cheek pouch showing the glycocalyx. Photo was taken during normal blood flow. (Courtesy of Charmaine Henry.)

Diffusion of Lipid-insoluble Molecules Is Restricted to the Pores

The mean size of the pores can be calculated by measurement of the diffusion rate of an uncharged molecule whose free diffusion coefficient is known. Movement of solutes across the endothelium is complex and involves corrections for attractions between solute and solvent molecules, interactions between solute molecules, pore configuration, and the charge on the molecules relative to the charge on the endothelial cells. It is not simply a question of random thermal movements of molecules down a concentration gradient.

When compared to the movement of water across the intact endothelium, solutes exhibit some degree of restriction based on molecular size. Molecules larger than about 60,000 MW do not penetrate the endothelium, whereas those smaller than 60,000 MW penetrate at a rate that is inversely proportional to their size. This filtering effect is thought to be due to the restrictive size of the pore and to a fiber matrix within it. However, the glycocalyx, a 0.5-μm layer lining the luminal side of the endothelium, may also serve as a molecular filter. The glycocalyx is shown in Figure 7-7 where it appears as a clear area between the luminal endothelial mem-

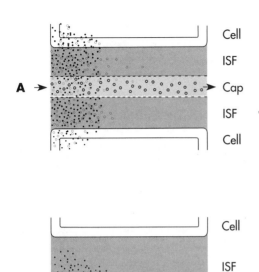

Cell

ISF

A → Cap

ISF

Cell

Cell

ISF

B → Cap

ISF

Cell

Figure 7-8 ■ **Flow- and diffusion-limited transport from capillaries *(Cap)* to tissue. A, Flow-limited transport. The smallest water-soluble inert tracer particles *(black dots)* reach negligible concentrations after passing only a short distance down the capillary. Larger particles *(blue circles)* with similar properties travel farther along the capillary before reaching insignificant intracapillary concentrations. Both substances cross the interstitial fluid *(ISF)* and reach the parenchymal tissue *(cell)*. Because of their size, more of the smaller particles are taken up by the tissue cells. The largest particles *(black circles)* cannot penetrate the capillary pores and hence do not escape from the capillary lumen except by pinocytotic vesicle transport. An increase in the volume of blood flow or an increase in capillary density increases tissue supply for the diffusible solutes. Note that capillary permeability is greater at the venous end of the capillary (and especially in the venule, not shown) because of the larger number of pores in this region. B, Diffusion-limited transport. When the distance between the capillaries and the parenchymal tissue is large as a result of edema or low capillary density, diffusion becomes a limiting factor in the transport of solutes from capillary to tissue even at high rates of capillary blood flow.**

brane and the red cell that was moving through the capillary.

For small molecules, such as water, NaCl, urea, and glucose, the capillary pores offer little restriction to diffusion (low **reflection coefficient,** see p 166) and diffusion is so rapid that the mean concentration gradient across the capillary endothelium is extremely small. With small molecules, the only limitation to net movement across the capillary wall is the rate at which blood flow transports the molecules to the capillary **(flow limited).**

When transport across the capillary is flow limited, the concentration of a small molecule solute in the blood reaches equilibrium with its concentration in the interstitial fluid near the origin of the capillary from the cognate

arteriole. If an inert small molecule tracer is infused intraarterially, its concentration falls to negligible levels near the arterial end of the capillary (Figure 7-8, *A*). If the flow is large, the small molecule tracer will be detectable farther downstream in the capillary. A somewhat larger molecule moves farther along the capillary before reaching an insignificant concentration in the blood, and the number of still larger molecules that enter the arterial end of the capillary and cannot pass through the capillary pores is the same as the number leaving the venous end of the capillary (Figure 7-8, *A*).

With large molecules, diffusion across the capillaries becomes the limiting factor **(diffusion limited).** In other words, capillary permeability to a large molecule solute limits its transport across the capillary wall (Figure 7-8, *A*). The diffusion of small lipid-insoluble molecules is so rapid that diffusion becomes limiting in blood-tissue exchange only when the distances-between capillaries and parenchymal cells are large (e.g., tissue edema or very low capillary density) (Figure 7-8, *B*).

Lipid-soluble Molecules Pass Directly Through the Lipid Membranes of the Endothelium and the Pores

The lipid-soluble molecules move with great rapidity between blood and tissue. The degree of lipid solubility (oil-to-water partition coefficient) provides a good index of the ease of transfer of lipid molecules through the endothelium.

Oxygen and carbon dioxide are both lipid soluble and readily pass through the endothelial cells. Calculations based on (1) the diffusion coefficient for O_2, (2) capillary density and diffusion distances, (3) blood flow, and (4) tissue O_2 consumption indicate that the O_2 supply of normal tissue at rest and during activity is not limited by diffusion or the number of open capillaries.

Measurements of Po_2 and saturation of blood in the microvessels indicate that, in many tissues, O_2 saturation at the entrance of the capillaries has already decreased to a saturation of about 80% as a result of diffusion of O_2 from arterioles and small arteries. Also, CO_2 loading and the resultant intravascular shifts in the oxyhemoglobin dissociation curve occur in the precapillary vessels. Hence direct flux of O_2 and CO_2 occurs between adjacent arterioles, venules, and possibly arteries and veins (**countercurrent exchange**), in addition to gas exchange at the level of the capillaries. This countercurrent exchange of gas represents a diffusional shunt of gas around the capillaries, and at low blood flow rates, it may limit the supply of O_2 to the tissue.

Capillary Filtration Is Regulated by the Hydrostatic and Osmotic Forces Across the Endothelium

The direction and magnitude of the movement of water across the capillary wall are determined by the algebraic sum of the hydrostatic and osmotic pressures that exist across the membrane. An increase in intracapillary hydrostatic pressure favors movement of fluid from the vessel to the interstitial space, whereas an increase in the concentration of osmotically active particles within the vessels favors movement of fluid into the vessels from the interstitial space.

Hydrostatic Forces The hydrostatic pressure (blood pressure) within the capillaries is not constant and depends on arterial pressure, venous pressure, and precapillary and postcapillary vessel resistances. An increase in small artery and arterial or venous pressure elevates capillary hydrostatic pressure, whereas a reduction in each has the opposite effect. An increase in arteriolar resistance or closure of arteries reduces capillary pressure, whereas greater venous resistance (venules and veins) increases capillary pressure.

Hydrostatic pressure is the principal force in capillary filtration. However, changes in the venous resistance affect capillary hydrostatic pressure more than do changes in arteriolar resistance. A given change in venous pressure produces a greater effect on capillary hydrostatic pressure than the same change in arterial pressure, and about 80% of an increase in venous pressure is transmitted back to the capillaries.

Despite the fact that capillary hydrostatic pressure (P_c) is variable from tissue to tissue (even within the same tissue), average values, obtained from many direct measurements in human skin, are about 32 mm Hg at the arterial end of the capillaries and 15 mm Hg at the venous end of the capillaries at the level of the heart (Figure 7-9). When a person stands, the hydrostatic pressure is higher in the legs and lower in the head.

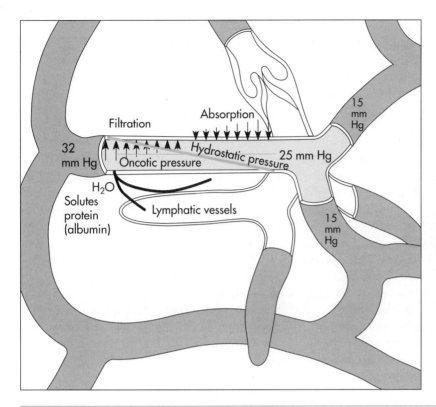

Figure 7-9 ▪ **Schematic representation of the factors responsible for filtration and absorption across the capillary wall and the formation of lymph.**

Tissue pressure, or more specifically interstitial fluid pressure (P_i) outside the capillaries, opposes capillary filtration, and it is $P_c - P_i$ that constitutes the hydrostatic driving force for filtration. In the normal (nonedematous) state of the subcutaneous tissue, P_i is close to zero or slightly negative (-1 to -4 mm Hg), so that P_c essentially represents the hydrostatic driving force.

Osmotic Forces *The key factor that restrains fluid loss from the capillaries is the osmotic pressure of the plasma proteins*—usually termed **colloid osmotic pressure** or **oncotic pressure** (π_p). The total osmotic pressure of plasma is about 6000 mm Hg, whereas the oncotic pressure is only about 25 mm Hg. However, this small oncotic pressure plays an important role in fluid exchange across the capillary wall, because the plasma proteins are essentially confined to the intravascular space, whereas the

electrolytes that are responsible for the major fraction of plasma osmotic pressure are practically equal in concentration on both sides of the capillary endothelium. The relative permeability of solute to water influences the actual magnitude of the osmotic pressure. The **reflection coefficient** (σ) is the relative impediment to the passage of a substance through the capillary wall. The reflection coefficient of water is zero and that of albumin (to which the endothelium is almost impermeable) is 1. Filterable solutes have reflection coefficients between 0 and 1. Also, different tissues have different reflection coefficients for the same molecule, and therefore movement of a given solute across the endothelial wall varies with the tissue. The true oncotic pressure (π) is defined by

$$\pi = \sigma RT(C_i - C_o) \qquad (3)$$

where
σ = Reflection coefficient
R = Gas constant
T = Absolute temperature
C_i and C_o = Solute (albumin) concentration, respectively, inside and outside the capillary

Of the plasma proteins, albumin is preponderate in determining oncotic pressure. The average albumin molecule (molecular weight 69,000) is approximately half the size of the average globulin molecule (molecular weight 150,000) and is present in almost twice the concentration as the globulins (4.5 versus 2.5 g/dl of plasma). Albumin also exerts a greater osmotic force than can be accounted for solely on the basis of the number of molecules dissolved in the plasma. Therefore it cannot be completely replaced by inert substances of appropriate molecular size such as dextran. This additional osmotic force becomes disproportionately greater at high concentrations of albumin (as in plasma) and is weak to absent in dilute solutions of albumin (as in interstitial fluid). The reason for this behavior of albumin is its negative charge at the normal blood pH and the attraction and retention of cations (principally Na^+) in the vascular compartment (the **Gibbs-Donnan effect**). Furthermore, albumin binds a small number of chloride ions, which increases its negative charge and hence its ability to retain more sodium ions inside the capillaries. The small increase in electrolyte concentration of the plasma over that of the interstitial fluid produced by the negatively charged albumin enhances its osmotic force to that of an ideal solution containing a solute of molecular weight of 37,000. If albumin did indeed have a molecular weight of 37,000, it would not be retained by the capillary endothelium because of its small size, and obviously could not function as a counterforce to capillary hydrostatic pressure. If, however, albumin did not have an enhanced osmotic force, it would require a concentration of about 12 g of albumin/dl of plasma to achieve a plasma oncotic pressure of 25 mm Hg. Such a high albumin concentration would greatly increase blood viscosity and the resistance to blood flow through the vascular system.

Some albumin escapes from the capillaries and enters the interstitial fluid, where it exerts an osmotic force of up to about 30% of plasma oncotic pressure.

This observation of a higher interstitial fluid (ISF) oncotic pressure than previously thought prompted the conclusion that filtration occurs in diminishing amounts along the entire length of the capillary in skin and skeletal muscle during steady state conditions. Abrupt reductions in capillary hydrostatic pressure can cause transient reabsorption of fluid from the ISF compartment, but with time plasma proteins continue to leak out of the capillaries, and this leakage plus removal of water from the ISF compartment by the lymphatics concentrates the ISF proteins and changes absorption to filtration.

Balance of Hydrostatic and Osmotic Forces

The relationship between hydrostatic pressure and oncotic pressure, and the role of these forces in regulating fluid passage across the capillary endothelium, were expounded by Starling in 1896 and constitute the **Starling hypothesis.** It can be expressed by the equation

$$Q_f = k[(P_c + \pi_i) - (P_i + \pi_p)] \qquad (4)$$

where Q_f = Fluid movement across the capillary wall
P_c = Capillary hydrostatic pressure
P_i = Interstitial fluid hydrostatic pressure
π_p = Plasma oncotic pressure
π_i = Interstitial fluid oncotic pressure
k = Filtration constant for capillary membrane

Filtration occurs when the algebraic sum is positive; absorption occurs when it is negative.

Classically, it has been thought that filtration occurs at the arterial end of the capillary and absorption at its venous end because of the gradient of hydrostatic pressure along the capillary. This may be true for the idealized capillary, as depicted in Figure 7-9, but direct observations have revealed that many capillaries show only filtration, whereas others show only absorption. In some vascular beds (e.g., the renal glomerulus) hydrostatic pressure in the capillary is high enough to result in filtration along the entire length of the capillary. In other vascular beds (e.g., the intestinal mucosa), the hydrostatic and oncotic forces are such that absorption occurs along the whole capillary.

As discussed earlier in this chapter, capillary pressure is variable and depends on several factors, the principal one being the contractile state of the precapillary vessel. In the normal steady state, arterial pressure, venous pressure, postcapillary resistance, interstitial fluid hydrostatic and oncotic pressures, and plasma oncotic pressure are relatively constant, and a change in precapillary resistance is the determining factor with respect to fluid movement across the wall for any given capillary. Because water moves so quickly across the capillary endothelium, the hydrostatic and osmotic forces are nearly in equilibrium along the entire capillary. Hence filtration and absorption in the normal state occur at very small degrees of imbalance of pressure across the capillary wall. Only a small percentage (2%) of the plasma flowing through the vascular system is filtered. Some is reabsorbed, and the rest is returned to the circulating blood via the lymphatic system.

In the lungs the mean capillary hydrostatic pressure is only 8 to 10 mm Hg, the plasma oncotic pressure is 25 mm Hg, and the lung interstitial fluid pressure is approximately 15 mm Hg, (-2 to -4 mm Hg). However, interstitial fluid oncotic pressure is 16 to 20 mg Hg. Hence pulmonary lymph is formed and consists of fluid that is osmotically drawn out of the capillaries by the plasma protein that escapes through the capillary endothelium.

BOX 7-3

In pathological conditions, such as left ventricular failure or stenosis of the mitral valve, pulmonary capillary hydrostatic pressure may exceed plasma oncotic pressure. When this occurs, it may cause pulmonary edema, a condition that seriously interferes with gas exchange in the lungs.

The Capillary Filtration Coefficient Is a Convenient Method to Estimate the Rate of Fluid Movement Across the Endothelium

The rate of fluid movement across the capillary membrane (Q_f) depends not only on the algebraic sum of the hydrostatic and osmotic forces across the endothelium (ΔP), but also on the area of the capillary wall available for filtration (A_m), the distance across the capillary wall (Δx), the viscosity of the filtrate (η), and the filtration constant of the membrane (k). These factors may be expressed by the equation

$$Q_f = \frac{kA_m\Delta P}{\eta\Delta x} \quad (5)$$

The dimensions are units of flow per unit of pressure gradient across the capillary wall per unit of capillary surface area. This expression, which describes the flow of fluid through a membrane (pores), is essentially Poiseuille's law for flow through tubes (p 118).

Because the thickness of the capillary wall and the viscosity of the filtrate are relatively constant, they can be included in the filtration constant, k, and if the area of the capillary membrane is not known, the rate of filtration can be expressed per unit weight of tissue. Hence the equation can be simplified to

$$Q_f = k_t\Delta P \quad (6)$$

where k_t is the capillary filtration coefficient for a given tissue, and the units for Q_f are milliliters per minute per 100 g of tissue per millimeter of mercury pressure.

In any given tissue the filtration coefficient per unit area of capillary surface, and hence capillary permeability, is not changed by different physiological conditions, such as arteriolar dilation and capillary distension, or by such adverse conditions as hypoxia, hypercapnia, or reduced pH.

BOX 7-4

With capillary injury (toxins, severe burns), capillary permeability increases, as indicated by the filtration coefficient, and significant amounts of fluid and protein leak out of the capillaries into the interstitial space. The escaped protein enhances the oncotic pressure of the interstitial fluid, which leads to additional fluid loss and dehydration. One of the important therapeutic measures in the treatment of extensive burns is replacement of fluid and plasma proteins.

Because capillary permeability is constant under normal conditions, the filtration coefficient can be used to determine the relative number of open capillaries (total capillary surface area available for filtration in tissue). For example, increased metabolic activity of contracting skeletal muscle induces relaxation of precapillary resistance vessels with opening of more capillaries (**capillary recruitment,** resulting in an increased filtering surface area).

Disturbances in Hydrostatic-Osmotic Balance Changes in arterial pressure per se may have little effect on filtration because the change in pressure may be countered by adjustments of the precapillary resistance vessels (autoregulation, p 180), so that hydrostatic pressure in the open capillaries remains the same.

BOX 7-5

With severe reduction in arterial pressure, as may occur in hemorrhage, there may be arteriolar constriction mediated by the sympathetic nervous system and a fall in venous pressure resulting from the blood loss. These changes will lead to a decrease in capillary hydrostatic pressure. Furthermore, the low blood pressure in hemorrhage causes a decrease in blood flow (and hence O_2 supply) to the tissue, with the result that vasodilator metabolites accumulate and induce relaxation of arterioles. Precapillary vessel relaxation is also engendered by the reduced transmural pressure (autoregulation, p 180). As a consequence of these several factors, absorption predominates over filtration and occurs at a larger capillary surface area. This is one of the compensatory mechanisms employed by the body to restore blood volume (p 278).

An increase in venous pressure alone, as occurs in the feet when one changes from the lying to the standing position, would elevate capillary pressure and enhance filtration. However, the increase in transmural pressure causes precapillary vessel closure (myogenic mechanism, p 278) so that the capillary filtration coefficient actually decreases. This reduction in capillary surface available for filtration protects against the extravasation of large amounts of fluid into the interstitial space (edema).

BOX 7-6

With prolonged standing, particularly when associated with some elevation of venous pressure in the legs (such as that caused by pregnancy) or with sustained increases in venous pressure (as seen in congestive heart failure), filtration is greatly enhanced and exceeds the capacity of the lymphatic system to remove the capillary filtrate from the interstitial space (see also Figure 9-19).

A large amount of fluid can move across the capillary wall in a relatively short time. In a normal individual the filtration coefficient (k_t) for the whole body is about 0.0061 ml/min/100 g of tissue/mm Hg. For a 70-kg man, elevation of venous pressure of 10 mm Hg for 10 minutes would increase filtration from capillaries by 342 ml. This would not lead to edema formation because the fluid is returned to the vascular compartment by the lymphatic vessels. When edema does develop, it usually appears in the dependent parts of the body, where the hydrostatic pressure is greatest, but its location and magnitude are also determined by the type of tissue. Loose tissues, such as the subcutaneous tissue around the eyes or in the scrotum, are more prone to collect larger quantities of interstitial fluid than are firm tissues, such as muscle, or encapsulated structures, such as the kidney.

The vascular endothelial growth factors (VEGFs) (of which there are at least 6) induce angiogenesis but also elicit vasodilation and increased permeability of the endothelium. These properties of the VEGFs must be taken into consideration when the exciting prospects of using VEGFs in promoting angiogenesis in poorly perfused myocardium or inhibiting angiogenesis in the treatment of malignant tumors are investigated.

Pinocytosis Enables Large Molecules to Cross the Endothelium

Some transfer of substances across the capillary wall can occur in tiny pinocytotic vesicles (pinocytosis). These vesicles (see Figures 7-5 and 7-6), formed by a pinching off of the surface membrane, can take up substances on one side of the capillary wall, move by thermal kinetic energy across the endothelial cell, and deposit their contents at the other side. The amount of material that can be transported in this way is very small relative to that moved by diffusion. However, pinocytosis may be responsible for the movement of large lipid-insoluble molecules (30 nm) between blood and interstitial fluid. The number of pinocytotic vesicles in endothelium varies with the tissue (muscle > lung > brain) and increases from the arterial to the venous end of the capillary.

■ THE LYMPHATICS RETURN THE FLUID AND SOLUTES THAT ESCAPE THROUGH THE ENDOTHELIUM TO THE CIRCULATING BLOOD

The terminal vessels of the lymphatic system consist of a widely distributed closed-end network of highly permeable lymph capillaries similar in appearance to blood capillaries. However, they are generally lacking in tight junctions between endothelial cells, and possess fine filaments that anchor them to the surrounding connective tissue. With muscular contraction, these fine strands distort the lymphatic vessel to open spaces between the endothelial cells and permit the entrance of protein and large particles and cells present in the interstitial fluid. The lymph capillaries drain into larger vessels that finally enter the right and left subclavian veins at their junctions with the respective internal jugular veins. Only cartilage, bone, epi-

---

BOX 7-7

The concentration of the plasma proteins may also change in different pathological states and thus alter the osmotic force and movement of fluid across the capillary membrane. The plasma protein concentration is increased in dehydration (e.g., water deprivation, prolonged sweating, severe vomiting, and diarrhea), and water moves by osmotic forces from the tissues to the vascular compartment. In contrast, the plasma protein concentration is reduced in **nephrosis** (a renal disease in which there is loss of protein in the urine), and edema may occur.

thelium, and tissues of the central nervous system are devoid of lymphatic vessels. The plasma capillary filtrate is returned to the circulation by virtue of tissue pressure, facilitated by intermittent skeletal muscle activity, contractions of the lymphatic vessels, and an extensive system of one-way valves. In this respect, they resemble the veins, although even the larger lymphatic vessels have thinner walls than the corresponding veins and contain only a small amount of elastic tissue and smooth muscle.

The volume of fluid transported through the lymphatics in 24 hours is about equal to an animal's total plasma volume, and the protein returned by the lymphatics to the blood in a day is about one fourth to one half of the circulating plasma proteins. This is the only means whereby protein (albumin) that leaves the vascular compartment can be returned to the blood because back diffusion into the capillaries cannot occur against the large albumin concentration gradient. Were the protein not removed by the lymph vessels, it would accumulate in the interstitial fluid and act as an oncotic force to draw fluid from the blood capillaries to produce edema. In addition to returning fluid and protein to the vascular bed, the lymphatic system filters the lymph at the lymph nodes and removes foreign particles, such as bacteria. The largest lymphatic vessel, the **thoracic duct,** in addition to draining the lower extremities, returns protein lost through the permeable liver capillaries and carries substances absorbed from the gastrointestinal tract, principally fat in the form of chylomicrons, to the circulating blood.

Lymph flow varies considerably, being almost nil from resting skeletal muscle and increasing during exercise in proportion to the degree of muscular activity. It is increased by any mechanism that enhances the rate of blood capillary filtration, for example, increased capillary pressure or permeability or decreased plasma oncotic pressure.

BOX 7-8

When either the volume of interstitial fluid exceeds the drainage capacity of the lymphatics or the lymphatic vessels become blocked, as may occur in certain disease states such as **elephantiasis** (caused by **filariasis,** a worm infestation) interstitial fluid accumulates (edema) chiefly in the more compliant tissues (e.g., subcutaneous tissue).

Summary

- Blood flow through the capillaries is chiefly regulated by contraction and relaxation of the arterioles (resistance vessels).
- The capillaries, which consist of a single layer of endothelial cells, can withstand high transmural pressure by virtue of their small diameter. According to the law of Laplace, T (wall tension) = P (transmural pressure) × r (radius of the capillary).
- The endothelium is the source of an endothelium-derived relaxing factor (EDRF—

identified as nitric oxide) and prostacyclin, which relax vascular smooth muscles.
- Movement of water and small solutes between the vascular and interstitial fluid compartments occurs through capillary pores mainly by diffusion but also by filtration and absorption.
- Because the rate of diffusion is about 40 times greater than the blood flow in the tissue, exchange of small lipid-insoluble molecules is flow limited. The larger the molecules, the

slower is the diffusion, until with large molecules the lipid-insoluble molecules become diffusion limited. Molecules larger than about 70,000 kd are essentially confined to the vascular compartment.

- Lipid-soluble substances such as CO_2 and O_2 pass directly through the lipid membranes of the capillary, and the ease of transfer is directly proportional to the degree of lipid solubility of the substance.
- Capillary filtration and absorption are described by the Starling equation: Fluid movement $= k[(P_c + \pi_i) - (P_i + \pi_p)]$ where $P_c =$ capillary hydrostatic pressure; $P_i =$ interstitial fluid hydrostatic pressure; $\pi_i =$ interstitial fluid oncotic pressure; $\pi_p =$ plasma oncotic pressure. Filtration occurs when the algebraic sum is positive; absorption occurs when it is negative.

- Large molecules can move across the capillary wall in vesicles formed from the lipid membrane of the capillaries by a process called pinocytosis.
- Fluid and protein that have escaped from the blood capillaries enter the lymphatic capillaries and are transported via the lymphatic system back to the blood vascular compartment.

■ BIBLIOGRAPHY

1. Aukland K: Why don't our feet swell in the upright position? *News Physiol Sci* 9:214, 1994.
2. Aukland K, Reed RK: Interstitial-lymphatic mechanisms in the control of extracellular fluid volume. *Physiol Rev* 73:1, 1993.
3. Bates DO, Lodwick D, Williams B: Vascular endothelial growth factor and microvascular permeability. *Microcirculation* 6:83, 1999.
4. Curry FE: Regulation of water and solute exchange in microvessel endothelium: studies in single perfused capillaries. *Microcirculation* 1:11, 1994.
5. Davies PF: Flow-mediated endothelial mechanotransduction. *Physiol Rev* 75:519, 1995.
6. Furchgott RF, Vanhoutte PM: Endothelium-derived relaxing and contracting factors. *FASEB J* 3:2007, 1989.
7. Levick JR, Mortimer PS: Fluid "balance" between microcirculation and interstitium in skin and other tissues: revision of the classical filtration-reabsorption scheme. *Prog Appl Microcirc* 23:42, 1999.
8. Lewis DH, editor: Symposium on lymph circulation. *Acta Physiol Scand Suppl* 463:9, 1979.
9. Luscher TF, Vanhoutte PM: *The endothelium: modulator of cardiovascular function*, Boca Raton, FL, 1990, CRC Press.
10. Michel CC, Neal CR: Openings through endothelial cells associated with increased microvascular permeability. *Microcirculation* 6:45, 1999.
11. Pries AR, Secomb TW, Gessner T, et al: Resistance to blood flow in microvessels in vivo. *Circ Res* 75:904, 1994.
12. Rippe B, Haraldsson B: Transport of macromolecules across microvascular walls: the two-pore theory. *Physiol Rev* 74:163, 1994.
13. Starling EH: On the absorption of fluids from the connective tissue spaces. *J Physiol* 19:312, 1896.
14. Vink H, Duling BR: The capillary endothelial surface layer selectively reduces plasma solute distribution volume. *Am J Physiol* 2000.
15. Welsh DG, Segal SS: Endothelial and smooth muscle cell conduction in arterioles controlling blood flow. *Am J Physiol* 274:H178, 1998.
16. Xia J, Duling BR: Patterns of excitation-contraction coupling in arterioles: dependence on time and concentration. *Am J Physiol* 274:H323, 1998.

■ CASE 7-1

HISTORY

A 45-year-old man with a long history of alcoholism (averaging a liter of whiskey per day) was admitted to the hospital as an emergency because of vomiting of blood and fainting. In the past few months, he noted progressive anorexia, fatigue, jaundice, generalized itching, and abdominal swelling. Physical examination revealed a semicomatose man with pallor, jaundice, and ascites. Blood pressure was 90/40, heart rate was 100, and hematocrit was 35. Liver function tests indicated severe liver damage. The diagnosis was advanced cirrhosis of the liver. Immediate treatment was transfusion with three units of blood. The following pressures were noted:

Mesenteric capillary hydrostatic pressure (estimated)	44 mm Hg
Plasma oncotic pressure	23 mm Hg
Pressure in peritoneal cavity	8 mm Hg
Peritoneal fluid oncotic pressure	2 mm Hg

QUESTIONS

1. The transcapillary pressure that was responsible for the ascites was
   a. 11 mm Hg
   b. 21 mm Hg
   c. 8 mm Hg
   d. 15 mm Hg
   e. 13 mm Hg
2. After lost blood was replaced by transfusion, the treatment for his condition was
   a. Dialysis
   b. High fat diet
   c. Portal-caval shunt
   d. Cholecystectomy
   e. Erythromycin
3. The substance mainly responsible for the oncotic pressure of the patient's plasma is
   a. Sodium
   b. Albumin
   c. Chloride
   d. Globulin
   e. Potassium

■ CASE 7-2

HISTORY

A 25-year-old man suffered third-degree burns over the upper three quarters of his body in a fire in his home. Several hours elapsed before he reached the hospital. On admission, he was in a shocklike state. Heart rate was 110, blood pressure was 90/70, and hematocrit was 55%. Blood analysis revealed a sodium level of 145 mEq/L, a potassium level of 4 mEq/l, a chloride level of 105 mEq/l, and an albumin level of 3/5 g/dl.

QUESTIONS

1. The most effective treatment is an intravenous infusion of
   a. Saline
   b. Whole blood
   c. 5% glucose
   d. Dextran
   e. Plasma
2. After several months of treatment with extensive artificial skin grafts, the patient was able to walk and to resume an almost normal life. After prolonged standing, he noted slight ankle swelling but no ecchymoses in his feet. Capillaries in his feet did not rupture when he stood because
   a. Arterioles reflexively constrict and prevent exposure of the capillaries to high pressure.
   b. Tissue pressure rises and opposes an increase in capillary pressure.
   c. Total capillary cross-sectional area is large enough to distribute the pressure and thereby compensate for the high intracapillary pressure.
   d. Capillary diameter is so small that the capillary wall tension is low.
   e. Capillaries constrict by a myogenic mechanism.

8

The Peripheral Circulation and Its Control

Objectives

1. Indicate the intrinsic and extrinsic (neural and humoral) factors that regulate peripheral blood flow.

2. Explain autoregulation of blood flow and the myogenic mechanism for local adjustments of blood flow.

3. Elucidate metabolic regulation of blood flow.

4. Explain the role of the sympathetic nerves in blood flow regulation.

5. Describe vascular reflexes in the control of blood flow.

6. Describe the role of humoral agents in the regulation of blood flow.

THE FUNCTION OF THE HEART AND large blood vessels is to pump and carry blood to the tissues of the body, but the distribution of blood to the regions of the body where it is needed and away from where it is not needed rests with the small arteries and arterioles. *The regulation of peripheral blood flow is essentially under dual control: centrally by the nervous system, and locally in the tissues by the conditions in the immediate vicinity of the blood vessels.* The relative importance of the central and local control mechanisms is not the same in all tissues. In some areas of the body, such as the skin and the splanchnic regions, neural regulation of blood flow predominates, whereas in others, such as the heart and the brain, local factors are dominant.

The small arteries and arterioles that regulate the blood flow throughout the body are called the **resistance vessels.** These vessels offer the greatest resistance to flow of blood pumped to the tissues by the heart and thereby are important in the maintenance of arterial blood pressure. Smooth muscle fibers are the main component of the walls of the resistance vessels (see Figure 1-1). Hence the vessel lumen can be varied from complete obliteration, by strong contraction of the smooth muscle with infolding of the endothelial lining, to maximal dilation, by full relaxation of the smooth muscle. At any given time some resistance vessels are closed by partial contraction (tone) of the arteriolar smooth muscle. If all the resistance vessels in the body dilated simultaneously, blood pressure

175

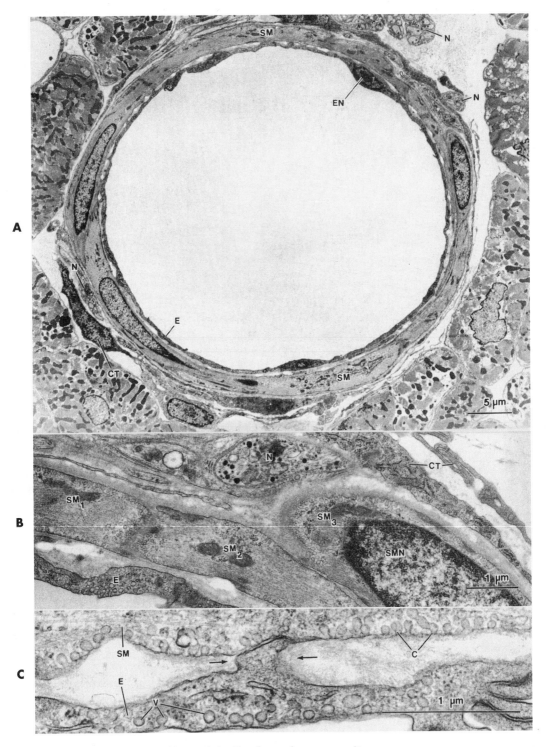

Figure 8-1 ■ For legend see opposite page.

Figure 8-1 ▪ A, Low-magnification electron micrograph of an arteriole in cross section (inner diameter of approximately 40 mm) in cat ventricle. The wall of the blood vessel is composed largely of vascular smooth muscle cells *(SM)* whose long axes are directed approximately circularly around the vessel. A single layer of endothelial cells *(E)* forms the innermost portion of the blood vessel. Connective tissue elements *(CT)*, such as fibroblasts and collagen, make up the adventitial layer at the periphery of the vessel; nerve bundles also appear in this layer *(N)*. EN, Endothelial cell nucleus. B, Detail of the wall of the blood vessel in A. This field contains a single endothelial layer *(E)*, the medial smooth muscle layer (three smooth muscle cell profiles: SM_1, SM_2, SM_3), and the adventitial layer (containing nerves *[N]* and connective tissue *[CT]*). SMN, Smooth muscle nucleus. C, Another region of the arteriole, showing the area in which the endothelial *(E)* and smooth muscle *(SM)* layers are apposed. A projection of an endothelial cell *(between arrows)* is closely applied to the surface of the overlying smooth muscle, forming a "myoendothelial junction." Plasmalemmal vesicles are prominent in both the endothelium *(V)* and the smooth muscle cell (where such vesicles are known as "caveolae" *[C]*).

---

would fall precipitously. Passive stretch of the microvessels by an increase in intravascular pressure decreases vascular resistance, whereas a decrease in intravascular pressure increases vascular resistance by recoil of the stretched vascular muscle.

▪ CONTRACTION AND RELAXATION OF ARTERIOLAR VASCULAR SMOOTH MUSCLE REGULATE PERIPHERAL BLOOD FLOW

Vascular smooth muscle is responsible for the control of total peripheral resistance, arterial and venous tone, and the distribution of blood flow throughout the body. The smooth muscle cells are small, mononucleate, and spindle shaped. They are generally arranged in helical or circular layers around the larger blood vessels and in a single circular layer around arterioles (Figure 8-1, *A* and *B*). Also, parts of endothelial cells project into the vascular smooth muscle layer (**myoendothelial junctions**) at various points along the arterioles (Figure 8-1, *C*). These projections suggest a

functional interaction between endothelium and adjacent vascular smooth muscle.

In general, the close association between action potentials and contraction observed in skeletal and cardiac muscle cells cannot be demonstrated in vascular smooth muscle. Also, vascular smooth muscle lacks transverse tubules.

Graded changes in membrane potential are often associated with increases or decreases in force. Contractile activity is generally elicited by neural or humoral stimuli. The behavior of smooth muscle in different vessels varies. For example, some vessels, particularly in the portal or mesenteric circulation, contain longitudinally oriented smooth muscle that is spontaneously active and shows action potentials that are correlated with the contractions and the electrical coupling between cells.

The vascular smooth muscle cells contain large numbers of thin actin filaments and comparatively small numbers of thick myosin filaments. These filaments are aligned in the long axis of the cell but do not form visible sarcomeres with striations. Nevertheless, the sliding filament mechanism is believed to operate in this tissue, and phosphorylation of crossbridges regulates their rate of cycling. Compared with skeletal muscle, the smooth muscle contracts very slowly, develops high forces, maintains force for long periods with low adenosine triphosphate (ATP) utilization, and operates over a considerable range of lengths under physiological conditions. Cell-to-cell conduction is via gap junctions as occurs in cardiac muscle (see p 56).

The interaction between myosin and actin, leading to contraction, is controlled by the myoplasmic Ca^{++} concentration as in other muscles, but the molecular mechanism whereby Ca^{++} regulates contraction differs. For example, smooth muscle lacks troponin and fast sodium channels. The increased myoplasmic Ca^{++} that elicits contraction can come through voltage-gated calcium channels (**electromechanical coupling**) and through receptor-mediated calcium channels (**pharmacomechanical coupling**) in the sarcolemma, and by release from the sarcoplasmic reticulum (Figure 8-2). The cells relax when intracellular free Ca^{++} is pumped back into the sarcoplasmic reticulum and is extruded from the cell by the calcium pump in the cell membrane and by the Na-Ca exchanger.

The response to humoral stimuli (pharmacomechanical coupling) occurs without evidence of electrical excitation and is the predominant mechanism for eliciting contraction of vascular smooth muscle. In the category of pharmacologic stimuli that cause contraction or relaxation are such substances as catecholamines, histamine, acetylcholine, serotonin, angiotensin, adenosine, nitric oxide (NO), CO_2, K^+, H^+, and prostaglandins (see Figure 7-4).

As illustrated in Figure 8-2, an agonist activates receptors in the vascular smooth muscle membrane. These receptors in turn activate phospholipase C in a reaction coupled to guanine nucleotide binding proteins (G proteins). The phospholipase C hydrolyzes phosphatidyl inositol bisphosphate in the membrane to yield diacylglycerol and inositol trisphosphate; the latter causes the release of Ca^{++} from the sarcoplasmic reticulum. The Ca^{++} binds to calmodulin, which in turn binds to myosin light chain kinase. This activated Ca^{++}-calmodulin-myosin kinase complex phosphorylates the myosin crossbridges, which initiates contraction. Dephosphorylation of the crossbridges by myosin phosphatase and reduction in the cytoplasmic Ca^{++} by uptake into the sarcoplasmic reticulum and extrusion by the Ca^{++} pump and the Na-Ca exchange produces relaxation (Figure 8-2).

Finally, the sensitivity of the contractile regulatory apparatus to Ca^{++} is increased by agonists. The mechanism for this enhanced sensitivity is still unclear but appears to involve G proteins. Local environmental changes alter the contractile state of vascular smooth muscle, and alterations such as increased temperature or increased carbon dioxide levels induce relaxation of this tissue.

Most of the arteries and veins of the body are supplied to different degrees solely by fibers of the sympathetic nervous system. These nerve fibers exert a tonic effect on the blood vessels, as evidenced by the fact that cutting or freezing the sympathetic nerves to a vascular bed (such as muscle) results in an increase in blood flow. Activation of the sympathetic nerves either directly or reflexly (pp 186 and 187) enhances vascular resistance. In contrast to the sympathetic nerves, the parasympathetic nerves tend to decrease vascular resistance, but they innervate only a small fraction of the blood vessels in the body, mainly in certain viscera and pelvic organs.

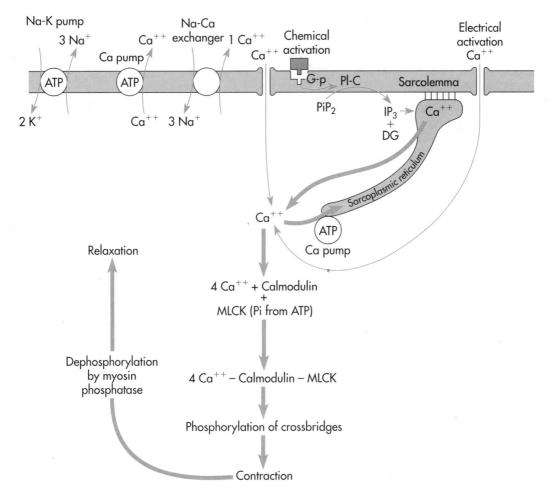

Figure 8-2 ■ **Excitation-contraction coupling in vascular smooth muscle. Calcium can enter the cell via electrically activated channels (electromechanical coupling) or via receptor-operated channels (chemical activation, termed *pharmacomechanical coupling*) in the sarcolemma. Calcium is also re-leased from the sarcoplasmic reticulum in response to inositol trisphosphate *(IP₃)* stimulation and is taken back into the sarcoplasmic reticulum by a calcium pump. Calcium is extruded from the cell by a calcium pump and by the Na-Ca exchanger. *G-p,* Guanine nucleotide binding protein; *Pl-C,* phos-pholipase C; *PiP₂,* phosphatidyl inositol bisphosphate; *DG,* diacylglycerol; *MLCK,* myosin light chain kinase.**

■ INTRINSIC (LOCAL) CONTROL OF PERIPHERAL BLOOD FLOW

Autoregulation and the Myogenic Mechanism Tend to Keep Blood Flow Constant in the Face of Changes in Perfusion Pressure

In a number of different tissues the blood flow is adjusted to the existing metabolic activity of the tissue. Furthermore, imposed changes in perfusion pressure (arterial blood pressure) at constant levels of tissue metabolism, as measured by oxygen consumption, are met with vascular resistance changes that maintain almost a constant blood flow. This mechanism is commonly referred to as **autoregulation** of blood flow and is illustrated graphically in Figure 8-3. In the skeletal muscle preparation from which these data were gathered, the muscle was completely isolated from the rest of the animal and was in a resting state. From a control pressure of 100 mm Hg, the pressure was abruptly increased or de-

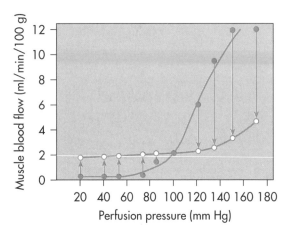

Figure 8-3 ■ Pressure-flow relationship in the skeletal muscle vascular bed of the dog. Closed circles represent the flows obtained immediately after abrupt changes in perfusion pressure from the control level *(point where lines cross).* **Open circles represent the steady-state flows obtained at the new perfusion pressure.** (Redrawn from Jones RD, Berne RM: *Circ Res* 14:126, 1964.)

creased, and the blood flows observed immediately after changing the perfusion pressure are represented by the closed circles. Maintenance of the altered pressure at each new level was followed within 30 to 60 seconds by a return of flow to or toward the control levels; the open circles represent these steady-state flows. Over the pressure range of 20 to 120 mm Hg, the steady-state flow is relatively constant. Calculation of resistance across the vascular bed (pressure/flow) during steady-state conditions indicates that with elevation of perfusion pressure, the resistance vessels constricted, whereas with reduction of perfusion pressure, they dilated.

The reason for this constancy of blood flow in the presence of an altered perfusion pressure is not known, but it appears to be explained best by the **myogenic mechanism.**

According to the myogenic mechanism, the vascular smooth muscle contracts in response to an increase in transmural pressure stretch and relaxes in response to a decrease in transmural pressure. Therefore the initial flow increment produced by an abrupt increase in perfusion pressure that passively distends the blood vessels would be followed by a return of flow to the previous control level by contraction of the smooth muscles of the resistance vessels.

An example of a myogenic response is shown in Figure 8-4. Arterioles isolated from the hearts of young pigs were cannulated at each end, and the transmural pressure (intravascular pressure minus extravascular pressure) and flow through the arteriole could be adjusted to desired levels. With no flow through the arteriole, successive increases of transmural pressure elicited progressive decreases in the vessel diameter (Figure 8-4, *A*). This response was independent of the endothelium because it was identical in intact vessels and in vessels denuded of endothelium (Figure 8-4, *B*). Arterioles that were relaxed by direct action of nitroprusside on the vascular smooth muscle showed only a passive increase in diameter when transmural pressure was increased. How vessel distension elicits contraction is unsettled, but because stretch of vascular smooth muscle elevates intracellular Ca^{++}, it has been proposed that an increase in transmural pressure activates membrane calcium channels.

Because blood pressure is reflexly maintained at a fairly constant level under normal conditions, it would be expected that operation of a myogenic mechanism would be minimized.

However, when a person changes position (from lying to standing), a large change in transmural pressure occurs in the lower extremities. The precapillary vessels constrict in response to this imposed stretch, which results in cessation of flow in most capillaries. After flow stops, capillary filtration diminishes until the increase in plasma oncotic pressure and the increase in interstitial fluid pressure balance the elevated capillary hydrostatic pressure produced by changing from a horizontal to a vertical position (see Chapters 7 and 9).

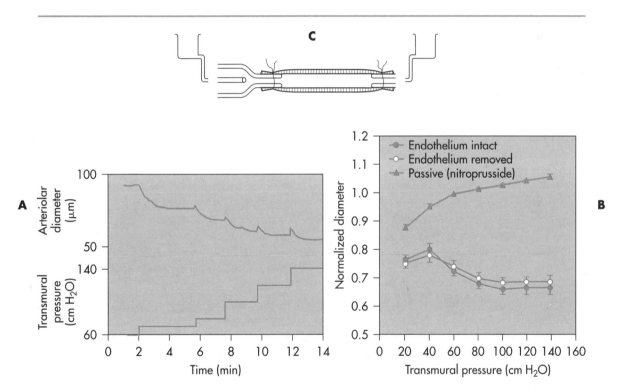

Figure 8-4 ■ A, **Constriction of an isolated cardiac arteriole in response to increases in transmural pressure without flow through the blood vessel. B, Constrictor response of the arteriole to an increase in transmural pressure is unaffected by removal of its endothelium. C, Diagram of cannulated arteriole. When the smooth muscle is relaxed by nitroprusside, the arteriole is passively distended by the increase in transmural pressure.** (Redrawn from Kuo L, Davis MJ, Chilian WM: *Am J Physiol* 259:H1063, 1990.)

BOX 8-1

If arteriolar resistance did not increase with standing, the hydrostatic pressure in the lower parts of the legs would reach such high levels that large volumes of fluid would pass from the capillaries into the interstitial fluid compartment and produce edema.

The Endothelium Actively Regulates Blood Flow

Stimulation of the endothelium can elicit a vasoactive response of the vascular smooth muscle. To demonstrate this response, transmural pressure is kept constant in an isolated arteriole, and intravascular pressure is increased by raising a perfusion fluid reservoir connected to one end of an arteriole and simultaneously lowering a reservoir connected to the other end of the arteriole by an equal distance. This maneuver increases the longitudinal pressure gradient along the vessel, and vasodilation occurs (Figure 8-5, *A*). The vasodilation is presumably caused by the NO (see p 159), which is released from the endothelium in response to the shear stress consequent to the increase in velocity of flow. If the arteriole is denuded of endothelium, the dilation of the vessel in response to increased flow is abolished (Figure 8-5, *B*).

Tissue Metabolic Activity Is the Main Factor in the Local Regulation of Blood Flow

According to the metabolic mechanism, any intervention that results in an O_2 supply that is inadequate for the requirements of the tissue gives rise to the formation of vasodilator metabolites. These metabolites are released from the tissue and act locally to dilate the resistance vessels. When the metabolic rate of the tissue increases or the O_2 delivery to the tissue decreases, more vasodilator substance is released and the metabolite concentration in the tissue increases.

Many substances have been proposed as mediators of metabolic vasodilation. Some of the earliest ones suggested are lactic acid, CO_2, and hydrogen ions. However, the decrease in vascular resistance induced by supernormal concentrations of these dilator agents falls considerably short of the dilation observed under physiological conditions of increased metabolic activity.

Changes in O_2 tension can evoke changes in the contractile state of vascular smooth muscle; an increase in Po_2 elicits contraction, and a decrease in Po_2, relaxation. If significant reductions in the intravascular Po_2 occur before the arterial blood reaches the resistance vessels (diffusion through the arterial and arteriolar walls, p 166), small changes in O_2 supply or consumption could elicit contraction or relaxation of the resistance vessels. However, direct measurements of Po_2 at the resistance vessels indicate that over a wide range of Po_2 (11 to 343 mm Hg), there is no correlation between O_2 tension and arteriolar diameter. Furthermore, if Po_2 were directly responsible for vascular smooth muscle tension, one would not expect to find a parallelism between the duration of arterial occlusion and the duration of the reactive hyperemia (flow above control level on release of an arterial occlusion) (Figure 8-6). With either short occlusions (5 to 10 seconds) or long occlusions (1 to 3 minutes), the venous blood becomes bright red (well oxygenated) within 1 or 2 seconds after release of the arterial occlusion, and hence the smooth muscle of the resistance vessels must be exposed to a high Po_2 in each instance. Nevertheless, the longer occlusions result in longer periods of reactive hyperemia. These observations are more compatible with the release of a vasodilator metabolite from the tissue than with a direct effect of Po_2 on the vascular smooth muscle.

Potassium ions, inorganic phosphate, and interstitial fluid osmolarity can also induce vasodilation. Because K^+ and phosphate are released and osmolarity is increased during skeletal

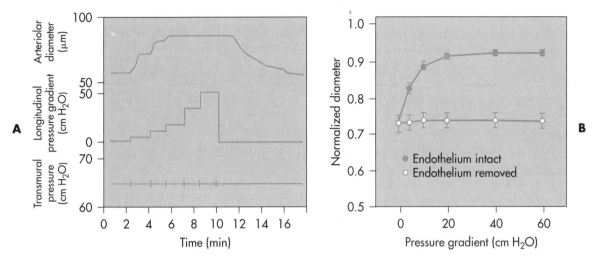

A

B

Figure 8-5 ■ A, **Flow-induced vasodilation in an isolated cardiac arteriole at constant transmural pressure. Flow was increased progressively by increasing the pressure gradient in the long axis of the arteriole (longitudinal pressure gradient). B, Flow-induced vasodilation is abolished by removal of the endothelium of the arteriole.** (Redrawn from Kuo L, Davis MJ, Chilian WM: *Am J Physiol* 259:H1063, 1990.)

muscle contraction, it has been proposed that these factors contribute to **active hyperemia** (increased blood flow caused by enhanced tissue activity). However, significant increases of phosphate concentration and osmolarity are not consistently observed during muscle contraction, and they may produce only transient increases in blood flow. Therefore they are not likely candidates as mediators of the vasodilation observed with muscular activity. Potassium release occurs with the onset of skeletal muscle contraction or an increase in cardiac activity, and could be responsible for the initial decrease in vascular resistance observed with exercise or increased cardiac work. However, K^+ release is not sustained, despite continued arteriolar dilation throughout the period of enhanced muscle activity. Therefore some other agent must serve as mediator of the vasodilation associated with the greater metabolic activity of the tissue. Reoxygenated venous blood obtained from active cardiac and skeletal muscles under steady-state conditions of exercise does not elicit vaso-

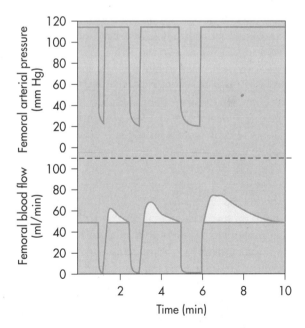

Figure 8-6 ■ **Reactive hyperemia in the hind limb of the dog after 15-, 30-, and 60-s occlusions of the femoral artery.** (Berne RM: Unpublished observations.)

dilation when infused into a test vascular bed. It is difficult to see how oxygenation of the venous blood could alter its K^+ or phosphate content or its osmolarity and thereby destroy its vasodilator effect.

Adenosine, which is involved in the regulation of coronary blood flow, may also participate in the control of the resistance vessels in skeletal muscle. In addition, NO and prostaglandins appear to play a role in flow-induced dilation of isolated perfused arterioles. Wild type (WT) mice and mice with deletion of the gene for encoding endothelial NO synthase, knock-out (KO) mice, showed the same degree of arteriolar dilation to enhanced flow. N^n-nitro-L-arginine methyl ester, an inhibitor of NO synthase, partially reduced the increased flow response in WT mice but had no effect on the response in KO mice. However, indomethacin, an inhibitor of prostaglandins, elicited partial reduction of flow-induced dilation in WT mice but abolished the response in KO mice. Combined administration of L-arginine and indomethacin abolished flow-induced dilation in the WT and in the KO mice.

Thus there are a number of candidates for the role of mediator of metabolic vasodilation, and the relative contribution of each of the various factors remains the subject for future investigation. Several factors may be involved in any given vascular bed, and different factors preponderate in different tissues.

Metabolic control of vascular resistance by the release of a vasodilator substance is predicated on the existence of basal vessel tone. This tonic activity, or **basal tone,** of the vascular smooth muscle is readily demonstrable, but, in contrast to tone in skeletal muscle, it is independent of the nervous system. The factor responsible for basal tone in blood vessels is not known, but one or more of the following factors may be involved: (1) an expression of myogenic activity in response to the stretch imposed by the blood pressure, (2) the high O_2 tension of

arterial blood, (3) the presence of calcium ions, or (4) some unknown factor in plasma, because addition of plasma to the bathing solution of isolated vessel segments evokes partial contraction of the smooth muscle.

If arterial inflow to a vascular bed is stopped for a few seconds to several minutes, the blood flow, on release of the occlusion, immediately exceeds the flow before occlusion and only gradually returns to the control level (**reactive hyperemia).** This is illustrated in Figure 8-6: blood flow to the leg was stopped by clamping the femoral artery for 15, 30, and 60 seconds. Release of the 60-second occlusion resulted in a peak blood flow 70% greater than the control flow, with a return to control flow within about 110 seconds. When this same experiment is performed in humans by inflating a blood pressure cuff on the upper arm, dilation of the resistance vessels of the hand and forearm, immediately after release of the cuff, is evident from the bright red color of the skin and the fullness of the veins. Within limits the peak flow, and particularly the duration of the reactive hyperemia, are proportional to the duration of the occlusion (Figure 8-6). If the extremity is exercised during the occlusion period, reactive hyperemia is increased. These observations, and the close relationship that exists between metabolic activity and blood flow in the unoccluded limb, are consonant with a metabolic mechanism in the local regulation of tissue blood flow.

When the vascular smooth muscle of the arterioles relaxes in response to vasodilator metabolites released by a decrease in the oxygen supply/oxygen demand ratio of the tissue, resistance may diminish in the arteries that feed these arterioles. This results in a greater blood flow than that produced by arteriolar dilation alone. Two possible mechanisms can account for this coordination of arterial and arteriolar dilation. First, vasodilation in the microvessels is propagated, and when initiated in the arterioles, it can propagate from arterioles back to arteries. Second, the metabolite-mediated dilation of the arterioles accelerates blood flow in the feeder arteries. This increases the shear stress on the arterial endothelium and thereby induces vasodilation.

BOX 8-2

Disease of the arterial walls can lead to obstruction of the arteries and symptoms, called **intermittent claudication** when it occurs in the legs. The symptoms consist of leg pain when walking or climbing stairs, which is relieved by rest. The disease is called **thromboangiitis obliterans** and is seen most frequently in men who are smokers. With minimal walking, the resistance vessels become maximally dilated by local metabolite release; when the oxygen demand of the muscles increases with further walking, blood flow cannot increase sufficiently to meet the muscle needs for oxygen, and pain caused by muscle ischemia results.

■ EXTRINSIC CONTROL OF PERIPHERAL BLOOD FLOW IS MEDIATED MAINLY BY THE SYMPATHETIC NERVOUS SYSTEM

Impulses Arising in the Medulla Descend in the Sympathetic Nerves to Increase Vascular Resistance

Several regions in the medulla influence cardiovascular activity. Some of the effects of stimulation of the dorsal lateral medulla (**pressor region**) are vasoconstriction, cardiac acceleration, and enhanced myocardial contractility. Caudal and ventromedial to the pressor region is a zone that produces a decrease in blood pressure on stimulation. This **depressor** area exerts its effect by direct spinal inhibition and by inhibition of the medullary pressor region. These areas constitute a center, not in an anatomical sense in that a discrete group of cells is discernible, but in a physiological sense in that stimulation of the pressor region produces the responses mentioned previously. From the vasoconstrictor regions, fibers descend in the spinal cord and synapse at different levels of the thoracolumbar region (T1 to L2 or L3). Fibers from the intermediolateral gray matter of the cord emerge with the ventral roots but leave the motor fibers to join the paravertebral sympathetic chains through the white communicating branches. These preganglionic white (myelinated) fibers may pass up or down the sympathetic chains to synapse in the various ganglia within the chains or in certain outlying ganglia. Postganglionic gray branches (unmyelinated) then join the corresponding segmental spinal nerves and accompany them to the periphery to innervate the arteries and veins. Postganglionic sympathetic fibers from the various ganglia join the large arteries and accompany them as an investing network of fibers to the resistance (small arteries and arterioles) and capacitance vessels (veins).

The vasoconstrictor regions are tonically active, and reflexes or humoral stimuli that enhance this activity result in an increase in frequency of impulses reaching the terminal branches to the vessels, where a constrictor neurohumor (**norepinephrine**) is released and elicits constriction (α-adrenergic effect) of the resistance vessels. Inhibition of the vasoconstrictor areas reduces their tonic activity and hence diminishes the frequency of impulses in the efferent nerve fibers, resulting in vasodilation. In this manner, neural regulation of the peripheral circulation is accomplished primarily by alteration of the number of impulses passing down the vasoconstrictor fibers of the sympathetic nerves to the blood vessels. The vasomotor regions may show rhythmic changes in tonic activity manifested as oscillations of arterial pressure. Some occur at the frequency of respiration (**Traube-Hering waves**) and are caused by an increase in sympathetic impulses to the resistance vessels coincident with inspiration.

Others are independent of, and at a lower frequency than, respiration **(Mayer waves).**

Sympathetic Nerves Regulate the Contractile State of Resistance and Capacitance Vessels

The vasoconstrictor fibers of the sympathetic nervous system supply the arteries, arterioles, and veins, but neural influence on the larger vessels is of far less functional importance than it is on the arterioles and small arteries. Capacitance vessels are more responsive to sympathetic nerve stimulation than are resistance vessels; they reach maximal constriction at a lower frequency of stimulation than do the resistance vessels. However, capacitance vessels do not possess β-adrenergic receptors, nor do they respond to vasodilator metabolites. Norepinephrine is the neurotransmitter released at the sympathetic nerve terminals in the blood vessels, and many factors, such as circulating hormones and particularly locally released substances, modify the liberation of norepinephrine from the vesicles of the nerve terminals.

The response of the resistance and capacitance vessels to stimulation of the sympathetic fibers is illustrated in Figure 8-7. At constant arterial pressure, sympathetic fiber stimulation evoked a reduction of blood flow (constriction of the resistance vessels) and a decrease in blood volume of the tissue (constriction of the capacitance vessels). The abrupt decrease in tissue volume is caused by movement of blood out of the capacitance vessels and out of the hindquarters of the cat, whereas the late, slow, progressive decline in volume (to the right of the arrow) is caused by movement of extravascular fluid into the capillaries and hence away from the tissue. The loss of tissue fluid is a consequence of the lowered capillary hydrostatic pressure brought about by constriction of the resistance vessels, with establishment of a new equilibrium of the forces responsible for filtration and absorption across the capillary wall (see p 168).

At basal tone, approximately one third of the blood volume of a tissue can be mobilized on stimulation of the sympathetic nerves at physiological frequencies. The basal tone is very low in capacitance vessels; with veins denervated,

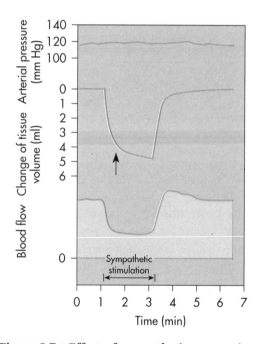

Figure 8-7 ■ **Effect of sympathetic nerve stimulation (2 Hz) on blood flow and tissue volume in the hindquarters of the cat. The arrow denotes the change in slope of the tissue volume curve where the volume decrease caused by emptying of capacitance vessels ceases and loss of extravascular fluid becomes evident.** (Redrawn from Mellander S: *Acta Physiol Scand* 50[suppl 176]:1-86, 1960.)

only small increases in volume are obtained with maximal doses of acetylcholine. Therefore the blood volume at basal tone is close to the maximal blood volume of the tissue. More blood can be mobilized from the skin than from the muscle capacitance vessels, in part because of greater sensitivity of the skin vessels to sympathetic stimulation, but also because basal tone is lower in skin vessels than in muscle vessels. Therefore in the absence of neural influence, the skin capacitance vessels contain more blood than do the muscle capacitance vessels.

Blood is mobilized from capacitance vessels in response to physiological stimuli. In exercise, activation of the sympathetic nerve fibers produces constriction of veins and hence augments the cardiac filling pressure. In **arterial hypotension,** as induced by hemorrhage, the capacitance vessels constrict and thereby aid in overcoming the associated decrease in central venous pressure. In addition, the resistance vessels constrict in **hemorrhage shock** and thereby assist in the restoration of arterial pressure (see Chapter 12). Furthermore, extravascular fluid is mobilized by a greater reabsorption of fluid from the tissues into the capillaries in response to the lowered capillary hydrostatic pressure caused by the lower arterial pressure.

In brief, neural and humoral stimuli can exert similar or dissimilar effects on different segments of the vascular tree, and in so doing can alter blood flow, tissue blood volume, and extravascular volume to meet the physiological requirements of the organism.

Parasympathetic Nervous System Only Innervates Blood Vessels in the Cranial and Sacral Regions of the Body

The efferent fibers of the cranial division of the parasympathetic nervous system supply blood vessels of the head and viscera, whereas fibers of the sacral division supply blood vessels of the genitalia, bladder, and large bowel. Skeletal muscle and skin do not receive parasympathetic innervation. Because only a small proportion of the resistance vessels of the body receive parasympathetic fibers, the effect of these cholinergic fibers on total vascular resistance is small.

Epinephrine and Norepinephrine Are the Main Humoral Factors That Affect Vascular Resistance

Epinephrine and norepinephrine exert a profound effect on the peripheral blood vessels. In skeletal muscle, epinephrine in low concentrations dilates resistance vessels (**β-adrenergic effect**) and in high concentrations produces constriction (**α-adrenergic effect**). In skin, only vasoconstriction is obtained with epinephrine, whereas in all vascular beds the primary effect of norepinephrine is vasoconstriction. When stimulated, the adrenal gland can release epinephrine and norepinephrine into the systemic circulation. However, under physiological conditions, the effect of catecholamine release from the adrenal medulla is of lesser importance than norepinephrine release produced by sympathetic nerve activation.

The Vascular Reflexes Are Responsible for Rapid Adjustments of Blood Pressure

Areas of the medulla that mediate sympathetic and vagal effects are under the influence of neural impulses arising in the baroreceptors, chemoreceptors, hypothalamus, cerebral cortex, and skin. These areas of the medulla are also affected by changes in the blood concentrations of CO_2 and O_2.

Arterial Baroreceptors The **baroreceptors** (or **pressoreceptors**) are stretch receptors located in the carotid sinuses (slightly widened areas of the internal carotid arteries at their points of origin from the common carotid arteries) and in the aortic arch (Figure 8-8). Impulses arising in the carotid sinus travel up the sinus nerve to the glossopharyngeal nerve and, via the latter, to the nucleus of the **tractus solitarius (NTS)** in the medulla. The NTS is the site

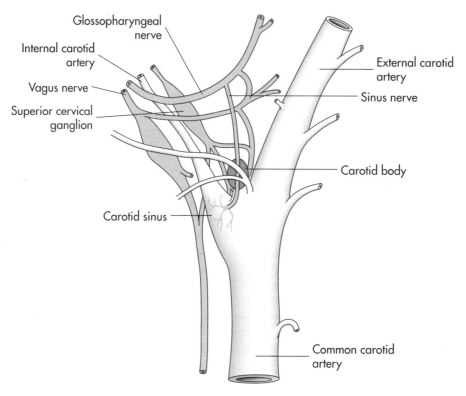

Glossopharyngeal
nerve

Internal carotid
artery

Vagus nerve

Superior cervical
ganglion

External carotid
artery

Sinus nerve

Carotid body

Carotid sinus

Common carotid
artery

Figure 8-8 ■ **Diagrammatic representation of the carotid sinus and carotid body and their innerva-tion in the dog.** (Redrawn from Adams WE: *The comparative morphology of the carotid body and carotid sinus,* Springfield, IL, 1958, Charles C Thomas.)

of central projection of the chemoreceptors and baroreceptors. Stimulation of the NTS inhibits sympathetic nerve impulses to the peripheral blood vessels **(depressor effect),** whereas lesions of the NTS produce vasoconstriction **(pressor effect).** Impulses arising in the pressoreceptors of the aortic arch reach the NTS via afferent fibers in the vagus nerves. *The pressoreceptor nerve terminals in the walls of the carotid sinus and aortic arch respond to the stretch and deformation of the vessel induced by the arterial pressure.* The frequency of firing is enhanced by an increase in blood pressure and diminished by a reduction in blood pressure. An increase in impulse frequency, as oc-

curs with a rise in arterial pressure, inhibits the vasoconstrictor regions, resulting in peripheral vasodilation and a lowering of blood pressure. Bradycardia, elicited by stimulation of the vagal nuclei in the medulla, contributes to a lowering of the blood pressure.

The carotid sinus and aortic baroreceptors are not equipotent in their effects on peripheral resistance in response to nonpulsatile alterations in blood pressure. The carotid sinus baroreceptors are more sensitive than those in the aortic arch. Changes in pressure in the carotid sinus evoke greater alterations in systemic arterial pressure than do equivalent changes in aortic arch pressure. However, with pulsatile

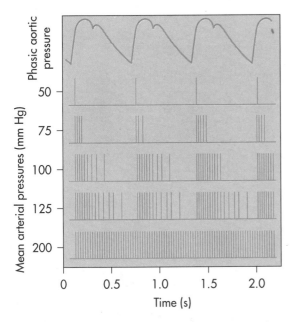

Figure 8-9 ■ **Relationship of phasic aortic blood pressure in the firing of a single afferent nerve fiber from the carotid sinus at different levels of mean arterial pressure.**

changes in blood pressure, the two sets of baroreceptors respond similarly.

The carotid sinus with the sinus nerve intact can be isolated from the rest of the circulation and perfused by either a donor animal or an artificial perfusion system. Under these conditions, changes in the pressure within the carotid sinus are associated with reciprocal changes in the blood pressure of the experimental animal. The receptors in the walls of the carotid sinus show some adaptation and therefore are more responsive to constantly changing pressures than to sustained constant pressures. This is illustrated in Figure 8-9, which shows that at normal levels of mean blood pressure (about 100 mm Hg) a barrage of impulses from a single fiber of the sinus nerve is initiated in early systole by the pressure rise, and only a few spikes are observed during late systole and early diastole. At

lower pressures these phasic changes are even more evident, but the overall frequency of discharge is reduced. The blood pressure threshold for eliciting sinus nerve impulses is about 50 mm Hg, and a maximal sustained firing is reached at around 200 mm Hg. Because the pressoreceptors show some degree of adaptation, their response at any level of mean arterial pressure is greater with a large than with a small pulse pressure. This is illustrated in Figure 8-10, which shows the effects of damping pulsations in the carotid sinus on the frequency of firing in a fiber of the sinus nerve and on the systemic arterial pressure. When the pulse pressure in the carotid sinuses is reduced with an air chamber, but mean pressure remains constant, the rate of electrical impulses recorded from a sinus nerve fiber decreases and the systemic arterial pressure increases. Restoration of the pulse pressure in the carotid sinus restores the frequency of sinus nerve discharge and systemic arterial pressure to control levels (Figure 8-10).

The resistance increases that occur in the peripheral vascular beds in response to reduced pressure in the carotid sinus vary from one vascular bed to another and thereby produce a redistribution of blood flow. For example, in the dog the resistance changes elicited by altering carotid sinus pressure around the normal operating sinus pressure are greatest in the femoral vessels, less in the renal, and least in the mesenteric and celiac vessels. Furthermore, the sensitivity of the carotid sinus reflex can be altered. Local application of norepinephrine or stimulation of sympathetic nerve fibers to the carotid sinuses enhances the sensitivity of the receptors in the sinus so that a given increase in intrasinus pressure produces a greater depressor response. A decrease in baroreceptor sensitivity occurs in hypertension when the carotid sinus becomes stiffer and less deformable as a result of the high intraarterial pressure. Under these conditions a given increase in carotid sinus pressure elicits a

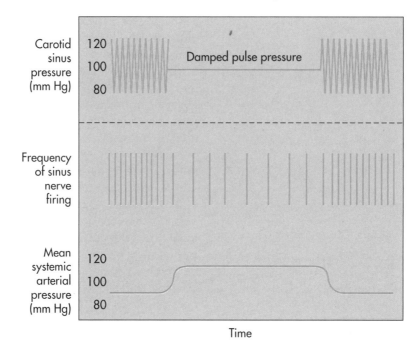

Figure 8-10 ■ **Effect of reducing pulse pressure in the vascularly isolated perfused carotid sinuses** *(top record)* **on impulses recorded from a fiber of a sinus nerve** *(middle record)* **and on mean systemic arterial pressure** *(bottom record)*. **Mean pressure in the carotid sinuses** *(horizontal line, top record)* **is held constant when pulse pressure is damped.**

smaller decrement in systemic arterial pressure than it does at normal levels of blood pressure. In other words, the set point of the baroreceptors is raised in hypertension so that the threshold is increased and the receptors are less sensitive to change in transmural pressure.

As would be expected, denervation of the carotid sinus can produce temporary, and in some instances prolonged, hypertension.

The arterial baroreceptors play a key role in short-term adjustments of blood pressure when relatively abrupt changes in blood volume, cardiac output, or peripheral resistance (as in exercise) occur. However, *long-term control of blood pressure—that is, over days, weeks, and longer—is determined by the fluid balance of*

the individual, namely, the balance between fluid intake and fluid output. By far the single most important organ in the control of body fluid volume, and hence of blood pressure, is the kidney. With overhydration excessive fluid intake is excreted, whereas with dehydration there is a marked reduction in urine output.

BOX 8-4

In some individuals the carotid sinus is quite sensitive to pressure. Hence tight collars or other forms of external pressure over the region of the carotid sinus may elicit marked hypotension and fainting.

Cardiopulmonary Baroreceptors In addition to the carotid sinus and aortic baroreceptors, there are cardiopulmonary receptors with vagal and sympathetic afferent and efferent nerves. These cardiopulmonary reflexes are tonically active and can alter peripheral resistance with changes in intracardiac, venous, or pulmonary vascular pressures. The receptors are located in the atria, ventricles, and pulmonary vessels.

The atria contain two types of receptors: those activated by the tension developed during atrial contraction (**A receptors**) and those activated by the stretch of the atria during atrial filling (**B receptors**). Stimulation of these atrial receptors sends impulses up vagal fibers to the vagal center in the medulla. Consequently, the sympathetic activity is decreased to the kidney and increased to the SA node. These changes in sympathetic activity increase renal blood flow, urine flow, and heart rate.

Activation of the cardiopulmonary receptors can also lower blood pressure reflexly by inhibiting the vasoconstrictor center in the medulla. Stimulation of the receptors inhibits angiotensin, aldosterone, and vasopressin (antidiuretic hormone) release; interruption of the reflex pathway has the opposite effects. Changes in urine volume elicited by changes in cardiopulmonary baroreceptor activation are important in the regulation of blood volume. For example, a decrease in blood volume (hypovolemia), as occurs in hemorrhage, enhances sympathetic vasoconstriction in the kidney and increases secretion of renin, angiotensin, aldosterone, and antidiuretic hormone. The renal vasoconstriction (primarily afferent arteriolar) reduces glomerular filtration and increases renin release from the kidney. Renin acts on a plasma substrate to form angiotensin, which increases aldosterone release from the adrenal cortex that in turn enhances retention

of NaCl. The enhanced release of antidiuretic hormone increases water reabsorption. The net result is retention of salt and water by the kidney and a sensation of thirst. Angiotensin II (formed from angiotensin I by converting enzyme) also raises systemic arteriolar tone.

The Peripheral Chemoreceptors Are Stimulated by Decreases in Blood Oxygen Tension and pH and by Increases in Carbon Dioxide Tension

The peripheral chemoreceptors consist of small, highly vascular bodies in the region of the aortic arch (aortic bodies) and the carotid bodies just medial to the carotid sinuses (Figure 8-8). Although they are primarily concerned with the regulation of respiration, the chemoreceptors reflexly influence the vasomotor regions to a minor degree. A reduction in arterial blood O_2 tension (Pao_2) stimulates the chemoreceptors, and the consequent increase in the number of impulses in the afferent nerve fibers from the carotid and aortic bodies stimulates the vasoconstrictor regions. This action increases tone of the resistance and capacitance vessels.

Stimulation of the peripheral chemoreceptors by increased arterial blood CO_2 tension ($Paco_2$) and reduced pH elicit a reflex response that is quite small compared with the direct effect of **hypercapnia** (high $Paco_2$) and hydrogen ions on the vasomotor regions in the medulla. When hypoxia and hypercapnia coexist (asphyxia), the stimulation of the chemoreceptors is greater than the sum of the two gas stimuli when they act alone. The effects of asphyxia on blood pressure, heart rate, and respiration are shown in Figure 8-11 (see also Figures 4-14 and 4-15).

When the chemoreceptors are simultaneously with a reduction in pressure in the baroreceptors, the chemoreceptors potentiate the vasoconstriction observed in the periph-

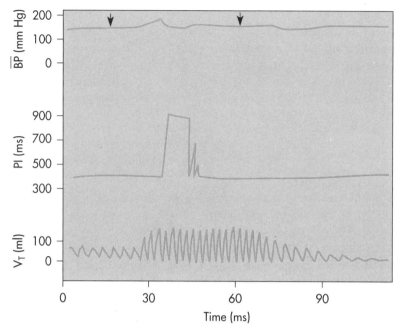

Figure 8-11 ■ **Effects of stimulation of the isolated perfused carotid body chemoreceptors at constant carotid sinus perfusion pressure, by substituting hypoxic hypercapnic blood (Po_2, 31.1 mm Hg; Pco_2, 84.9 mm Hg; pH, 7.242) for arterial blood (Po_2, 140.4 mm Hg; Pco_2, 42.1 mm Hg; pH, 7.33) between arrows. Note that the bradycardia was transient. The increase in pulse interval *(PI)* indicates a decrease in heart rate. The enhanced respiratory response *(bottom record)* abolishes bradycardia and can produce tachycardia, especially with sustained stimulation of the carotid body receptors (see Figures 4-14 and 4-15). $\overline{BP}$, Mean arterial blood pressure; V_T, tidal volume.** (Redrawn from Daly MdeB, Kouner PI, Angell-James JE, et al: *Clin Exp Pharmacol Physiol* 5:511, 1978.)

eral vessels. However, when the baroreceptors and chemoreceptors are stimulated together (e.g., high carotid sinus pressure and low Pao_2), the effects of the baroreceptors predominate.

BOX 8-5

Chemoreceptors with sympathetic afferent fibers are present in the heart. These cardiac chemoreceptors are activated by ischemia and transmit the precordial pain **(angina pectoris)** associated with an inadequate blood supply to the myocardium.

The Central Chemoreceptors Are Quite Sensitive to Changes in $Paco_2$

Increases of $Paco_2$ stimulate chemosensitive regions of the medulla and elicit vasoconstriction and increased peripheral resistance. Reduction in $Paco_2$ below normal levels (as with hyperventilation) decreases the degree of tonic activity of these areas in the medulla, thereby decreasing peripheral resistance. The chemosensitive regions are also affected by changes in pH. A lowering of blood pH stimulates, and a rise in blood pH inhibits, these areas. These effects of changes in $Paco_2$ and blood pH possibly operate through changes in cerebrospinal fluid pH, as appears to be the case for the respiratory center.

Oxygen tension has relatively little direct effect on the medullary vasomotor region. The primary effect of hypoxia is reflexly mediated via the carotid and aortic chemoreceptors. Moderate reduction of Pao_2 stimulates the vasomotor region, but severe reduction depresses vasomotor activity in the same manner that other areas of the brain are depressed by very low O_2 tensions.

BOX 8-6

At high altitudes the low Pao_2 stimulates the peripheral chemoreceptors to increase the rate and depth of respiration. This is the main mechanism involved in an attempt to restore the oxygen supply to the body.

Other Vascular Reflexes

Hypothalamus Optimal function of the cardiovascular reflexes requires the integrity of the pontine and hypothalamic structures. Furthermore, these structures are responsible for behavioral and emotional control of the cardiovascular system. Stimulation of the anterior hypothalamus produces a fall in blood pressure and bradycardia, whereas stimulation of the posterolateral region of the hypothalamus produces a rise in blood pressure and tachycardia. The hypothalamus also contains a temperature-regulating center that affects the skin vessels. Stimulation by cold applications to the skin or by cooling of the blood perfusing the hypothalamus results in constriction of the skin vessels and heat conservation, whereas warm stimuli result in cutaneous vasodilation and enhanced heat loss (see Chapter 11).

Cerebrum The cerebral cortex can also exert a significant effect on blood flow distribution in the body. Stimulation of the motor and premotor areas can affect blood pressure; usually a pressor response is obtained. However, vasodilation and depressor responses may be evoked

(e.g., blushing or fainting) in response to an emotional stimulus.

BOX 8-7

Cerebral ischemia, which may occur because of excessive pressure exerted by an expanding intracranial tumor, results in a marked increase in peripheral vasoconstriction. The stimulation is probably caused by a local accumulation of CO_2 and reduction of O_2, and possibly by excitation of intracranial baroreceptors. With prolonged, severe ischemia, central depression eventually supervenes and blood pressure falls.

Skin and Viscera Painful stimuli can elicit either pressor or depressor responses, depending on the magnitude and location of the stimulus. Distension of the viscera often evokes a depressor response, whereas painful stimuli on the body surface usually evoke a pressor response.

Pulmonary Reflexes Inflation of the lungs reflexly induces systemic vasodilation and a decrease in arterial blood pressure. Conversely, collapse of the lungs evokes systemic vasoconstriction. Afferent fibers that mediate this reflex are carried by the vagus nerves. Their stimulation by stretch of the lungs inhibits the vasomotor areas. The magnitude of the depressor response to lung inflation is directly related to the degree of inflation and to the existing level of vasoconstrictor tone; the greater the vascular tone, the greater the hypotension produced by lung inflation.

■ BALANCE BETWEEN EXTRINSIC AND INTRINSIC FACTORS IN REGULATION OF PERIPHERAL BLOOD FLOW

Dual control of the peripheral vessels by intrinsic and extrinsic mechanisms makes possible a number of vascular adjustments that enable the body to direct blood flow to areas where the need is greater and away from areas where the

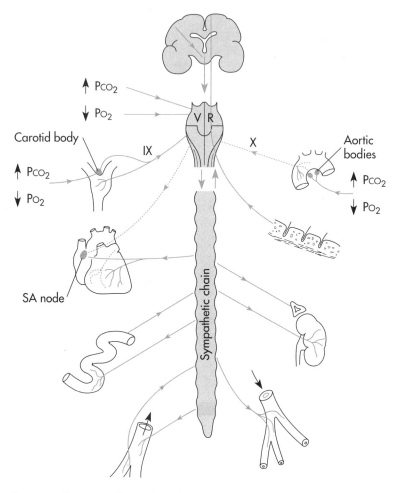

Figure 8-12 ■ Schematic diagram illustrating the neural input and output of the vasomotor region *(VR). IX,* Glossopharyngeal nerve; *X,* vagus nerve.

need is less. The relative potency of extrinsic and intrinsic mechanisms is constant in some tissues, whereas in other tissues the ratio is changeable, depending on the state of activity of that tissue.

In the brain and the heart, both vital structures with very limited tolerance for a reduced blood supply, intrinsic flow-regulating mechanisms are dominant.

BOX 8-8

Massive discharge of the vasoconstrictor region over the sympathetic nerves, which might occur in severe, acute hemorrhage, has negligible effects on the cerebral and cardiac resistance vessels, whereas skin, renal, and splanchnic blood vessels become greatly constricted.

In the skin the extrinsic vascular control is dominant. Not only do the cutaneous vessels participate strongly in a general vasoconstrictor discharge, but they also respond selectively through hypothalamic pathways to subserve the heat loss and heat conservation function required in body temperature regulation. However, intrinsic control can be demonstrated by local changes of temperature that can modify or override the central influence on resistance and capacitance vessels.

In skeletal muscle the interplay and changing balance between extrinsic and intrinsic mechanisms can be clearly seen. In resting skeletal muscle, neural control (vasoconstrictor tone) is dominant, as can be demonstrated by the large increment in blood flow that occurs immediately after section of the sympathetic nerves to the tissue. In anticipation of and at the start of exercise, such as running, blood flow increases in the leg muscles. After the onset of exercise the intrinsic flow-regulating mechanisms elicit vasodilation in the active muscles because of the local increase in metabolites. Vasoconstriction occurs in the inactive muscles as a manifestation of the general sympathetic discharge associated with exercise. However, the constrictor impulses that reach the resistance vessels of the active muscles are overridden by the local metabolic effect that dilates them. Hence operation of this dual control mechanism provides increased blood flow where it is required and shunts it away from the inactive areas.

Similar effects may be achieved with an increase in Pa_{CO_2}. Normally, the hyperventilation associated with exercise keeps Pa_{CO_2} at normal levels. However, were Pa_{CO_2} to increase, a generalized vasoconstriction would occur because of stimulation of the medullary vasoconstrictor region by CO_2. In the active muscles, where the CO_2 concentration is highest, the smooth muscle of the arterioles would relax in response to the local P_{CO_2}. Factors affecting and affected by the vasomotor region are summarized in Figure 8-12.

Summary

- The arterioles, often referred to as the resistance vessels, are important in the regulation of blood flow through their cognate capillaries. The smooth muscle, which makes up a major fraction of the walls of the arterioles, contracts and relaxes in response to neural and humoral stimuli.
- Most tissues show autoregulation of blood flow, a phenomenon characterized by a constant blood flow in the face of a change in perfusion pressure. A logical explanation of autoregulation is the myogenic mechanism whereby an increase in transmural pressure elicits a contractile response, whereas a decrease in transmural pressure elicits relaxation.
- The striking parallelism between tissue blood flow and tissue oxygen consumption indicates that blood flow is largely regulated by a metabolic mechanism. A decrease in the oxygen supply/oxygen demand ratio of a tissue releases one or more vasodilator metabolites that dilate arterioles and thereby enhance the oxygen supply.
- Neural regulation of blood flow is mainly accomplished by the sympathetic nervous system. Sympathetic nerves to blood vessels are tonically active; inhibition of the vasoconstrictor center in the medulla reduces peripheral vascular resistance. Stimulation of the sympathetic nerves constricts resistance and capacitance (veins) vessels.

- Blood vessels in the head, viscera, and genitalia are supplied by the cranial and sacral divisions of the parasympathetic nervous system, as well as by the sympathetic nervous system. Parasympathetic activity usually induces vasodilation, but the effect is generally weak.
- The baroreceptors (pressoreceptors) in the internal carotid arteries and aorta are tonically active and regulate blood pressure on a moment-to-moment basis. Stretch of these receptors by an increase in arterial pressure reflexly inhibits the vasoconstrictor center in the medulla and induces vasodilation, whereas a decrease in arterial pressure disinhibits the vasoconstrictor center and induces vasoconstriction.
- The carotid baroreceptors predominate over those in the aorta and both respond more vigorously to pulsatile (stretch) than they do to steady (nonpulsatile) pressure; they adapt to an imposed constant pressure.

- Baroreceptors are also present in the cardiac chambers and large pulmonary vessels (cardiopulmonary baroreceptors); they have less influence on blood pressure but they participate in blood volume regulation.
- Peripheral chemoreceptors (carotid and aortic bodies) and central chemoreceptors in the medulla oblongata are stimulated by a decrease in blood oxygen tension (Pa_{O_2}) and an increase in blood carbon dioxide tension (Pa_{CO_2}). Stimulation of these chemoreceptors increases the rate and depth of respiration but also produces peripheral vasoconstriction.
- Peripheral resistance, and hence blood pressure, can be affected by stimuli arising in the skin, viscera, lungs, and brain.
- The combined effect of neural and local metabolic factors is to distribute blood to active tissues and divert it from inactive tissues. In vital structures, such as the heart and brain and in contracting skeletal muscle, the metabolic factors predominate over the neural factors.

■ BIBLIOGRAPHY

1. Berg BR, Cohen KD, Sarelius IH: Direct coupling between blood flow and metabolism at the capillary level in striated muscle. *Am J Physiol* 272:H2693, 1997.
2. Berne RM, Knabb RM, Ely SW, et al: Adenosine in the local regulation of blood flow: a brief overview. *Fed Proc* 42:3136, 1983.
3. Cowley AW Jr: Long-term control of blood pressure. *Physiol Rev* 72:231, 1992.
4. Hainsworth R: Reflexes from the heart. *Physiol Rev* 71:617, 1991.
5. Hickner RC, Fisher JS, Ehsani AA, et al: Role of nitric oxide in skeletal muscle blood flow at rest and during dynamic exercise in humans. *Am J Physiol* 273:H405, 1997.
6. Hirst GDS, Edwards FR: Sympathetic neuroeffector transmission in arteries and arterioles. *Physiol Rev* 69:546, 1989.
7. Kuo L, Davis JJ, Chilian WM: Endothelium-dependent flow-induced dilation of isolated coronary arterioles. *Am J Physiol* 259:H1063, 1990.
8. Marshall JM: Peripheral chemoreceptors and cardiovascular regulation. *Physiol Rev* 74:543, 1994.
9. Monos E, Berczi V, Nadasy G: Local control of veins: biomechanical, metabolic, and humoral aspects. *Physiol Rev* 75:611, 1995.
10. Persson PB: Modulation of cardiovascular control mechanisms and their interaction. *Physiol Rev* 76:193, 1996.
11. Somlyo AP, Somlyo AV: *Smooth muscle structure and function.* In Fozzard HA, Haber E, Jennings RB, et al, editors: *The heart and cardiovascular system, scientific foundations,* ed 2, New York, 1991, Raven Press.
12. Sun D, Huang A, Smith CJ, et al: Enhanced release of prostaglandins to flow-induced arteriolar dilation in eNOs knockout mice. *Circ Res* 85:288, 1999.
13. Zucker IH, Gilmore JP, editors: *Reflex control of the circulation,* Boca Raton, FL, 1991, CRC Press.

■ CASE 8-1

HISTORY

A 40-year-old man sees his physician because of pain in the calves of both legs when he walks moderate distances; the pain is especially noticeable when he walks uphill or when he climbs stairs. The onset of the pain was insidious and has progressively increased in frequency and severity. He has had no other symptoms. He eats a normal diet, has two cocktails before dinner, and has smoked two packs of cigarettes per day for the past 22 years. Physical examination was essentially normal except for the absence of pulses in the dorsalis pedis and posterior tibial arteries in both legs. Arteriography revealed a narrowing of the major arteries of both lower legs. He was diagnosed as having thromboangiitis obliterans, a severe progressive obstructive disease of large arteries.

QUESTIONS

1. At rest the arterioles in the lower legs show
   a. Myogenic constriction
   b. Metabolic dilation
   c. Autoregulation
   d. Myogenic dilation
   e. Metabolic constriction
2. His physician would probably recommend
   a. He stop smoking
   b. A vasodilation drug
   c. Bilateral sympathectomy of the lower extremities
   d. Application of heat to the lower legs 3 to 4 times daily
   e. A vasoconstrictor drug

■ CASE 8-2

HISTORY

A 72-year-old man was admitted to the hospital for repeated brief episodes of loss of consciousness.

QUESTIONS

1. Which of the following diagnoses should <u>not</u> be considered?
   a. Carotid sinus hypersensitivity
   b. Complete heart block
   c. Orthostatic hypotension
   d. Atrial or ventricular tachycardia
   e. Diabetic coma
2. The electrocardiogram indicated supraventricular (atrial) tachycardia (SVT) as the cause of his syncope, a rare complication of SVT. Which of the following would *not* be prescribed for treatment of his dysrhythmia?
   a. Intravenous adenosine
   b. Valsalva's maneuver
   c. Digitalis
   d. Carotid sinus massage
   e. Electrical ablation of the atrial ectopic focus

CHAPTER 9

Control of Cardiac Output: Coupling of Heart and Blood Vessels

Objectives

1. Describe the principal determinants of cardiac output.

2. Describe the principal determinants of cardiac preload and afterload.

3. Explain the mechanical coupling between the heart and blood vessels.

4. Explain the effects of gravity on venous function.

FOUR FACTORS CONTROL CARDIAC output: heart rate, myocardial contractility, preload, and afterload (Figure 9-1). Heart rate and myocardial contractility are strictly **cardiac factors.** They are characteristics of the cardiac tissues, although they are modulated by various neural and humoral mechanisms. Preload and afterload, however, depend on the characteristics of both the heart and the vascular system. *On the one hand, preload and afterload are important determinants of cardiac output. On the other hand, preload and afterload are themselves determined by the cardiac output and by certain vascular characteristics.* Preload and afterload may be designated **coupling factors,** because they constitute a functional coupling between the heart and blood vessels.

To understand the regulation of cardiac output, it is important to appreciate the nature of the coupling between the heart and the vascular system. Graphic techniques have been developed to analyze the interactions between the cardiac and vascular components of the circulatory system. The graphic analysis involves two simultaneous functional relationships between **cardiac output** and **central venous pressure** (i.e., the pressure in the right atrium and thoracic venae cavae).

The curve that defines one of these relationships will be called the **cardiac function curve.** It is an expression of the well-known Frank-Starling relationship (see Chapters 3 and 4) and reflects the dependence of cardiac output on preload (i.e., central venous, or right atrial, pressure). *The cardiac function curve is a characteristic of the heart itself* and it has been studied in hearts completely isolated from the rest of the circulatory system.

The second curve, which we will call the **vascular function curve,** defines the depen-

199

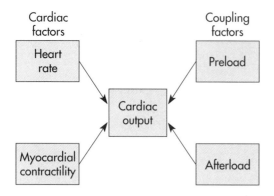

Figure 9-1 ■ The four factors that determine cardiac output.

dence of central venous pressure on cardiac output. This relationship depends only on certain vascular system characteristics, namely, peripheral resistance, arterial and venous compliances, and blood volume. *The vascular function curve is entirely independent of the characteristics of the heart,* and it could be evaluated even if the heart were replaced by a mechanical pump.

■ THE VASCULAR FUNCTION CURVE RELATES CENTRAL VENOUS PRESSURE TO CARDIAC OUTPUT

The vascular function curve is independent of the Frank-Starling relationship. *The vascular function curve defines the changes in central venous pressure evoked by changes in cardiac output;* that is, central venous pressure is the **dependent variable** (or **response**), and cardiac output is the **independent variable** (or **stimulus**). This contrasts with the cardiac function curve, for which central venous pressure (or preload) is the independent variable and cardiac output is the dependent variable.

The simplified model of the circulation illustrated in Figure 9-2 helps explain how cardiac output determines the level of central venous pressure. The essential components of the cardiovascular system have been lumped into four

elements. The right and left sides of the heart, as well as the pulmonary vascular bed, are considered simply as a **pump,** much as that employed during open heart surgery. The high-resistance microcirculation is designated the **peripheral resistance.** Finally, the compliance of the system is subdivided into two components, the **arterial compliance,** C_a, and the **venous compliance,** C_v. As defined in Chapter 6, compliance (C) is the increment of volume (ΔV) accommodated per unit change of pressure (ΔP); that is,

$$C = \Delta V/\Delta P \tag{1}$$

The venous compliance is about 20 times as great as the arterial compliance. In the example to follow, the ratio of C_v to C_a will be set at 19:1 to simplify certain calculations. Thus if it were necessary to add x ml of blood to the arterial system to produce a 1 mm Hg increment in arterial pressure, it would be necessary to add 19x ml of blood to the venous system to raise venous pressure by the same amount.

To illustrate why central venous pressure varies inversely with cardiac output, let us first give our model certain characteristics that resemble those of an average adult person (Figure 9-2, *A*). Let the flow (Q_h) generated by the heart (i.e., cardiac output) be 5 L/min; let mean arterial pressure, P_a, be 102 mm Hg; and let central venous pressure, P_v, be 2 mm Hg. The peripheral resistance, R, is the ratio of pressure difference ($P_a - P_v$) to flow (Q_r) through the resistance vessels; this ratio equals 20 mm Hg/L/min. An arteriovenous pressure difference of 100 mm Hg is sufficient to force a flow (Q_r) of 5 L/min through a peripheral resistance of 20 mm Hg/L/min; this flow (peripheral runoff) is precisely equal to the flow (Q_h) generated by the heart. From heartbeat to heartbeat, the volume (V_a) of blood in the arteries and the volume (V_v) of blood in the veins remain constant because the volume of blood transferred from the veins to the arteries by the

A Control state

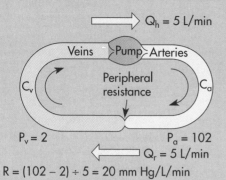

$$Q_h = 5 \text{ L/min}$$

Veins ⟩ Pump ⟩ Arteries

C_v

Peripheral resistance

C_a

$P_v = 2$ $P_a = 102$

$$Q_r = 5 \text{ L/min}$$

$$R = (102 - 2) \div 5 = 20 \text{ mm Hg/L/min}$$

Control state. The flow (Q_r) across the peripheral resistance is equal to the flow (Q_h) generated by the heart. The mean arterial pressure (P_a) is 102 mm Hg, the central venous pressure (P_v) is 2 mm Hg, and the peripheral resistance is 20 mm Hg/L/min.

B Beginning of cardiac arrest

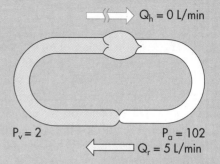

$$Q_h = 0 \text{ L/min}$$

$P_v = 2$ $P_a = 102$

$$Q_r = 5 \text{ L/min}$$

At the very beginning of cardiac arrest (i.e., $Q_h = 0$ L/min), P_a and P_v have not yet changed. Hence Q_r is still 5 L/min through a resistance of 20 mm Hg/L/min. Because of the disparity between Q_h and Q_r, P_a will begin to decrease rapidly and P_v will begin to rise rapidly.

C Cardiac arrest: steady state

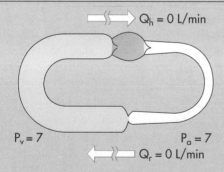

$$Q_h = 0 \text{ L/min}$$

$P_v = 7$ $P_a = 7$

$$Q_r = 0 \text{ L/min}$$

When the effects of cardiac arrest have attained the steady state, P_a will have fallen to 7 mm Hg and P_v will have risen to the same value. Because $P_a - P_v = 0$, flow across the resistance will cease (i.e., $Q_r = 0$).

D Beginning of cardiac resuscitation

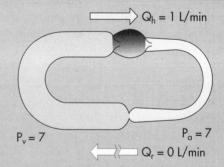

$$Q_h = 1 \text{ L/min}$$

$P_v = 7$ $P_a = 7$

$$Q_r = 0 \text{ L/min}$$

The heart is resuscitated and it begins to pump at a constant value of $Q_h = 1$ L/min. At the very beginning of resuscitation, P_a and P_v have not had time to change, and therefore Q_r is still 0 L/min. Because Q_h exceeds Q_r by 1 L/min, P_a will rise rapidly and P_v will fall rapidly. A new equilibrium will be attained when P_a increases to 26 mm Hg and P_v falls to 6 mm Hg. When $P_a - P_v = 20$ mm Hg, the flow (Q_r) through the resistance will be 1 L/min, which equals the cardiac output (Q_h).

Figure 9-2 ■ **Simplified model of the cardiovascular system, consisting of a pump, arterial compliance (C_a), peripheral resistance, and venous compliance (C_v).**

heart equals the volume of blood that flows from the arteries through the resistance vessels and into the veins.

Figure 9-2, *B* illustrates the status of the circulation at the very beginning of an episode of cardiac arrest, i.e., $Q_h = 0$. Initially, the volumes of blood in the arteries (V_a) and veins (V_v) have not had time to change. The arterial and venous pressures depend on V_a and V_v, respectively. Therefore these pressures are identical to the respective pressures in panel *A* (i.e., $P_a = 102$ and $P_v = 2$). The arteriovenous pressure gradient of 100 mm Hg will force a flow (the peripheral runoff) of 5 L/min through the peripheral resistance of 20 mm Hg/L/min. Although cardiac output now equals 0 L/min, the flow through the microcirculation transiently equals 5 L/min. In other words, the potential energy stored in the arteries by the previous pumping action of the heart causes blood to be transferred from arteries to veins, initially at the control rate, even though the heart can no longer transfer blood from the veins into the arteries.

As time passes, the blood volume in the arteries progressively decreases and the blood volume in the veins progressively increases. Because the vessels are elastic structures, arterial pressure falls gradually and venous pressure rises gradually. This process will continue until the arterial and venous pressures become equal (Figure 9-2, *C*). Once this condition is reached, the flow (Q_r) from the arteries to the veins through the resistance vessels will be zero, as is the cardiac output (Q_h).

At zero flow equilibrium (Figure 9-2, *C*), the pressure attained in the arteries and veins depends on the relative compliances of these vessels. Had the arterial (C_a) and venous (C_v) compliances been equal, the decline in P_a would have been equal to the rise in P_v because the decrement in arterial volume equals the increment in venous volume (principle of conservation of mass). P_a and P_v would have both attained the average of P_a and P_v in panels *A* and *B*, i.e., $P_a = P_v = (102 + 2)/2 = 52$ mm Hg.

However, the veins are much more compliant than the arteries; the compliance ratio is approximately equal to the ratio ($C_v : C_a = 19$) that we have assumed for the model. Hence the transfer of blood from arteries to veins at equilibrium would induce a fall in arterial pressure 19 times as great as the concomitant rise in venous pressure. As Figure 9-2, *C* shows, P_v would increase by 5 mm Hg (from 2 to 7 mm Hg), whereas P_a would fall by $19 \times 5 = 95$ mm Hg (from 102 to 7 mm Hg). This equilibrium pressure that prevails in the circulatory system in the absence of flow is often referred to as the **mean circulatory pressure,** or **static pressure.** The pressure in the static system reflects the total volume of blood in the system and the overall compliance of the entire system.

The example of cardiac arrest in Figure 9-2 provides the basis for understanding the vascular function curves. Two important points on the curve have already been derived, as shown in Figure 9-3. One point *(A)* represents the normal operating status (depicted in Figure 9-2, *A*). At that point, when cardiac output was 5 L/min, P_v was 2 mm Hg. Then, when flow stopped (cardiac output = 0), P_v became 7 mm Hg at equilibrium; this pressure is the mean circulatory pressure, P_{mc}.

The inverse relation between central venous pressure and cardiac output in Figure 9-3 simply denotes that when cardiac output is suddenly decreased, the peripheral runoff from arteries to veins is temporarily greater than the rate at which the heart pumps it from the veins back into the arteries. During that transient period, a net volume of blood is translocated from arteries to veins; hence, P_a falls and P_v rises.

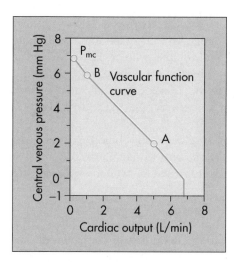

Figure 9-3 ■ **Changes in central venous pressure produced by changes in cardiac output. The mean circulatory pressure (or static pressure), P_{mc}, is the equilibrium pressure throughout the cardiovascular system when cardiac output is 0. Points B and A represent the values of venous pressure at cardiac outputs of 1 and 5 L/min, respectively.**

An example of a sudden increase in cardiac output, but with peripheral resistance remaining constant, will illustrate how a third point (B) on the vascular function curve is derived. Consider that the arrested heart is suddenly restarted and immediately begins pumping blood from the veins into the arteries at a rate of 1 L/min (Figure 9-2, D). When the heart first begins to beat, the arteriovenous pressure gradient is zero, and hence no blood flows from the arteries into the veins. When beating has just resumed, blood is being depleted from the veins at the rate of 1 L/min, and the arterial volume is being repleted at the same rate. Hence P_v begins to fall and P_a begins to rise. Because of the difference in compliances, P_a will rise 19 times more rapidly than P_v will fall.

The resulting pressure gradient will cause blood to flow through the resistance. If the heart maintains a constant output of 1 L/min, P_a will continue to rise and Pv will continue to fall until the pressure gradient becomes 20 mm Hg. This gradient will force a flow of 1 L/min through a resistance of 20 mm Hg/L/min. This gradient will be achieved by a 19 mm Hg rise (to 26 mm Hg) in P_a and a 1 mm Hg fall (to 6 mm Hg) in P_v. This equilibrium value of $P_v = 6$ mm Hg for a cardiac output of 1 L/min also appears (B) on the vascular function curve of Figure 9-3. It reflects a net transfer of blood from the venous to the arterial side of the circuit after the heart has been restarted, and a consequent reduction of P_v.

The reduction of P_v that can be achieved by an increase in cardiac output is limited. At some critical maximal value of cardiac output, sufficient fluid will be translocated from the venous to the arterial side of the circuit to reduce P_v below the ambient pressure. In a system of very distensible vessels, such as the venous system, the vessels will collapse when the intravascular pressure falls below the extravascular pressure. This venous collapse constitutes an impediment to venous return to the heart. Hence it will limit the maximal value of cardiac output to 7 L/min in this example (see Figure 9-3), regardless of the capabilities of the pump. For readers interested in the mathematical derivation of these results, the basic equations are presented in the next section.

Mathematical Analysis of the Vascular Function Curve

From the definition of peripheral resistance (see Chapter 5):

$$R = (P_a - P_v)/Q_r \qquad (2)$$

where R is resistance, P_a is arterial pressure, P_v is venous pressure, and Q_r is blood flow through the resistance vessels.

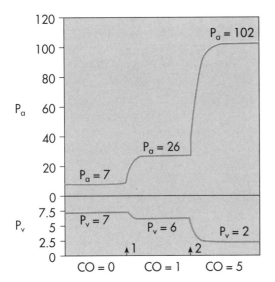

Figure 9-4 ■ **Changes in arterial** (P_a) **and venous** (P_v) **pressures in the circulatory model shown in Figure 9-3. The total peripheral resistance is 20 mm Hg/L/min, and the ratio of** C_v **to** C_a **is 19:1. The cardiac output (CO) is 0 to the left of arrow** *1*. **It is increased to 1 L/min at arrow** *1*, **and to 5 L/min at arrow** *2*.

At equilibrium, Q_r equals cardiac output, Q_h. Assume that R = 20 and that Q_h had been 0, but that it had then been increased to a constant value of 1 L/min (Figure 9-4, arrow *1*). If we solve equation 2 for P_a when the system is in equilibrium (i.e., $Q_r = Q_h$):

$$P_a = P_v + Q_r R = P_v + (1 \times 20) \tag{3}$$

Thus P_a will increase to a value 20 mm Hg greater than P_v. It will continue to be 20 mm Hg above Pv, as long as the pump output is maintained at 1 L/min and the peripheral resistance remains at 20 mm Hg/L/min.

We can calculate what the actual changes in P_a and P_v will be when Q_r attains a constant value of 1 L/min. The arterial volume increment needed to achieve the required level of P_a depends entirely on the arterial compliance,

C_a. For a rigid arterial system (low compliance), this volume will be small; for a distensible system, the volume will be large. Whatever the magnitude, however, the change in volume represents the translocation of some quantity of blood from the venous to the arterial side of the circuit.

For a given total blood volume, any increment in arterial volume (ΔV_a) must equal the decrement in venous volume (ΔV_v); that is,

$$\Delta V_a = - \Delta V_v \tag{4}$$

From the definition of compliance,

$$C_a = \Delta V_a / \Delta P_a \tag{5}$$

and

$$C_v = \Delta V_v / \Delta P_v \tag{6}$$

By substitution into equation 4,

$$\frac{\Delta P_v}{\Delta P_a} = - \frac{C_a}{C_v} \tag{7}$$

Given that C_v is 19 times as great as C_a, the increment in P_a will be 19 times as great as the decrement in P_v; that is,

$$\Delta P_a = -19\Delta P_v \tag{8}$$

To calculate the absolute values of P_a and P_v, let ΔP_a represent the difference between the prevailing P_a and the mean circulatory pressure (P_{mc}); that is, let

$$\Delta P_a = P_a - P_{mc} \tag{9}$$

and let ΔP_v represent the difference between the prevailing P_v and the mean circulatory pressure.

$$\Delta P_v = P_v - P_{mc} \tag{10}$$

Substituting these values for ΔP_a and ΔP_v into equation 8:

$$P_a - P_{mc} = -19 (P_v - P_{mc}) \tag{11}$$

By solving equations 3 and 11 simultaneously:

$$P_a = P_{mc} + 19 \qquad (12)$$

and

$$P_v = P_{mc} - 1 \qquad (13)$$

Hence for a mean circulatory pressure of 7 mm Hg, P_a increases to 26 mm Hg and P_v decreases to 6 mm Hg when Q_h increases from 0 to 1 L/min (Figure 9-4). These pressure changes provide the required arteriovenous pressure gradient of 20 mm Hg.

If the pump output is abruptly increased to a constant level of 5 L/min (Figure 9-4, arrow *2*) and peripheral resistance remains constant at 20 mm Hg/L/min, an additional volume of blood again will be translocated from the venous to the arterial side of the circuit. It will progressively accumulate in the arteries until P_a reaches a level of 100 mm Hg above P_v, as shown by substitution into equation 3:

$$P_a = P_v + Q_rR = P_v + (5 \times 20) \qquad (14)$$

By solving equations 11 and 14 simultaneously, we find that P_a rises to a value of 95 mm Hg above P_{mc}, and P_v falls to a value 5 mm Hg below P_{mc}. In Figure 9-4, therefore, P_v declines to 2 mm Hg and P_a rises to 102 mm Hg. The resulting pressure gradient of 100 mm Hg will force a cardiac output of 5 L/min through a constant peripheral resistance of 20 mm Hg/L/min.

The following equation for P_v as a function of Q_r in the model is derived from equations 2, 7, 9, and 10 above:

$$P_v = -\frac{RC_a}{C_a + C_v} Q_r + P_{mc} \qquad (15)$$

Note that the slope depends only on R, C_a and C_v. Note also that when $Q_r = 0$, $P_v = P_{mc}$; that is, at zero flow, P_v equals the mean circulatory pressure.

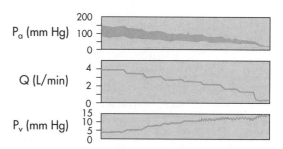

Figure 9-5 ■ **Changes in arterial (P_a) and central venous (P_v) pressures produced by changes in systemic blood flow (Q_r) in a canine right-heart bypass preparation. Stepwise changes in Q_r were produced by altering the rate of a mechanical pump.** (From Levy MN: *Circ Res* 44:739, 1979.)

Venous Pressure Depends on Cardiac Output

Experimental and clinical observations have shown that changes in cardiac output do indeed evoke the alterations in P_a and P_v that have been predicted above for our simplified model. In an experiment on an anesthetized dog, for example, a mechanical pump was substituted for the right ventricle (Figure 9-5). As the cardiac output, Q, was diminished in a series of small steps, P_a fell and P_v rose.

BOX 9-1

Similarly, a major coronary artery may suddenly become occluded in a human patient. The resultant acute **myocardial infarction (death of myocardial tissue)** often diminishes cardiac output, which is attended by a fall in arterial pressure and a rise in central venous pressure.

Blood Volume

The vascular function curve is affected by variations in total blood volume. During circulatory standstill (zero cardiac output), the mean circulatory pressure depends only on total vascular compliance and blood volume, as stated previously. Thus for a given vascular compliance the mean circulatory pressure will be increased when the blood volume is expanded (**hypervolemia**) and decreased when the blood volume is diminished (**hypovolemia**). This is illustrated by the Y-axis intercepts in Figure 9-6, where the mean circulatory pressure is 5 mm Hg after hemorrhage and 9 mm Hg after transfusion, as compared with the value of 7 mm Hg at the normal blood volume (**normovolemia**).

From Figure 9-6 it is also apparent that the cardiac output at which $P_v = 0$ varies directly with the blood volume. Therefore the maximal value of cardiac output becomes progressively more limited as the total blood volume is

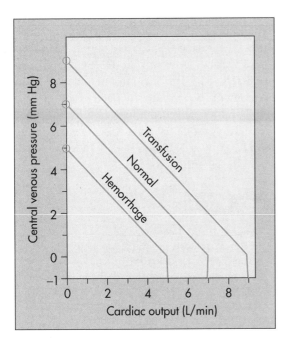

Figure 9-6 ■ **Effects of increased blood volume** (*transfusion curve*) **and of decreased blood volume** (*hemorrhage curve*) **on the vascular function curve. Similar shifts in the vascular function curve are produced by increases and decreases, respectively, in venomotor tone.**

reduced. However, the pressure ($P_v = 0$) at which the veins collapse (sharp change in slope of the vascular function curve) is not altered appreciably by changes in blood volume. This pressure depends only on the pressure surrounding the central veins.

Furthermore, the differences in P_v during hypervolemia, normovolemia, and hypovolemia in the static system are preserved at each level of cardiac output such that the vascular function curves parallel each other (Figure 9-6). To illustrate, consider the example of hypervolemia, in which the mean circulatory pressure is 9 mm Hg. In Figure 9-6, both P_a and P_v would be 9 mm Hg, instead of 7 mm Hg, when the cardiac output is zero. With a sudden increase in cardiac output to 1 L/min (at arrow *1*, Figure 9-4), if the peripheral resistance was still 20 mm Hg/L/min, an arteriovenous pressure gradient of 20 mm Hg would still be necessary for 1 L/min to flow through the resistance vessels. This does not differ from the example for normovolemia. Assuming the same ratio of C_v to C_a of 19:1, the pressure gradient would be achieved by a 1 mm Hg decline in P_v and a 19 mm Hg rise in P_a. Hence a change in cardiac output from 0 to 1 L/min would evoke the same 1 mm Hg reduction in P_v irrespective of the blood volume, as long as C_a, C_v, and the peripheral resistance were independent of blood volume. Equation 15 also discloses that the slope of the vascular function curve remains constant as long as R, C_v, and C_a do not change.

Venomotor Tone

The effects of changes in venomotor tone on the vascular function curve closely resemble those for changes in blood volume. In Figure 9-6, for example, the transfusion curve could just as well represent increased venomotor tone, whereas the hemorrhage curve could represent decreased tone. During circulatory standstill, for a given blood volume, the pressure within the vascular system will rise as the tension exerted by the smooth muscle within the vascular walls increases. It is principally the arteriolar and venous smooth muscle that is under any notable nervous or humoral control. The fraction of the blood volume located within the arterioles is very small, whereas the blood volume in the veins is large (see Table 1-1). Therefore if blood volume remains constant, only changes in venous tone can alter the mean circulatory pressure appreciably. Hence mean circulatory pressure rises with increased venomotor tone and falls with diminished tone.

Experimentally, the pressure attained shortly after abrupt circulatory standstill is usually above 7 mm Hg, even when blood volume is normal. This is attributable to the generalized venoconstriction elicited by cerebral ischemia, activation of the arterial and central chemoreceptors, and reduced excitation of the arterial baroreceptors. If resuscitation is not successful, this reflex response subsides as central nervous activity ceases. At normal blood volume the mean circulatory pressure usually approaches a value close to 7 mm Hg.

Blood Reservoirs

Venoconstriction is considerably greater in certain regions of the body than in others. In effect, large vascular beds that undergo appreciable venoconstriction constitute blood reservoirs. The vascular bed of the skin is one of the major blood reservoirs in humans. Blood loss evokes profound subcutaneous venoconstriction, which produces the characteristic pale appearance of the skin in people who have lost a substantial amount of blood. The resulting diversion of blood away from the skin liberates several hundred milliliters of blood to be perfused through more vital regions. The vascular beds of the liver, lungs, and spleen are also important blood reservoirs. In the dog the spleen

is packed with red blood cells and can constrict to a small fraction of its normal size. During hemorrhage, this mechanism autotransfuses blood of high erythrocyte content into the general circulation. However, in humans the volume changes of the spleen are considerably smaller (see also Chapter 12).

Peripheral Resistance

The changes in the vascular function curve induced by changes in arteriolar tone are shown in Figure 9-7. The arterioles contain only about 3% of the total blood volume (see Table 1-1). Changes in the contractile state of these vessels do not significantly alter the mean circulatory pressure, as stated previously. Thus the family of vascular function curves that represent different peripheral resistances converges at a common point on the ordinate.

At any given cardiac output, P_v varies inversely with the arteriolar tone, all other factors remaining constant. Arteriolar constriction suffi-

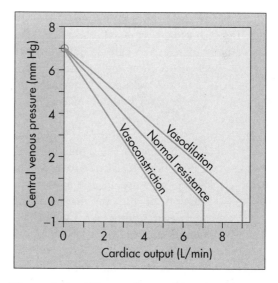

Figure 9-7 ■ **Effects of arteriolar vasodilation and vasoconstriction on the vascular function curve.**

cient to double the peripheral resistance will cause a twofold rise in P_a (see Chapter 6). In the example shown in Figure 9-4, a change in the cardiac output from 0 to 1 L/min (arrow *1*) caused P_a to rise from 7 to 26 mm Hg, an increment of 19 mm Hg. If peripheral resistance had been twice as great, the same change in cardiac output would have evoked twice as great an increment in P_a.

To achieve this greater rise in P_a, twice as great an increment in blood volume would be required on the arterial side of the circulation, if the arterial compliance remained constant. Given a constant total blood volume, this larger arterial volume signifies a corresponding reduction in venous volume. Hence the decrement in venous volume would be twice as great when the peripheral resistance was doubled.

If venous compliance remained constant, a twofold reduction in venous volume would be reflected by a twofold decline in P_v. Therefore in Figure 9-4, an increase in cardiac output from 0 L/min to 1 L/min (arrow *1*) would have caused a 2 mm Hg decrement in P_v, to a level of 5 mm Hg, instead of the 1 mm Hg decrement that occurred with normal peripheral resistance. Similarly, greater increases in cardiac output would have evoked proportionately greater decrements in P_v under conditions of increased peripheral resistance than with normal levels of resistance.

This relationship between the peripheral resistance and the decrement in P_v, together with the failure of peripheral resistance to affect the mean circulatory pressure, accounts for the clockwise rotation of the vascular function curves with increased peripheral resistance (see Figure 9-7). Conversely, arteriolar vasodilation is associated with a counterclockwise rotation from the same vertical axis intercept. A higher maximal level of cardiac output is attainable when the resistance vessels are dilated than when they are constricted.

■ CARDIAC OUTPUT AND VENOUS RETURN ARE CLOSELY ASSOCIATED

Except for small, transient disparities, the heart is unable to pump any more blood than is delivered to it through the venous system. Similarly, because the circulatory system is a closed circuit, the venous return must equal the cardiac output over any appreciable time interval. The flow around the entire closed circuit depends on the capability of the pump, the characteristics of the circuit, and the total volume of fluid in the system. Cardiac output and venous return are simply two terms for the flow around the closed circuit. Cardiac output is the volume of blood being pumped by the heart per unit time. Venous return is the volume of blood returning to the heart per unit time. At equilibrium, these two flows are equal.

The techniques of circuit analysis will be applied in an effort to gain some insight into the control of flow around the circuit. Acute changes in cardiac contractility, peripheral resistance, or blood volume may transiently affect cardiac output and venous return disparately. Except for such brief disparities, however, such factors simply alter flow around the entire circuit. Whether one thinks of that flow as "cardiac output" or "venous return" is irrelevant. Many authors have ascribed a reduction in cardiac output during some intervention, such as hemorrhage, to a decrease in venous return. Such an explanation, however, may be a blatant example of circular reasoning. Hemorrhage reduces flow around the entire circuit, for reasons to be elucidated. To attribute the reduction in cardiac output to a curtailment of venous return is equivalent to ascribing the decrease in total blood flow to a decrease in total blood flow!

■ THE HEART AND VASCULATURE ARE COUPLED FUNCTIONALLY

In accordance with Starling's law of the heart, cardiac output is intimately dependent on the right atrial (or central venous) pressure. Furthermore, right atrial pressure is approximately equal to right ventricular end-diastolic pressure, because the normal tricuspid valve constitutes a low resistance junction between the right atrium and ventricle. In the discussion to follow, graphs of cardiac output as a function of central venous pressure (P_v) will be called **cardiac function curves.** Extrinsic regulatory influences may be expressed as shifts in such curves, as indicated previously (see Figure 4-19).

A typical cardiac function curve is plotted on the same coordinates as a normal vascular function curve in Figure 9-8. *The cardiac function curve is plotted according to the usual convention;* that is, the variable (P_v) plotted along the abscissa is the **independent variable** (stimulus), and the variable (cardiac output) plotted along the ordinate is the **dependent variable** (response). In accordance with the Frank-Starling mechanism, *the cardiac function curve reveals that a rise in P_v causes an increase in cardiac output.*

Conversely, *the vascular function curve describes an inverse relationship between cardiac output and P_v;* that is, a rise in cardiac output causes a reduction in P_v. P_v is the dependent variable (or response) and cardiac output is the independent variable (or stimulus) for the vascular function curve. By convention, P_v should be scaled along the Y axis and cardiac output should be scaled along the X axis. Note that this convention is observed for the vascular function curves displayed in Figures 9-3, 9-6, and 9-7.

However, to include the vascular function curve on the same set of coordinate axes with the cardiac function curve (see Figure 9-8), it is necessary to violate the plotting convention for one of these curves. *We arbitrarily violated the convention for the vascular function curve. Note that the vascular function curve in Figure 9-8 reflects how P_v (scaled along the X axis)*

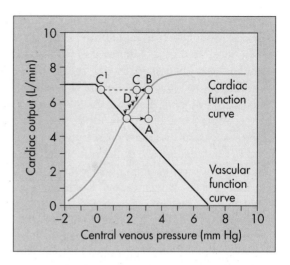

Figure 9-8 ■ **Typical vascular and cardiac function curves plotted on the same coordinate axes. Note that to plot both curves on the same graph, it is necessary to reverse the X and Y axes for the vascular function curves shown in Figures 9-3, 9-6, and 9-7. The coordinates of the equilibrium point, at the intersection of the cardiac and vascular function curves, represent the stable values of cardiac output and central venous pressure at which the system tends to operate. Any perturbation (e.g., when venous pressure is suddenly increased to point *A*) institutes a sequence of changes in cardiac output and venous pressure that restore these variables to their equilibrium values.**

varies in response to a change of cardiac output (scaled along the Y axis).

The **equilibrium point** of a system represented by a given pair of cardiac and vascular function curves is defined by the intersection of these two curves. The coordinates of this equilibrium point represent the values of cardiac output and P_v at which such a system tends to operate. Only transient deviations from such values for cardiac output and P_v are possible, as long as the given cardiac and vascular function curves accurately describe the system.

The tendency for the cardiovascular system to operate about such an equilibrium point may best be illustrated by examining its response to a sudden perturbation. Consider the changes elicited by a sudden rise in P_v from the equilibrium point to point A in Figure 9-8. Such a change might be induced by rapid injection, during ventricular diastole, of a given volume of blood on the venous side of the circuit, accompanied by withdrawal of an equal volume from the arterial side so that total blood volume would remain constant.

As defined by the cardiac function curve, this elevated P_v would increase cardiac output (A to B) during the very next ventricular systole. The increased cardiac output, in turn, would result in the net transfer of blood from the venous to the arterial side of the circuit, with a consequent reduction in P_v.

In one heartbeat, the reduction in P_v would be small (B to C) because the heart would transfer only a tiny fraction of the total venous blood volume over to the arterial side. Because of this reduction in P_v, the cardiac output during the very next beat diminishes (C to D) by an amount dictated by the cardiac function curve. Because D is still above the intersection point, the heart will pump blood from the veins to the arteries at a rate greater than that at which the blood will flow across the peripheral resistance from arteries to veins. Hence P_v will continue to fall. This process will continue in diminishing steps until the point of intersection is reached. Only one specific combination of cardiac output and venous pressure (denoted by the coordinates of the point of intersection) will satisfy simultaneously the requirements of the cardiac and vascular function curves.

Myocardial Contractility

Combinations of cardiac and vascular function curves help explain the effects of alterations in ventricular contractility. In Figure 9-9 the lower

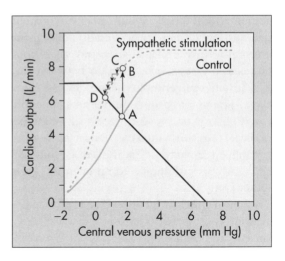

Figure 9-9 ■ **Enhancement of myocardial contractility, as by cardiac sympathetic nerve stimulation, causes the equilibrium values of cardiac output and P_v to shift from the intersection (point A) of the control vascular and cardiac function curves** (*continuous lines*) **to the intersection (point D) of the same vascular function curve with the cardiac function curve** (*dashed line*) **that represents enhanced myocardial contractility.**

cardiac function curve represents the control state, whereas the upper curve reflects an improved contractility. This pair of curves is analogous to the family of ventricular function curves shown in Figure 4-19. The enhancement of ventricular contractility might be achieved by electrical stimulation of the cardiac sympathetic nerves. If the effects of such stimulation were restricted to the heart, the vascular function curve would be unaffected. Therefore one vascular function curve would suffice, as shown in Figure 9-9.

During the control state the equilibrium values for cardiac output and P_v are designated by point A. Cardiac sympathetic nerve stimulation would abruptly raise cardiac output to point B, because of the enhanced contractility, before P_v would change appreciably. However, this high cardiac output would increase the net transfer of blood from the venous to the arterial side of the circuit, and consequently P_v would then begin to fall (point *C*). Cardiac output would continue to fall until a new equilibrium point *(D)* was reached; this point is located at the intersection of the vascular function curve with the new cardiac function curve. The new equilibrium point *(D)* lies above and to the left of the control equilibrium point *(A)*. This shift reveals that sympathetic stimulation evokes a greater cardiac output at a lower level of P_v.

Such a change accurately describes the true response. In the experiment depicted in Figure 9-10, the left stellate ganglion was stimulated between the two arrows. During stimulation, aortic flow (cardiac output) rose quickly to a peak value and then fell gradually to a steady-state value significantly greater than the control level. The increased aortic flow was accompanied by reductions in right and left atrial pressures (P_{RA} and P_{LA}). The initial abrupt rise in cardiac output in this experiment represents the shift from *A* to *B* in Figure 9-9, whereas the subsequent, more gradual reductions in cardiac output and atrial pressure in the experiment represent the progressive shift from *B* to *D*.

Blood Volume

Changes in blood volume affect the vascular function curve in the manner shown in Figure 9-6. To understand the circulatory alterations evoked by a given change in blood volume, the appropriate cardiac function curve should be plotted along with the vascular function curves that represent the control and experimental states.

Figure 9-11 illustrates the response to a blood transfusion. Equilibrium point *B,* which denotes the values for cardiac output and P_v after trans-

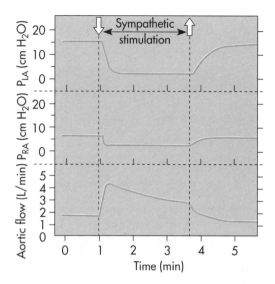

Figure 9-10 ■ During electrical stimulation of the left stellate ganglion (containing cardiac sympathetic nerve fibers), aortic blood flow increased while pressures in the left atrium (P_{LA}) and right atrium (P_{RA}) diminished. These data conform with the conclusions derived from Figure 9-9, in which the equilibrium values of cardiac output and venous pressure are observed to shift from point *A* to point *D* during cardiac sympathetic nerve stimulation. (Redrawn from Sarnoff SJ, Brockman SK, Gilmore JP, et al: *Circ Res* 8:1108, 1960.)

fusion, lies above and to the right of the control equilibrium point *A.* Thus transfusion increases both cardiac output and P_v. Hemorrhage has the opposite effect. Mechanistically, the change in ventricular filling pressure (central venous pressure) evoked by a given change in blood volume alters cardiac output by changing the sensitivity of the contractile proteins to the prevailing level of intracellular Ca^{++}, as explained in Chapters 3 and 4. Pure increases or decreases in venomotor tone elicit responses analogous to those evoked by augmentations or reductions, respectively, of the total blood volume, for reasons discussed on page 206.

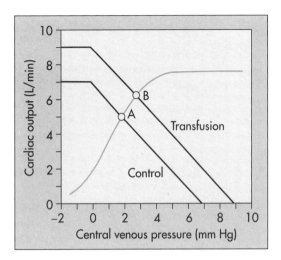

Figure 9-11 ■ After a blood transfusion, the vascular function curve is shifted to the right. Therefore cardiac output and venous pressure are both increased, as denoted by the translocation of the equilibrium point from *A* to *B*.

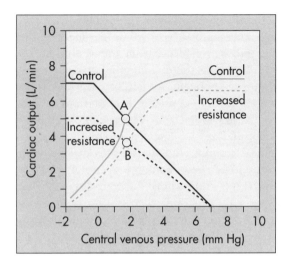

Figure 9-12 ■ An increase in peripheral resistance shifts the cardiac and vascular function curves downward. At equilibrium the cardiac output is less *(B)* when the peripheral resistance is high than when it is normal *(A)*.

Peripheral Resistance

Predictions concerning the effects of changes in peripheral vascular resistance are also complex because both the cardiac and vascular function curves shift. With increased peripheral resistance (Figure 9-12), the vascular function curve is rotated counterclockwise, but it converges to the same P_v-axis intercept as the control curve (see Figure 9-7); the direction of rotation differs in Figures 9-7 and 9-12 because the axes were switched for the vascular function curves in the two figures. The cardiac function curve is also shifted downward because (1) as peripheral resistance increases, arterial pressure (afterload) tends to rise, and (2) at any given P_v the heart is able to pump less blood against a greater afterload. Because the cardiac and vascular function curves are both displaced downward, the new equilibrium point, *B*, will fall below the control point, *A*.

Whether point *B* will fall directly below point *A* or will lie to the right or left of point *A* de-

pends on the magnitude of the shift in each curve. For example, if a given increase in peripheral resistance shifts the vascular function curve more than the cardiac function curve, equilibrium point *B* will fall below and to the left of *A;* that is, both cardiac output and P_v will diminish. Conversely, if the cardiac function curve is displaced more than the vascular function curve, point *B* will fall below and to the right of point *A;* that is, cardiac output will decrease but P_v will rise somewhat.

BOX 9-2

Heart Failure

Heart failure is the general term that refers to those conditions in which the heart is not able to provide adequate blood flow to the tissues of the body. Heart failure may be acute or chronic. Acute heart failure may be caused by toxic quantities of drugs and anesthetics or by certain pathological conditions, such as a sudden coronary artery occlusion. Chronic heart

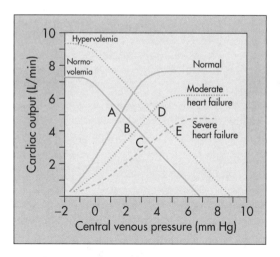

Figure 9-13 ■ **With moderate or severe heart failure, the cardiac function curves are shifted to the right. Before any change in blood volume, cardiac output decreases and central venous pressure rises (from control equilibrium point A to point B or point C). After the increase in blood volume that usually occurs in heart failure, the vascular function curve is shifted to the right. Hence central venous pressure may be elevated with no reduction in cardiac output (point D) or (in severe heart failure) with some diminution in cardiac output (point E).**

Heart Failure—cont'd

failure may occur in such conditions as essential hypertension or ischemic heart disease. In these various forms of heart failure, myocardial contractility is impaired. Consequently, the cardiac function curve is shifted downward and to the right, as depicted in Figure 9-13.

In **acute heart failure,** blood volume does not change immediately. Therefore the equilibrium point of the cardiac and vascular function curves will shift from the intersection of the normal curves (Figure 9-13, point *A*) to the intersection of the normal vascular function curve with a cardiac function curve that denotes impaired contractility (point *B* or *C*).

In **chronic heart failure,** both the cardiac function and vascular function curves shift. The vascular function curve shifts because of an increase in blood volume caused in part by fluid retention by the kidneys. The fluid retention is related to the concomitant reduction in glomerular filtration rate and to the increased secretion of aldosterone by the adrenal cortex. The resulting hypervolemia is reflected by a rightward shift of the vascular function curve, as shown in Figure 9-13. Hence with moderate degrees of heart failure, P_v will be elevated, but cardiac output will be approximately normal (point *D*). With more severe degrees of heart failure, P_v will be still higher, but cardiac output will be subnormal (point *E*).

■ THE RIGHT VENTRICLE REGULATES NOT ONLY PULMONARY BLOOD FLOW BUT ALSO CENTRAL VENOUS PRESSURE

Although the interrelations between cardiac output and central venous pressure are complicated and perplexing even in the simplified circulation model that includes just one pump and only the systemic circulation, the interrelations are much more complex when the systemic and pulmonary circulations and the left and right ventricles are included in the analysis. However,

the systemic and pulmonary vascular systems are important components of the cardiovascular systems in mammals, and therefore the more complete model does merit analysis.

Figure 9-14 shows a more complete, but still oversimplified, cardiovascular system model that contains two pumps in series (the left and right ventricles) and two vascular beds in series (the systemic and pulmonary vasculature). The series arrangement requires that the flows pumped by the two ventricles be virtually equal to each other over any substantial period; otherwise, the blood would ultimately accumulate in one or the other of the vascular systems. Because the cardiac function curves for the two ventricles differ substantially, the filling (atrial) pressures for the two ventricles must differ ap-

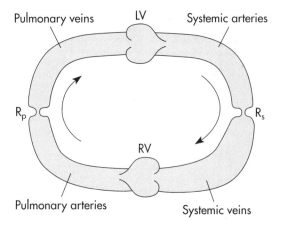

Figure 9-14 ▪ **Simplified cardiovascular system model that consists of left (*LV*) and right (*RV*) ventricles, systemic (*R$_s$*) and pulmonary (*R$_p$*) vascular resistances, systemic arterial and venous compliances, and pulmonary arterial and venous compliances.**

propriately to ensure equal stroke volumes (see Figure 4-20).

Two basic tenets about ventricular function are that the left ventricle is the pump that forces blood through the systemic vasculature, and the right ventricle is the pump that forces blood through the pulmonary vasculature. Although these assertions are essentially correct, it is still instructive to examine right ventricular function in more detail.

Consider the effect on the circulatory system model in Figure 9-14 if the right ventricle suddenly ceases to function as a pump, but instead serves as a passive, low-resistance conduit between the systemic veins and the pulmonary arteries. In such a circulatory system, the only pump would then be the left ventricle. The left ventricle would now be required to pump blood through two vascular resistances in series, namely, the systemic and pulmonary resistances (we shall consider the resistance of the right ventricle itself to be negligible).

Normally, pulmonary resistance is about 10% as great as systemic resistance. Because the two resistances are in series with one another, the total resistance would be 10% greater than the systemic resistance alone (see Chapter 5). In a normal cardiovascular system, a 10% increase in systemic vascular resistance would increase mean arterial pressure (and hence left ventricular afterload) by approximately 10%, which would not affect left ventricular function drastically. *However, when the 10% increase in total resistance is achieved by adding a small resistance (namely, the pulmonary resistance) downstream of the systemic resistance, and that resistance is separated from the systemic resistance by a large compliance (the combined systemic venous and pulmonary arterial compliance), the 10% increase in total resistance will then drastically affect the cardiovascular system.*

The simulated effects of inactivating the pumping action of the right ventricle in a hydraulic analog of the circulatory system are shown in Figure 9-15. In the model, the right and left ventricles generate cardiac outputs that vary directly with their respective filling pressures. Under control conditions, the output of the right ventricle (5 L/min) is equal to that of the left ventricle. The right ventricular pumping action causes the pressure in the pulmonary artery to exceed the pressure in the pulmonary veins by an amount that will force fluid through the pulmonary vascular resistance at a rate of 5 L/min.

When the right ventricle ceases pumping (arrow *1*), the systemic venous and pulmonary arterial systems become a common passive conduit with a large compliance; pulmonary arterial pressure decreases *(not shown)* and systemic venous pressure rises to a common value (5 mm Hg in Figure 9-15). At this low pressure, however, fluid flows from the pulmonary arteries to the pulmonary veins at a greatly reduced rate. At the same time, the left ventricle initially pumps fluid from the pulmonary veins to the systemic arteries at the control rate of 5 L/min. Hence pulmonary ve-

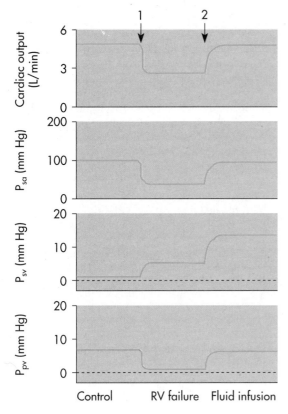

Figure 9-15 ■ **The changes in cardiac output, systemic arterial pressure (P_{sa}), systemic venous pressure (P_{sv}), and pulmonary venous pressure (P_{pv}), evoked by simulated right ventricular failure and by simulated fluid infusion in the circulatory model shown in Figure 9-14. At arrow *1,* the pumping action of the right ventricle was discontinued (simulated right ventricular failure) and the right ventricle served only as a low-resistance conduit. At arrow *2,* fluid volume was expanded and the right ventricle continued to serve only as a conduit.** (Modified from Furey SA, Zieske HA, Levy MN: *Am Heart J* 107:404, 1984.)

nous pressure drops precipitously. Because pulmonary venous pressure is the preload for the left ventricle, left ventricular (cardiac) output also drops abruptly. This effect in turn results in a rapid reduction in systemic arterial pressure. In summary, cessation of right ventricular pumping causes marked reductions in cardiac output, systemic arterial pressure, and pulmonary venous pressure, as well as a modest rise in systemic venous pressure (Figure 9-15).

Most of the hemodynamic problems induced by inactivating the right ventricle can be reversed by increasing the fluid (blood) volume of the system (arrow *2,* Figure 9-15). If fluid is added until pulmonary venous pressure (left ventricular preload) is raised to its control value, cardiac output and systemic arterial pressure are restored to normal, but systemic venous pressure is abnormally elevated. In a human subject, such a rise in systemic venous pressure may lead to the accumulation of fluid **(edema)** in the dependent regions of the body; such edema is characteristic of **right heart failure.**

Severe contractile failure of the right ventricle is the equivalent of overstressing the left ventricle by adding in series of relatively small (10%) hydraulic resistance (pulmonary vascular resistance) to the normal systemic vascular resistance. Ordinarily, increasing the systemic vascular resistance itself by 10% does not seriously stress the cardiovascular system. However, when the 10% additional resistance is downstream of the systemic venous bed (which has a very large compliance), it may diminish cardiac output drastically. The main compensatory response of the body is to increase blood volume, in part by renal retention of fluid and electrolytes. However, this compensatory response may lead to severe peripheral edema.

With these findings in mind, we might reassess the principal function of the right ventricle as follows. From the viewpoint of providing sufficient flow of blood to all the tissues in the body, the left ventricle alone is adequate to carry out this function; the operation of two ventricles in series is not essential to provide adequate blood flow to the tissues. *The crucial function of the right ventricle is therefore to prevent the rise in systemic venous (and pulmonary arterial) pressure that would be re-*

Any change in contractility that affects the two ventricles disparately will alter the distribution of blood volume in the two vascular systems. For example, if a coronary artery to the left ventricle becomes occluded suddenly, left ventricular contractility will be impaired and **left ventricular failure** will ensue. Instantaneously, left atrial pressure will not change perceptibly and the left ventricle will begin to pump a diminished flow. If the right ventricle is not affected by the acute coronary artery occlusion, the right ventricle will initially continue to pump the normal flow. The disparate right and left ventricular outputs will result in a progressive increase in left atrial pressure and a progressive decrease in right atrial pressure. Therefore left ventricular output will increase toward the normal value and the right ventricular output will fall below the normal value. This process will continue until the outputs of the two ventricles become equal to each other again. At this new equilibrium, the outputs of the two ventricles will be subnormal. The elevated left atrial pressure will be accompanied by an equally elevated pulmonary venous pressure, which can have serious clinical consequences. The high pulmonary venous pressure can increase lung stiffness and lead to respiratory distress by increasing the mechanical work of pulmonary ventilation. Furthermore, the high pulmonary venous pressure will elevate the hydrostatic pressure in the pulmonary capillaries, and hence may lead to transudation of fluid from the pulmonary capillaries to the pulmonary interstitium or into the alveoli themselves **(pulmonary edema).** The last of these consequences may be lethal.

In humans, **right heart failure** may be caused by occlusive disease predominantly of the coronary vessels to the right ventricle; these vessels are affected much less commonly than are the vessels to the left ventricle. The major hemodynamic effects of acute right heart failure are pronounced reductions in cardiac output and in arterial blood pressure, and the principal treatment consists of infusion of blood or plasma. Bypass of the right ventricle is not infrequently implemented surgically for patients with certain **congenital cardiac defects,** such as severe narrowing of the tricuspid valve or maldevelopment of the right ventricle. The effects of acute right heart failure or of right ventricular bypass are directionally similar to those predicted by the model study (Figure 9-15).

■ HEART RATE HAS AMBIVALENT EFFECTS ON CARDIAC OUTPUT

Cardiac output is the product of stroke volume and heart rate. The above analysis of the control of cardiac output was, in reality, restricted to the control of stroke volume, and the role of heart rate was neglected.

The effect of changes in heart rate on cardiac output will now be considered. The analysis is complex, because a change in heart rate alters the other three factors (preload, afterload, and contractility) that determine stroke volume (see Figure 9-1). An increase in heart rate, for example, would decrease the duration of diastole. Hence ventricular filling would be diminished; that is, preload would be reduced. If the proposed increase in heart rate did alter cardiac output, the arterial pressure would change; that is, afterload would be altered. Finally, the rise in heart rate would increase the net influx of Ca^{++} per minute into the myocardial cells, and this would enhance myocardial contractility (see Chapter 4).

quired to force the normal cardiac output through the pulmonary vascular resistance. By preventing the abnormal rise in systemic venous pressure, extensive dependent edema is averted.

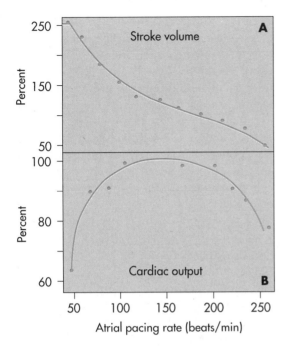

Figure 9-16 ▪ The changes in stroke volume (A) **and cardiac output** (B) **induced by changing the rate of atrial pacing in an anesthetized dog.** (Redrawn from Kumada M, Azuma T, Matsuda K: *Jpn J Physiol* 17:538, 1967.)

Heart rate has been varied by artificial pacing in many types of experimental preparations and in humans. The effects on cardiac output have usually resembled the experimental results shown in Figure 9-16. In that experiment, as the atrial pacing frequency was gradually increased in an anesthetized dog, the stroke volume progressively diminished (Figure 9-16, *A*). Presumably, the curtailment of stroke volume was induced by the abridged time for ventricular filling.

The change in cardiac output induced by a change in heart rate is influenced markedly by the actual level of the heart rate. In the experiment shown in Figure 9-16, for example, as the pacing frequency was increased within the range of 50 to 100 beats/min, an increase in heart rate augmented the cardiac output (Q_h). Presum-

ably, over this lower frequency range, the reduction in stroke volume (SV) evoked by a given increase in heart rate (HR) was proportionately less than the increase in heart rate itself; that is, because $Q_h = SV \times HR$, if a given increment in HR exceeds the induced decrement in SV, the induced Q_h will be greater than the initial Q_h.

Over the frequency range from about 100 to 200 beats/min, however, cardiac output was not affected appreciably by changes in pacing frequency (Figure 9-16, *B*). As the pacing frequency was increased, the stroke volume needed to decrease proportionately to the increase in heart rate.

Finally, at excessively high pacing frequencies (above 200 beats/min), increments in heart rate decreased the cardiac output. Therefore the induced decrement in SV must have exceeded the increment in HR over this high range of pacing frequencies. Although the relationship of Q_h to HR is characteristically that of an inverted U, the relationship varies quantitatively among subjects and among physiological states in any given subject.

Attribution of causation to observed correlations between cardiac output and heart rate should be made very cautiously. During physical exercise, for example, cardiac output and heart rate often rise proportionately, and stroke volume may change very little (see Chapter 12). The temptation is great to conclude that the increase in cardiac output must be caused by the observed increase in heart rate, because of the striking correlation between cardiac output and heart rate. However, Figure 9-16 emphasizes that, over a wide range of heart rates, a change in heart rate has little influence on cardiac output. Several studies on exercising subjects have confirmed that, even during exercise, changes in pacing frequency over a substantial frequency range do not alter cardiac output very much.

The principal increase in cardiac output during exercise must therefore be ascribed to (1)

The characteristic relationship between cardiac output and heart rate explains the urgent need for treatment of patients who have excessively slow or excessively fast heart rates. Profound **bradycardias** (slow rates) may occur as the result of a very slow sinus rhythm in patients with **sick sinus syndrome** or as the result of a slow idioventricular rhythm in patients with **complete atrioventricular block.** In either rhythm disturbance, the capacity of the ventricles to fill during a prolonged diastole is limited (often by the noncompliant pericardium). Hence cardiac output usually decreases substantially because the very slow heart rate cannot be overcome by a sufficiently great stroke volume. Consequently, these rhythm disturbances often require installation of an artificial pacemaker.

At the other end of the heart rate spectrum, excessively high heart rates in patients with **supraventricular** or **ventricular tachycardias** often require emergency treatment because their cardiac outputs may be critically low. In such patients, the filling time is so restricted at very high heart rates that small additional reductions in filling time elicit disproportionately severe reductions in filling volume. Reversion of the tachycardia to a more normal rhythm can usually be accomplished pharmacologically. However, **cardioversion,** which delivers a strong electrical current across the thorax or directly to the heart through an implanted device, may be required in emergencies.

the pronounced reduction in peripheral vascular resistance, (2) the positive inotropic effect of the increased sympathetic neural activity on the ventricular myocardium, and (3) the auxiliary pumping action of the contracting skeletal muscles, combined with the directional effects on blood flow effected by the venous valves (as explained toward the end of this chapter). The attendant changes in heart rate are not inconsequential, however. If the heart rate cannot increase normally during exercise, the augmentation of cardiac output and the capacity for exercise may be severely limited. The increase in heart rate does play a *permissive role* in augmenting cardiac output, even if it is not proper to assign it a primary, causative role. The mechanisms responsible for raising heart rate in precise proportion to the increase in cardiac output are undoubtedly neural in origin, but the specific components of the reflex arcs have not yet been elucidated.

■ ANCILLARY FACTORS AFFECT THE VENOUS SYSTEM AND CARDIAC OUTPUT

We have explained the interrelationships between central venous pressure and cardiac output in an oversimplified fashion, and we have described the effects evoked by changes in isolated variables. However, because many feedback control loops regulate the cardiovascular system, an isolated change in a single response rarely occurs. A change in blood volume, for example, reflexly alters cardiac function, peripheral resistance, and venomotor tone. Several auxiliary factors also regulate cardiac output. Such ancillary factors may be considered to modulate the more basic factors that we have considered above.

Gravity

Gravitational forces may affect cardiac output profoundly. It is not unusual for some soldiers standing at attention to faint because of reduced cardiac output. Gravitational effects are exaggerated in airplane pilots during pullouts from dives. The centrifugal force in the footward direction may be several times greater than the force of gravity. Such individuals characteristically black out momentarily during the maneuver, as blood is drained from the cephalic regions and pooled in the lower parts of the body.

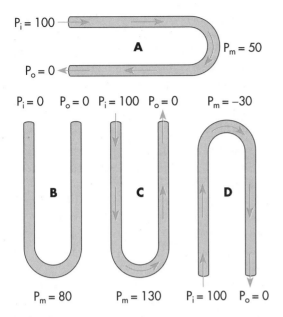

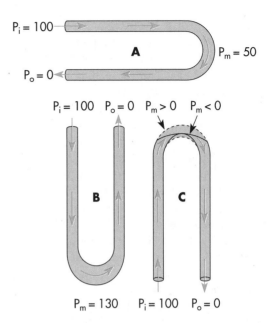

Figure 9-17 ■ Pressure distributions in rigid U tubes with constant internal diameters, all with the same dimensions. For a given inflow pressure ($P_i = 100$) and outflow pressure ($P_o = 0$), the pressure at the midpoint (P_m) depends on the orientation of the U tube, but the flow through the tube is independent of the orientation.

Figure 9-18 ■ In U tubes with a distensible section at the bend, even when inflow (P_i) and outflow (P_o) pressures are the same, the resistance to flow, and the fluid volume contained within each tube, vary with the orientation of the tube. P_m, Pressure at the midpoint of the tube.

The explanation for the reduction in cardiac output under such conditions is often specious. It is argued that when an individual is standing, the forces of gravity impede venous return from the dependent regions of the body. This statement is incomplete, however, because it ignores the facilitative counterforce on the arterial side of the same circuit.

In this sense the vascular system resembles a U tube. To comprehend the action of gravity on flow through such a system, the models depicted in Figures 9-17 and 9-18 will be analyzed. In Figure 9-17, all the U tubes represent rigid cylinders of constant diameter. With both limbs of the U tube oriented horizontally (*A*), the flow

depends only on the pressures at the inflow and outflow ends of the tube (P_i and P_o, respectively), the viscosity of the fluid, and the length and radius of the tube, in accordance with Poiseuille's equation (see Chapter 5). With a constant cross section, the pressure gradient will be uniform; hence the pressure midway down the tube (P_m) will equal the average of the inflow and outflow pressures.

When the U tube is oriented vertically (*B* to *D*), hydrostatic forces must be taken into consideration. In tube *B*, both limbs are open to atmospheric pressure and both ends are located at the same hydrostatic level; hence there is no flow. The pressure at the midpoint of the tube will simply be ρhg. The pressure will depend on the density of the fluid, ρ; the height of the U tube, h; and the acceleration of gravity, g. In the example, the length of the U tube is such that the midpoint pressure is 80 mm Hg.

Now consider tube C, where the tube is oriented the same as tube B, but where a 100 mm Hg pressure difference is applied across the two ends. The flow will precisely equal that in A because the pressure gradient, tube dimensions, and fluid viscosity are all the same. Gravitational forces are precisely equal in magnitude but opposite in direction in the two limbs of the U tube. Because the flow will be the same as that in A, there will be a pressure drop of 50 mm Hg at the midpoint due to the viscous losses resulting from flow. Furthermore, gravity will tend to increase pressure by 80 mm Hg at the midpoint, just as in tube B. The actual pressure at the midpoint of tube C will be the result of the viscous loss and hydrostatic gain, or 130 mm Hg in this example.

In D a pressure gradient of 100 mm Hg is applied to the same U tube, but the tube is oriented in the opposite direction. Gravitational forces will be so directed that the pressure at the midpoint will tend to be 80 mm Hg less than that at the end of the U tube. Viscous losses will still produce a 50 mm Hg pressure drop at the midpoint relative to P_i. With this orientation, pressure at the midpoint of the U tube will be 30 mm Hg below ambient pressure. Flow will be the same as in tubes A and C, for the reasons stated in relation to C.

In a system of rigid U tubes, gravitational effects will not alter the rate of fluid flow. However, experience shows that gravity does affect the cardiovascular system. The reason is that the vessels are distensible rather than rigid. To explain the gravitational effects, the pressures in a set of U tubes with distensible components (at the bends in the tubes of Figure 9-18) will be examined. In tubes A and B the pressure distributions will resemble those in tubes A and C, re-

spectively, in Figure 9-17. Because the pressure is higher at the bend of tube B than at the bend of tube A in Figure 9-18 and because the segments are distensible in this region, the distension at the bend in tube B will exceed that at the bend in tube A. The extent of the distension will depend on the compliance of these tube segments. Because flow varies directly with the tube diameter, the flow through B will exceed the flow through A for a given pressure difference applied at the ends.

Orienting a U tube with its bend downward actually increases rather than diminishes flow; how then is the observed impairment of cardiovascular function explained when the body is similarly oriented? The explanation is that the cardiovascular system is a closed circuit of constant fluid (blood) volume, whereas the U tube is an open conduit supplied by a fluid source of unlimited volume. In the dependent regions of the cardiovascular system, the distension will occur more on the venous than on the arterial side of the circuit because the venous compliance is so much greater than the arterial compliance. Such venous distension is readily observed on the back of the hands when the arms are allowed to hang down. The hemodynamic effects of such venous distension (**venous pooling**) resemble those caused by the hemorrhage of an equivalent volume of blood from the body. When an adult person shifts from a supine position to a relaxed standing position, 300 to 800 ml of blood are pooled in the legs. This may reduce cardiac output by about 2 L/min.

The compensatory adjustments to the erect position are similar to the adjustments to blood loss. For example, the diminished baroreceptor excitation reflexly speeds the heart, strengthens the cardiac contraction, and constricts the arterioles and veins. The baroreceptor reflex has a greater effect on the resistance than on the capacitance vessels. Warm ambient temperatures interfere with the compensatory vasomotor reactions, and the absence of muscular activity exaggerates the effects.

When the U tube is rotated so that the bend is directed upward (Figure 9-18, tube *C*), the effects are opposite to those that take place in tube *B*. The pressure at the bend of tube C would tend to be -30 mm Hg, just as in tube *D* of Figure 9-17. Because the ambient pressure exceeds the internal pressure, however, the distensible segment of tube *C* will collapse. Flow will then cease, and therefore the pressure decrease associated with viscous flow will not occur. In U tube *C*, when flow stops, the pressure at the top of each limb will be 80 mm Hg less than at the bottom (the hydrostatic pressure difference). Hence in the left, or inflow, limb the pressure will begin to rise rapidly from a negative value. If the tube remained collapsed at the bend, the pressure to the left of the collapsed segment would rapidly approach 20 mm Hg. However, as soon as this pressure exceeds ambient pressure (0 mm Hg), the collapsed tubing will be forced open and flow will begin. With the onset of flow, however, pressure at the bend will again drop below the ambient pressure. *Thus the tubing at the bend will flutter; that is, it will fluctuate between the open and closed states.*

When an arm is raised, the cutaneous veins in the hand and forearm collapse, for the reasons described previously. Fluttering does not occur here because the deeper veins are protected from collapse by being tethered to surrounding structures. This protection allows these deeper veins to accommodate the flow ordinarily carried by the collapsed superficial veins. The analogy would be to add a rigid tube (representing the deeper veins) in parallel with the collapsible tube (representing the superficial veins) at the bend of tube *C* in Figure 9-18. The collapsible tube would no longer flutter but would remain closed. All flow would occur through the rigid tube, just as in tube *D* in Figure 9-17.

Muscular Activity and Venous Valves

When a recumbent person stands but remains at rest, the pressure rises in the veins in the dependent regions of the body. The venous pressure in the legs increases gradually and does not reach an equilibrium value until almost 1 minute after standing. The slowness of this rise in P_v is attributable to the venous valves, which permit flow only toward the heart. When the person stands, the valves prevent blood in the veins from actually falling toward the feet. Hence the column of venous blood is supported at numerous levels by these valves; temporarily, the venous column consists of many discontinuous segments. However, blood continues to enter the column from many venules and small tributary veins, and the pressure continues to rise. As soon as the pressure in one segment exceeds that in the segment just above it, the intervening valve is forced open. Ultimately, all the valves are open and the column is continuous, similar to the state in the outflow limbs of the U tubes shown in Figures 9-17 and 9-18.

Precise measurement reveals that the final level of P_v in the feet during quiet standing is only slightly greater than that in a static column of blood extending from the right atrium to the feet. This indicates that the pressure drop

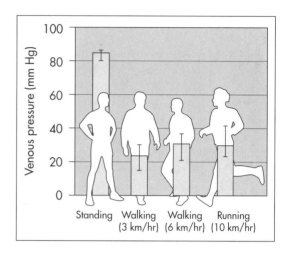

Figure 9-19 ■ **Mean pressures (± 95% confidence intervals) in the foot veins of 18 people during quiet standing, walking, and running.** (From Stick C, Jaeger H, Witzleb E: *J Appl Physiol* 72:2063, 1992.)

caused by blood flow from the foot veins to the right atrium is very small. This very low resistance justifies lumping all the veins as a common venous compliance in the circulatory system model illustrated in Figure 9-2.

When an individual who has been standing quietly begins to walk, the venous pressure in the legs decreases appreciably (Figure 9-19). Because of the intermittent venous compression exerted by the contracting leg muscles and because of the presence of the venous valves, blood is forced from the veins toward the heart (see Figure 11-2). Hence muscular contraction lowers the mean venous pressure in the legs and serves as an auxiliary pump. Furthermore, it prevents venous pooling and lowers capillary hy-

drostatic pressure. Thereby it reduces the tendency for edema fluid to collect in the feet during standing.

Respiratory Activity

The normal, periodic activity of the respiratory muscles causes rhythmic variations in vena caval flow. Thus respiration constitutes an auxiliary pump to promote venous return. Coughing, straining at stool, and other activities that require respiratory muscle exertion may affect cardiac output substantially.

The changes in blood flow in the superior vena cava during the normal respiratory cycle are shown in Figure 9-20. During respiration the reduction in intrathoracic pressure is transmitted to the lumina of the intrathoracic blood vessels. The reduction in central venous pressure during inspiration increases the pressure gradient between extrathoracic and intrathoracic veins. The consequent acceleration of venous return to the right atrium is displayed in Figure 9-20 as an increase in superior vena caval blood

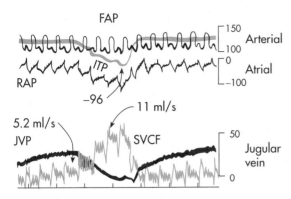

Figure 9-20 ■ **During a normal inspiration, intrathoracic *(ITP),* right atrial *(RAP),* and jugular venous *(JVP)* pressures decrease, and flow in the superior vena cava *(SVCF)* increases (from 5.2 to 11 ml/s). All pressures are in millimeters of water, except for femoral arterial pressure *(FAP),* which is in millimeters of mercury.** (Modified from Brecher GA: *Venous return,* New York, 1956, Grune & Stratton.)

flow from 5.2 ml/s during expiration to 11 ml/s during inspiration.

An exaggerated reduction in intrathoracic pressure achieved by a strong inspiratory effort against a closed glottis (called **Müller's maneuver**) does not increase venous return proportionately. The extrathoracic veins collapse near their entry into the chest when their internal pressures fall below the ambient level. As the veins collapse, flow into the chest momentarily stops. The cessation of flow raises pressure upstream, forcing the collapsed segment to open again. The process is repetitive; the venous segments adjacent to the chest alternately open and close.

During normal expiration, flow into the central veins decelerates. However, the mean rate of venous return during normal respiration exceeds the flow during a brief period of **apnea** (cessation of respiration). Hence normal inspiration apparently facilitates venous return more than normal expiration impedes it. In part, this

must be attributable to the valves in the veins of the extremities and neck. These valves prevent any reversal of flow during expiration. Thus the respiratory muscles and venous valves constitute an **auxiliary pump** for venous return.

Sustained expiratory efforts increase intrathoracic pressure and thereby impede venous return. Straining against a closed glottis (termed **Valsalva's maneuver**) regularly occurs during coughing, defecation, and heavy lifting. Intrathoracic pressures in excess of 100 mm Hg have been recorded in trumpet players, and pressures over 400 mm Hg have been observed during paroxysms of coughing. Such pressure increases are transmitted directly to the lumina of the intrathoracic arteries. After cessation of coughing the arterial blood pressure may fall precipitously because of the preceding impediment to venous return.

BOX 9-9

The intense, brief increases in intrathoracic pressure induced by coughing constitute an **auxiliary pumping mechanism** for the blood, despite its concurrent tendency to impede venous return momentarily. During certain diagnostic procedures, such as coronary angiography or electrophysiological testing, patients are at increased risk for **ventricular fibrillation.** Such patients have been trained to cough rhythmically on command. If ventricular fibrillation does occur, substantial arterial blood pressure increments are generated by each cough, and enough cerebral blood flow may be promoted to sustain consciousness and to preserve the viability of the cerebral tissues. The cough raises the intravascular pressure equally in intrathoracic arteries and veins. Blood is propelled through the extrathoracic tissues, however, because the increased pressure is transmitted to the extrathoracic arteries but not to the extrathoracic veins. The venous valves prevent transmission of the intrathoracic pressure to the extrathoracic veins.

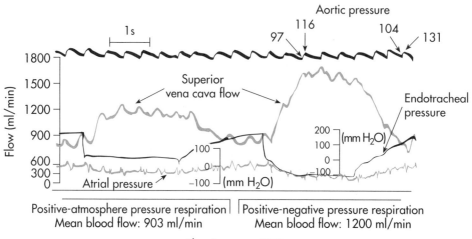

Figure 9-21 ■ **During intermittent positive-pressure respiration, the flow in the superior vena cava is approximately 30% greater when the lungs are deflated actively by applying negative endotracheal pressure *(right side)* than when they are allowed to deflate passively against atmospheric pressure *(left side).* (Modified from Brecher GA: *Venous return,* New York, 1956, Grune & Stratton.)

Artificial Respiration

In most forms of artificial respiration (mouth-to-mouth resuscitation, mechanical respiration), lung inflation is achieved by applying endotracheal pressures above atmospheric pressure, and expiration occurs by passive recoil of the thoracic cage. Thus lung inflation is attended by an appreciable rise in intrathoracic pressure. Vena caval flow decreases sharply during the phase of positive-pressure lung inflation (indicated by the progressive rise in endotracheal pressure in the central portion of Figure 9-21). When negative endotracheal pressure (indicated by the abrupt decrease in endotracheal pressure in the right half of Figure 9-21) is used to facilitate deflation, vena caval flow accelerates more than when the lungs are allowed to deflate passively (near the left border of Figure 9-21).

Summary

- Two important relationships between cardiac output (CO) and central venous pressure (P_v) prevail in the cardiovascular system. One applies to the heart and the other to the vascular system.
    - With respect to the heart, CO varies directly with P_v (or preload) over a very wide range of P_v. This relationship is represented by the cardiac function curve, and it expresses the Frank-Starling mechanism.
- With respect to the vascular system, P_v varies inversely with CO. This relationship is represented by the vascular function curve, and it reflects the fact that as CO increases, for example, a greater fraction of the total blood volume resides in the

arteries and a smaller volume resides in the veins.

- The principal mechanism that governs the cardiac function curve is the change in the affinity of the contractile proteins for calcium. This effect is evoked by changes in the cardiac filling pressure (preload).
- The principal factors that govern the vascular function curve are the arterial and venous compliances, the peripheral vascular resistance, and the total blood volume.
- The equilibrium values of CO and P_v that prevail under a given set of conditions are determined by the intersection of the cardiac and vascular function curves.
- At very low and very high heart rates, the heart is unable to pump an adequate CO. At the very low rates, the increment in filling during diastole cannot compensate for the small number of cardiac contractions per minute. At the very high rates, the large number of contractions per minute cannot compensate for the inadequate filling time.
- Gravity influences CO because the veins are so compliant, and substantial quantities of blood tend to pool in the veins of the dependent portions of the body.
- Respiration changes the pressure gradient between the intrathoracic and extrathoracic veins. Hence respiration serves as an auxiliary pump, which may alter the mean level of CO and may induce rhythmic changes in stroke volume during the various phases of the respiratory cycle.

■ BIBLIOGRAPHY

1. Aukland K: Why don't our feet swell in the upright position? *News Physiol Soc* 9:214, 1994.
2. Geddes LA, Wessale JL: Cardiac output, stroke volume, and pacing rate. *J Cardiovasc Electrophysiol* 2:408, 1991.
3. Jacob G, Ertl AC, Shannon JR, et al: Effect of standing on neurohumoral responses and plasma volume in healthy subjects. *J Appl Physiol* 84:914, 1998.
4. Lacolley PJ, Pannier BM, Cuche J-L, et al: Microgravity and orthostatic intolerance: carotid hemodynamics and peripheral responses. *Am J Physiol* 264:H588, 1993.
5. Monos E, Berczi V, Nadasy G: Local control of veins: biomechanical, metabolic, and humoral aspects. *Physiol Rev* 75:611, 1995.
6. Risöe C, Tan W, Smiseth OA: Effect of carotid sinus baroreceptor reflex on hepatic and splenic vascular capacitance in vagotomized dogs. *Am J Physiol* 266: H1528, 1994.
7. Rothe CF: Mean circulatory filling pressure: its meaning and measurement. *J Appl Physiol* 74:499, 1993.
8. Seymour RS, Hargens AR, Pedley TJ: The heart works against gravity. *Am J Physiol* 265:R715, 1993.
9. Sheriff DD, Zhou XP, Scher AM, et al: Dependence of cardiac filling pressure on cardiac output during rest and dynamic exercise in dogs. *Am J Physiol* 265:H316, 1993.
10. Shoukas AA: Overall systems analysis of the carotid sinus baroreceptor reflex control of the circulation. *Anesthesiology* 79:1402, 1993.
11. Smith JJ, editor: *Circulatory response to the upright posture,* Boca Raton, FL, 1990, CRC Press.
12. Stick C, Jaeger H, Witzleb E: Measurement of volume changes and venous pressure in the human lower leg during walking and running. *J Appl Physiol* 72:2063, 1992.
13. Tyberg JV: Venous modulation of ventricular preload. *Am Heart J* 123:1098, 1992.
14. Tyberg JV, Belenkie I, Manyari DE, et al: Ventricular interaction and venous capacitance modulate left ventricular preload. *Can J Cardiol* 12:1058, 1996.
15. Ursino M, Antonucci M, Belardinelli E: Role of active changes in venous capacity by the carotid baroreflex: analysis with a mathematical model. *Am J Physiol* 267:H2531, 1994.

■ CASE 9

HISTORY

A 44-year-old woman with severe cardiac failure caused by coronary artery disease was treated by cardiac transplantation. She recovered very well, and 1 month after surgery her cardiovascular function was entirely normal, even though her new heart was entirely denervated. About 3 months after surgery, she developed a bleeding duodenal ulcer and was estimated to have lost about 600 ml of blood in 1 hour. Her physician treated her with diet and antibiotics, and her ulcer was cured in about 2 weeks. The patient was healthy for 3 years, but then her strength and energy gradually diminished. Her physician determined that the cardiac transplant was slowly being rejected, and he began to treat her with a new drug that specifically increases myocardial contractility. Occasionally, the patient experienced brief periods of tachycardia with a rate of 250 beats/min; the electrocardiogram indicated that the tachycardia originated in the AV junction.

QUESTIONS

1. The acute blood loss from her duodenal ulcer would be expected to
   a. Decrease central venous pressure and increase cardiac output
   b. Increase central venous pressure and decrease mean arterial pressure
   c. Decrease central venous pressure and decrease cardiac output
   d. Increase mean arterial pressure and decrease cardiac output
   e. Decrease central venous pressure and increase aortic pulse pressure

2. Administration of a drug that acts specifically to improve myocardial contractility would
   a. Decrease central venous pressure and increase cardiac output
   b. Decrease central venous pressure and decrease mean arterial pressure
   c. Increase central venous pressure and increase aortic pulse pressure
   d. Decrease central venous pressure and decrease cardiac output
   e. Increase central venous pressure and increase arterial compliance

3. Strapping the patient to a tilt-table and tilting her to the vertical, head-up position would
   a. Increase the pressure in a foot vein and increase the central venous pressure
   b. Decrease the pressure in a foot vein and decrease the cardiac output
   c. Decrease the central venous pressure and increase the mean arterial pressure
   d. Decrease the pressure in a foot vein and decrease the arterial pulse pressure
   e. Increase the pressure in a foot vein and decrease the cardiac output

4. When the patient was experiencing the tachycardia, the critical hemodynamic changes would be expected to be
   a. An increase in mean arterial blood pressure and an increase in central venous pressure
   b. A decrease in stroke volume and a decrease in cardiac output
   c. An increase in stroke volume and an increase in aortic compliance
   d. An increase in central venous pressure and an increase in cardiac output
   e. A decrease in central venous pressure and an increase in arterial pulse pressure

CHAPTER 10

Coronary Circulation

Objectives

1. Delineate the physical, neural, and metabolic factors that affect coronary blood flow.

2. Explain the relative importance of these factors in the regulation of the coronary circulation.

3. Compare the oxygen requirements of the heart during pressure work versus volume work.

4. Explain the efficiency of the heart.

5. Describe the development of coronary collateral vessels.

■ FUNCTIONAL ANATOMY OF CORONARY VESSELS

The right and left coronary arteries, which arise at the root of the aorta behind the right and left cusps of the aortic valve, respectively, provide the entire blood supply to the myocardium. The right coronary artery supplies principally the right ventricle and atrium; the left coronary artery, which divides near its origin into the anterior descending and the circumflex branches, supplies principally the left ventricle and atrium, but there is some overlap. In humans the right coronary artery is dominant in 50% of individuals, the left coronary artery is dominant in another 20%, and the flow delivered by each main artery is about equal in the remaining 30%. The epicardial distribution of the coronary arteries and veins is illustrated in Figure 10-1.

After passage through the capillary beds, most of the venous blood returns to the right atrium through the coronary sinus, but some reaches the right atrium by way of the anterior coronary veins. There are also vascular communications directly between the vessels of the myocardium and the cardiac chambers; these make up the **arteriosinusoidal, arterioluminal,** and **thebesian vessels.** The arteriosinusoidal channels consist of small arteries or arterioles that lose their arterial structure as they penetrate the chamber walls and divide into irregular, endothelium-lined sinuses (50 to 250 μm). These sinuses anastomose with other sinuses and with capillaries, and communicate with the cardiac chambers. The arterioluminal vessels are small arteries or arterioles that open directly into the atria and ventricles. The thebesian vessels are small veins that connect capillary beds

227

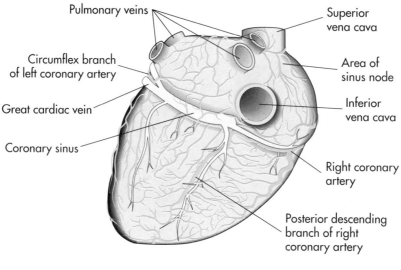

Pulmonary veins

Circumflex branch
of left coronary artery

Great cardiac vein

Coronary sinus

Superior
vena cava

Area of
sinus node

Inferior
vena cava

Right coronary
artery

Posterior descending
branch of right
coronary artery

POSTERIOR VIEW

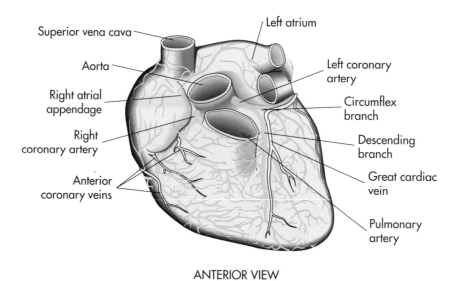

Superior vena cava

Aorta

Right atrial
appendage

Right
coronary artery

Anterior
coronary veins

Left atrium

Left coronary
artery

Circumflex
branch

Descending
branch

Great cardiac
vein

Pulmonary
artery

ANTERIOR VIEW

Figure 10-1 ▪ Anterior and posterior surfaces of the heart, illustrating the location and distribution
of the principal coronary vessels.

directly with the cardiac chambers and also communicate with cardiac veins and other thebesian veins. On the basis of anatomical studies, *intercommunication appears to exist among all the minute vessels of the myocardium in the form of an extensive plexus of subendocardial vessels.* However, the myocardium does not receive significant nutritional blood flow directly from the cardiac chambers.

■ CORONARY BLOOD FLOW IS REGULATED BY PHYSICAL, NEURAL, AND METABOLIC FACTORS

Physical Factors

The principal factor responsible for perfusion of the myocardium is the aortic pressure, which is generated by the heart itself. Changes in aortic pressure generally evoke parallel directional changes in coronary blood flow. However, alterations of cardiac work, produced by an increase or decrease in aortic pressure, have a considerable effect on coronary resistance. Increased metabolic activity of the heart results in a decrease in coronary resistance, and a reduction in cardiac metabolism produces an increase in coronary resistance. If a cannulated coronary artery is perfused by blood from a pressure-controlled reservoir, perfusion pressure can be altered without changing aortic pressure and cardiac work. Under these conditions, abrupt variations in perfusion pressure produce equally abrupt changes in coronary blood flow in the same direction. However, maintenance of the perfusion pressure at the new level is associated with a return of blood flow toward the level observed before the induced change in perfusion pressure (Figure 10-2). This phenomenon is an example of autoregulation of blood flow and is discussed in Chapter 8. Under normal conditions, blood pressure is kept within relatively narrow limits by the baroreceptor reflex mechanisms, so that *changes in coronary blood flow are mainly caused by caliber changes of the*

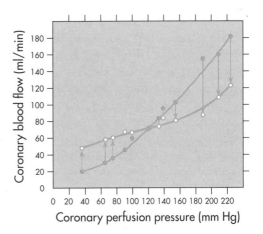

Figure 10-2 ■ **Pressure-flow relationships in the coronary vascular bed. At constant aortic pressure, cardiac output, and heart rate, coronary artery perfusion pressure was abruptly increased or decreased from the control level indicated by the point where the two lines cross. The closed circles represent the flows that were obtained immediately after the change in perfusion pressure; the open circles represent the steady-state flows at the new pressures. There is a tendency for flow to return toward the control level (autoregulation of blood flow), and this is most prominent over the intermediate pressure range (about 60 to 180 mm Hg).** (From Berne RM, Rubio R: Coronary circulation. In *Handbook of physiology*, Section 2: *The cardiovascular system—the heart*, vol 1, Bethesda, MD, 1979, American Physiological Society.)

coronary resistance vessels in response to metabolic demands of the heart.

In addition to providing the head of pressure to drive blood through the coronary vessels, the heart also influences its blood supply by the squeezing effect of the contracting myocardium on the blood vessels that course through it (**extravascular compression** or **extracoronary resistance**). This force is so great during early ventricular systole that blood flow, as measured in a large coronary artery that supplies the left ventricle, is briefly reversed. Maximal left coronary inflow occurs in early diastole, when the ventricles have relaxed and extravascular compression of the coronary vessels is virtually absent. This flow pattern is seen in the phasic coronary flow curve for the left coronary artery (Figure 10-3). After an initial reversal in early systole, left coronary blood flow follows the aortic pressure until early diastole, when it rises abruptly and then declines slowly as aortic pressure falls during the remainder of diastole.

BOX 10-1

The minimal extravascular resistance and absence of left ventricular work during diastole can be used to improve myocardial perfusion in patients with damaged myocardium and low blood pressure. The method is called **counterpulsation** and consists of the insertion of an inflatable balloon into the thoracic aorta through a femoral artery. The balloon is inflated during ventricular diastole and deflated during systole. This procedure enhances coronary blood flow during diastole by raising diastolic pressure at a time when coronary extravascular resistance is lowest. Furthermore, it reduces cardiac energy requirements by lowering aortic pressure (afterload) during ventricular ejection.

Left ventricular intramural pressure (pressure within the wall of the left ventricle) is greatest near the endocardium and least near the epicardium. However, under normal conditions, this pressure gradient does not impair endocardial blood flow because a greater blood flow to the endocardium during diastole compensates for the greater blood flow to the epicardium during systole. In fact, when 10-μm diameter radioactive spheres are injected into the coronary arteries, their distribution indicates that the blood flow to the epicardial and endocardial halves of the left ventricle is approximately equal (slightly higher in the endocardium) under normal conditions. Because extravascular compression is greatest at the endocardial surface of the ventricle, equality of epicardial and endocardial blood flow must mean that the tone of the endocardial resistance vessels is less than the tone of the epicardial vessels.

BOX 10-2

Under abnormal conditions, when diastolic pressure in the coronary arteries is low (such as in **severe hypotension, partial coronary artery occlusion,** or **severe aortic stenosis**), the ratio of endocardial to epicardial blood flow falls below a value of 1. This indicates that in the left ventricle blood flow to the endocardial regions is more severely impaired than that to the epicardial regions of the ventricle. Reduced blood flow to the endocardium is also reflected in an increase in the gradient of myocardial lactic acid and adenosine concentrations from epicardium to endocardium. For this reason, the myocardial damage observed in the left ventricle after occlusion of a major coronary artery is greater in the inner wall than in the outer wall of the ventricle.

Flow in the right coronary artery shows a similar pattern (see Figure 10-3), but because of the lower pressure developed during systole by the thin right ventricle, reversal of blood flow does not occur in early systole, and systolic blood flow constitutes a much greater proportion of total coronary inflow than it does in the left coronary artery.

The extent to which extravascular compression restricts coronary inflow can be readily seen when the heart is suddenly arrested in diastole or with the induction of ventricular fibrillation. Figure 10-4 depicts mean left coronary flow when the vessel was perfused with blood at a constant pressure from a reservoir. At the arrow in record

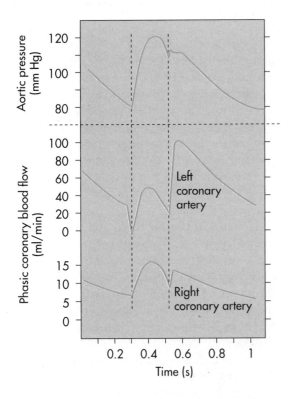

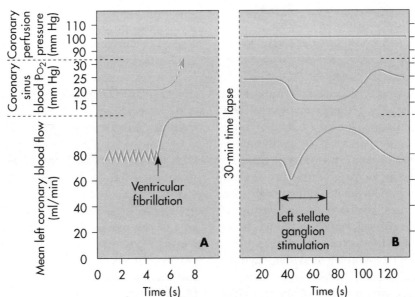

Figure 10-3 ■ Comparison of phasic coronary blood flow in the left and right coronary arteries.

Figure 10-4 ■ A, **Unmasking of the restricting effect of ventricular systole on mean coronary blood flow by induction of ventricular fibrillation during constant pressure perfusion of the left coronary artery.** B, **Effect of cardiac sympathetic nerve stimulation on coronary blood flow and coronary sinus blood O₂ tension in the fibrillating heart during constant pressure perfusion of the left coronary artery.** (From Berne RM: Unpublished observations.)

A, ventricular fibrillation was electrically induced and an immediate and substantial increase in blood flow occurred. Subsequent increase in coronary resistance over a period of 30 minutes reduced myocardial blood flow to below the level existing before induction of ventricular fibrillation (record *B,* before stellate ganglion stimulation).

Tachycardia and bradycardia have dual effects on coronary blood flow. A change in heart rate is accomplished chiefly by shortening or lengthening of diastole. With tachycardia the proportion of time spent in systole, and consequently the period of restricted inflow, increases. However, this mechanical reduction in mean coronary flow is overridden by the coronary dilation associated with the increased metabolic activity of the more rapidly beating heart. With bradycardia the opposite is true; coronary inflow is less restricted (more time in diastole), but the metabolic (O_2) requirements of the myocardium are also diminished.

Neural and Neurohumoral Factors

Stimulation of the sympathetic nerves to the heart elicits a marked increase in coronary blood flow. However, the increase in flow is associated with cardiac acceleration and a more forceful systole. The stronger myocardial contractions and the tachycardia (with the consequence that a greater proportion of time is spent in systole) tend to restrict coronary flow, whereas the increase in myocardial metabolic activity, as evidenced by the rate and contractility changes, tends to evoke dilation of the coronary resistance vessels. The increase in coronary blood flow observed with cardiac sympathetic nerve stimulation is the algebraic sum of these factors. In perfused hearts in which the mechanical effect of extravascular compression is eliminated by cardiac arrest or ventricular fibrillation, an initial coronary vasoconstriction is often observed with cardiac sympathetic nerve stimulation before the vasodilation attributable to the metabolic effect comes into play (Figure 10-4, *B*).

Furthermore, after the beta receptors are blocked to eliminate the chronotropic and inotropic effects, direct reflex activation of the sympathetic nerves to the heart increases coronary resistance. These observations indicate that *the main action of the sympathetic nerve fibers on the coronary resistance vessels is vasoconstriction.*

α- and β-adrenergic drugs and their respective blocking agents reveal the presence of alpha receptors (constrictors) and beta receptors (dilators) on the coronary vessels. Furthermore, the coronary resistance vessels participate in the baroreceptor and chemoreceptor reflexes, and there is sympathetic constrictor tone of the coronary arterioles that can be reflexly modulated. Nevertheless, coronary resistance is predominantly under local nonneural control.

Vagus nerve stimulation slightly dilates the coronary resistance vessels, and activation of the carotid and aortic chemoreceptors can elicit a small decrease in coronary resistance via the vagus nerves to the heart.

Reflexes originating in the myocardium and altering vascular resistance in peripheral systemic vessels, including the coronary vessels, have been conclusively demonstrated. However, the existence of extracardiac reflexes, with the coronary resistance vessels as the effector sites, has not been established.

Metabolic Factors

One of the most striking characteristics of the coronary circulation is the close parallelism between the level of myocardial metabolic activity and the magnitude of the coronary blood flow (Figure 10-5). This relationship is also found in the denervated heart or the completely isolated heart, regardless of whether the heart is beating or fibrillating.

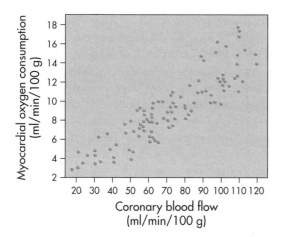

Figure 10-5 ■ Relationship between myocardial oxygen consumption and coronary blood flow during a variety of interventions that increased or decreased myocardial metabolic rate. (Redrawn from Berne RM, Rubio R: Coronary circulation. In *Handbook of physiology,* Section 2: *The cardiovascular system—the heart,* vol 1, Bethesda, MD, 1979, American Physiological Society.)

The link between cardiac metabolic rate and coronary blood flow remains unsettled. However, it appears that *a decrease in the ratio of oxygen supply to oxygen demand (whether produced by a reduction in oxygen supply or by an increment in oxygen demand) releases a vasodilator substance from the myocardium into the interstitial fluid, where it can relax the coronary resistance vessels.* As diagrammed in Figure 10-6, a decrease in arterial blood oxygen content, coronary blood flow, or both, or an increase in cardiac metabolic rate, decreases the oxygen supply/demand ratio. This causes the release of a vasodilator substance, such as adenosine, which dilates the arterioles, thereby adjusting oxygen supply to demand. A decrease in oxygen demand would reduce the vasodilator release and permit greater expression of basal tone.

Numerous agents, generally referred to as metabolites, have been suggested as mediators of the vasodilation observed with increased cardiac work.* Among the substances implicated are CO_2, O_2 (reduced O_2 tension), hydrogen ions (lactic acid), potassium ions, adenosine, prosta-

---

* Accumulation of vasoactive metabolites may also be responsible for reactive hyperemia, because the duration of coronary flow after release of the briefly occluded vessel is proportional within certain limits to the duration of the period of occlusion.

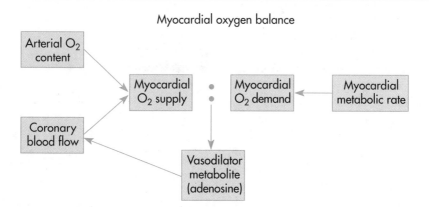

Figure 10-6 ■ Imbalance in the oxygen supply/oxygen demand ratio alters coronary blood flow by the rate of release of a vasodilator metabolite from the cardiomyocytes. A decrease in the ratio elicits an increase in vasodilator release, whereas an increase in the ratio has the opposite effect.

glandins, nitric oxide (NO), and opening of ATP-sensitive K^+ channels (K^+_{ATP}).

Of these agents, the key factors appear to be adenosine, NO, and opening of the K^+_{ATP}. However, the contribution of each of these factors, and their interaction under basal conditions and during increased myocardial activity, is complex and has not been clearly delineated. For example, at low concentrations adenosine appears to activate endothelial K^+_{ATP} channels and to enhance NO release, whereas at higher concentrations it acts directly on vascular smooth muscle by activating K^+_{ATP} channels. If all three agents are inhibited, coronary blood flow is reduced both at rest and during exercise, and contractile dysfunction and signs of myocardial ischemia become evident.

■ CARDIAC OXYGEN CONSUMPTION IS A FUNCTION OF THE WORK PERFORMED BY THE HEART

The volume of O_2 consumed by the heart is determined by the amount and type of activity of the myocardium. Under basal conditions, myocardial O_2 consumption is about 8 to 10 ml/min/100 g of heart. It can increase several-fold with exercise and decrease moderately under conditions such as hypotension and hypothermia. The cardiac venous blood is normally quite low in O_2 (about 5 ml/dl), and the myocardium can receive little additional O_2 by further O_2 extraction from the coronary blood. Therefore increased O_2 demands of the heart must be met primarily by an increase in coronary blood flow. When the heartbeat is arrested, as with administration of potassium, but coronary perfusion is maintained experimentally, O_2 consumption falls to 2 ml/min/100 g or less, which is still six to seven times greater than that for resting skeletal muscle.

Left ventricular work per beat (**stroke work**) is generally considered to be equal to the product of the stroke volume and the mean aortic pressure (afterload) against which the blood is ejected by the left ventricle. At resting levels of cardiac output the kinetic energy component is negligible. However, at high cardiac outputs, as in severe exercise, the kinetic component can account for up to 50% of total cardiac work. One can simultaneously halve the aortic pressure and double the cardiac output, or vice versa, and still arrive at the same value for cardiac work. However, *the O_2 requirements are greater for any given amount of cardiac work when a major fraction is pressure work as opposed to volume work.* An increase in cardiac output at a constant aortic pressure (volume work) is accomplished with a small increase in left ventricular O_2 consumption, whereas increased arterial pressure at constant cardiac output (pressure work) is accompanied by a large increment in myocardial O_2 consumption. Thus myocardial O_2 consumption may not correlate well with overall cardiac work. The magnitude and duration of left ventricular pressure do correlate with left ventricular O_2 consumption.

Work of the right ventricle is one seventh that of the left ventricle because pulmonary vascular resistance is much less than systemic vascular resistance.

BOX 10-3

The greater energy demand of pressure work compared with volume work is of great clinical importance, especially in **aortic stenosis,** in which left ventricular O_2 consumption is increased. The greater O_2 consumption is caused by the extra energy needed to overcome the resistance of the stenotic aortic valve. The clinical problem is usually complicated by a decreased coronary perfusion pressure because of the pressure drop across the narrowed orifice of the diseased aortic valve.

■ CARDIAC EFFICIENCY

As with an engine, the efficiency of the heart is calculated as the ratio of the work accomplished to the total energy utilized. Assuming an average O_2 consumption of 9 ml/min/100 g for the two ventricles, a 300-g heart consumes 27 ml O_2/min, which is equivalent to 130 small calories at a respiratory quotient of 0.82. Together the two ventricles do about 8 kg-m of work per minute, which is equivalent to 18.7 small calories. Therefore the gross efficiency is 14%.

$$\frac{18.7}{130} \times 100 = 14\%$$

The net efficiency is slightly higher (18%) and is obtained by subtracting the O_2 consumption of the nonbeating (asystolic) heart (about 2 ml/min/100 g) from the total cardiac O_2 consumption in the calculation of efficiency. It is thus evident that the efficiency of the heart as a pump is relatively low and is comparable with the efficiency of many mechanical devices used in everyday life. With exercise, efficiency improves because mean blood pressure shows little change, whereas cardiac output and work increase considerably without a proportional increase in myocardial O_2 consumption. The energy expended in cardiac metabolism that does not contribute to the propulsion of blood through the body appears in the form of heat. The energy of the flowing blood is also dissipated as heat, chiefly in passage of the blood through the resistance vessels.

■ DIMINISHED CORONARY BLOOD FLOW IMPAIRS CARDIAC FUNCTION

Most of the oxygen in the coronary arterial blood is extracted during one passage through the myocardial capillaries. Thus the supply of oxygen to the myocardial cells is **flow limited;** that is, any substantial reduction in coronary blood flow will curtail the delivery of oxygen to the myocardium, because the extraction of oxygen from each unit volume of blood is nearly maximal even under basal conditions.

In myocardial ischemia, intracellular acidosis occurs and Na^+ accumulates in the myocytes. The high H^+ concentration activates Na^+/H^+ exchange and H^+ is extruded from the cells in exchange for Na^+. In addition, the ischemia inhibits Na^+-K^+-ATPase, thereby reducing Na^+ extrusion. The increased intracellular Na^+ enhances Na^+/Ca^{++} exchange so that as Na^+ leaves the cells, Ca^{++} enters (see Figure 3-5). The result is Ca^{++} overload, which impairs myocardial contraction and can lead to cell death. Inhibition of Na^+/H^+ exchange or of Na^+/Ca^{++} exchange hastens recovery from ischemia during reperfusion.

BOX 10-4

Reductions in coronary blood flow (**myocardial ischemia**) may critically impair the mechanical and electrical behavior of the heart. Diminished coronary blood flow as a consequence of coronary artery disease (usually **coronary atherosclerosis**) is one of the most common causes of serious cardiac disease. The ischemia may be global (i.e., it affects an entire ventricle) or regional (i.e., it affects some fraction of the ventricle). The impairment of the mechanical contraction of the affected myocardium is produced not only by the diminished delivery of oxygen and metabolic substrates, but also by the accumulation of potentially deleterious substances (e.g., K^+, lactic acid, H^+) in the cardiac tissues. If the reduction of coronary flow to any region of the heart is sufficiently severe and prolonged, necrosis (death) of the affected cardiac cells will result.

Substantial but temporary mechanical dysfunction of the heart may occur if the reduction of coronary flow is neither too prolonged nor too severe to cause myocardial necrosis. A relatively brief period of severe ischemia, followed by reperfusion, may be associated with pronounced mechanical dysfunction (called **myocardial stunning**) of the heart, which eventually will fully recover.

Myocardial stunning can be prevented by preconditioning, which consists of one or more brief occlusions of a coronary artery before a prolonged occlusion that in the absence of the brief occlusions would impair contractile force. Preconditioning appears to involve adenosine release from the myocardium in short (minutes) responses and protein synthesis in the myocardium in late (2 to 3 days) responses. Protection from the ischemia-induced impairment of cardiac function can be achieved by chronic administration of dipyridamole, a drug that blocks cellular uptake of adenosine, which results in an increase in blood levels of adenosine. Administration of an adenosine A_1 receptor antagonist abolishes the protective action of dipyridamole.

BOX 10-5

Myocardial stunning may be evident in patients who have had an **acute coronary artery occlusion** (a so-called heart attack). If the patient is treated sufficiently early by **coronary bypass surgery** or **balloon angioplasty** and if adequate blood flow is restored to the ischemic region, the myocardial cells in this region may eventually recover fully. However, for many days or even weeks, the contractility of the myocardium in the affected region may be grossly subnormal.

■ **CORONARY COLLATERAL VESSELS DEVELOP IN RESPONSE TO IMPAIRMENT OF CORONARY BLOOD FLOW**

In the normal human heart there are virtually no functional intercoronary channels, whereas in the dog there are a few small vessels that link branches of the major coronary arteries. Abrupt

---

BOX 10-6

Myocardial hibernation also occurs mainly in patients with coronary artery disease. Their coronary blood flow is diminished persistently and significantly, and the mechanical function of the heart is impaired concomitantly. However, the metabolic activity of the heart does not reflect the extent of the ischemia; the process is called hibernation, because the downregulation of metabolism tends to preserve the viability of the cardiac tissues. If coronary blood flow is restored to normal by bypass surgery or angioplasty, mechanical function returns to normal.

---

occlusion of a coronary artery or one of its branches in a human or dog leads to ischemic necrosis and eventual fibrosis of the areas of myocardium supplied by the occluded vessel. However, if narrowing of a coronary artery occurs slowly and progressively over a period of days, weeks, or longer, collateral vessels develop and may furnish sufficient blood to the ischemic myocardium to prevent or reduce the extent of necrosis. The development of collateral coronary vessels has been extensively studied in dogs, and the clinical picture of coronary atherosclerosis, as it occurs in humans, can be simulated by gradual narrowing of the normal dog's coronary arteries. Collateral vessels develop between branches of occluded and nonoccluded arteries. They originate from preexisting arterioles that undergo proliferative changes of the endothelium and smooth muscle.

The stimulus to **arteriogenesis** is the shear stress caused by the enhanced blood flow velocity that occurs in the arterioles proximal to the site of occlusion. With occlusion of a coronary artery the pressure gradient along the proximal arterioles increases because of a greater perfusion pressure upstream from the occlusion. The stress-activated endothelium up-regulates expression of monocyte chemoattractant protein-1 (MCP-1), which attracts monocytes that then invade the arterioles. Other adhesion molecules and growth factors participate with MCP-1 in an inflammatory reaction and cell death in the potential collateral vessels. This is followed by remodeling and development of new and enlarged collateral vessels that are indistinguishable from normal arteries after several months.

Capillary proliferation is stimulated by vascular endothelial growth factor (VEGF), whose expression is upregulated by hypoxia. The enhanced production of VEGF is mediated in part by adenosine release caused by the hypoxia. Drug-induced chronic bradycardia can also enhance capillary density by greater expression of VEGF protein. However, the role of VEGF in development of collateral arterial vessels remains to be elucidated.

BOX 10-7

Numerous surgical attempts have been made to enhance the development of coronary collateral vessels. However, the techniques used do not increase the collateral circulation over and above that produced by coronary artery narrowing alone. When discrete occlusions or severe narrowing occur in coronary arteries, as in coronary atherosclerosis, the lesions can be bypassed with an artery (internal mammary) or a vein graft. In many cases the narrow segment can be dilated by inserting a balloon-tipped catheter into the diseased vessel via a peripheral artery and inflating the balloon. Distension of the vessel by balloon inflation (**angioplasty**) can produce a lasting dilation of a narrowed coronary artery, especially when a stent is inserted to maintain patency of the diseased vessel (Figure 10-7).

BOX 10-8

A number of drugs that induce coronary vasodilation are available and are used in patients with coronary artery disease to relieve **angina pectoris,** the chest pain associated with myocardial ischemia. Many of these compounds are organic nitrates and nitrites. They are not selective dilators of the coronary vessels, and the mechanism whereby they accomplish their beneficial effects has not been established. The arterioles in the ischemic heart that would dilate in response to the drugs are undoubtedly already maximally dilated by the ischemia responsible for the symptoms.

In fact, in a patient with marked narrowing of a coronary artery, administration of a vasodilator can fully dilate normal vessel branches parallel to the narrowed segment and reduce the head of pressure to the partially occluded vessel. This will further compromise blood flow to the ischemic myocardium and elicit pain and electrocardiographic changes indicative of tissue injury. This phenomenon is known as **coronary steal,** and it can be observed with vasodilator drugs such as dipyridamole, which acts by blocking cellular uptake and metabolism of endogenous adenosine. Nitrites and nitrates alleviate angina pectoris, at least partly, by reducing cardiac work and myocardial oxygen requirements by relaxing the great veins (decreased preload) and decreasing blood pressure (decreased afterload). In short, the reduction in pressure work and O_2 requirement must be greater than the reduction in coronary blood flow and O_2 supply consequent to the lowered coronary perfusion pressure. It has also been demonstrated that nitrites and endogenous NO dilate large coronary arteries and coronary collateral vessels, thus increasing blood flow to ischemic myocardium and alleviating precordial pain.

Cusps of aortic valve   Cardiac catheter

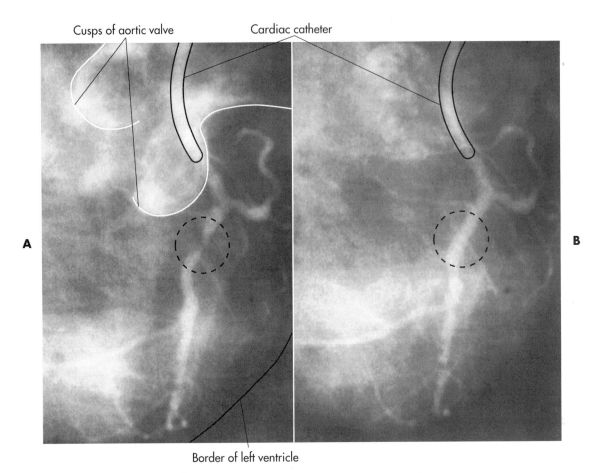

Border of left ventricle

Figure 10-7 ■ A, Angiogram (intracoronary radiopaque dye) of a person with marked narrowing of the circumflex branch of the left coronary artery *(encircled).* **Reflux of dye into the root of the aorta outlines two of the aortic valve cusps.** B, The same segment of the coronary artery after angioplasty. (Courtesy Dr. Eric R. Powers.)

Summary

- The physical factors that influence coronary blood flow are the viscosity of the blood, the frictional resistance of the vessel walls, the aortic pressure, and the extravascular compression of the vessels within the walls of the left ventricle. Left coronary blood flow is re-

stricted during ventricular systole as a result of extravascular compression, and flow is greatest during diastole when the intramyocardial vessels are not compressed.
- Neural regulation of coronary blood flow is much less important than is metabolic regula-

tion. Activation of the cardiac sympathetic nerves directly constricts the coronary resistance vessels. However, the enhanced myocardial metabolism caused by the associated increase in heart rate and contractile force produces vasodilation, which overrides the direct constrictor effect of sympathetic nerve stimulation. Stimulation of the cardiac branches of the vagus nerves slightly dilates the coronary arterioles.

- A striking parallelism exists between metabolic activity of the heart and coronary blood flow. A decrease in oxygen supply or an increase in oxygen demand apparently releases a vasodilator that decreases coronary resistance. Of the factors that can mediate this response, the key ones are adenosine, nitric oxide, and activation of the ATP-sensitive K^+ channels.

- Prolonged, severe reduction in coronary blood flow leads to myocardial cell necrosis and thereby impairs cardiac contraction. Moderate, sustained reductions in coronary blood flow may evoke myocardial hibernation, which is a reversible impairment of mechanical performance associated with a downregulation of cardiac metabolism. Transient periods of severe ischemia followed by reperfusion may induce myocardial stunning, which is a temporary stage of impaired mechanical performance by the heart.

- In response to gradual occlusion of a coronary artery, collateral vessels from adjacent unoccluded arteries develop and supply blood to the compromised myocardium distal to the point of occlusion.

- The stimulus for the development of coronary collateral arteries is the shear stress caused by the enhanced blood flow in arterioles proximal to the occlusion.

■ BIBLIOGRAPHY

1. Belardinelli L, Linden J, Berne RM: The cardiac effects of adenosine. *Prog Cardiovasc Dis* 32:73, 1989.
2. Bolli R: Myocardial "stunning" in man. *Circulation* 86:1671, 1992.
3. Buschmann I, Schaper W: Arteriogenesis versus angiogenesis: two mechanisms of vessel growth. *News Physiol Sci* 14:121, 1999.
4. Figueredo VM, Diamond I, Zhou H-Z, et al: Chronic dipyridamole therapy produces sustained protection against cardiac ischemia-reperfusion injury. *Am J Physiol* 277:H2091, 1999.
5. Gödecke A, Decking UKM, Ding Z, et al: Coronary hemodynamics in endothelial NO synthase knockout mice. *Circ Res* 82:186, 1998.
6. Gu J-W, Brady AL, Anand V, et al: Adenosine upregulates VEGF expression in cultured myocardial vascular smooth muscle. *Am J Physiol* 277:H595, 1999.
7. Hein TW, Kuo L: cAMP-independent dilation of coronary arterioles to adenosine: role of nitric oxide, G proteins, and K_{ATP} channels. *Circ Res* 85:634, 1999.
8. Imahashi K, Kusuoka H, Hashimoto K, et al: Intracellular sodium accumulation during ischemia as the substitute for reperfusion injury. *Circ Res* 84:1401, 1999.
9. Ishibashi Y, Duncker DJ, Zhang J, et al: ATP-sensitive K^+ channels, adenosine, and nitric oxide-mediated mechanisms account for coronary vasodilation during exercise. *Circ Res* 82:346, 1998.
10. Karmazyn M, Gan XT, Humphreys RA, et al: The myocardial Na^+-H^+ exchange: structure, regulation, and its role in heart disease. *Circ Res* 85:777, 1999.
11. Kusuoka H, Marban E: Cellular mechanisms of myocardial stunning. *Annu Rev Physiol* 54:243, 1992.
12. Marban E: Myocardial stunning and hibernation: the physiology behind the colloquialisms. *Circulation* 83:681, 1991.
13. Olsson RA, Bunger R, Spaan JAE: The coronary circulation. In Fozzard HA, Haber E, Jennings RB, editors: *The heart and cardiovascular system*, ed 2, New York, 1991, Raven Press.
14. Rizri A, Tang X-L, Qiu Y, et al: Increased protein synthesis is necessary for the development of late preconditioning against myocardial stunning. *Am J Physiol* 277:H874, 1999.
15. Zheng W, Brown MD, Brock TA, et al: Bradycardia-induced coronary angiogenesis is dependent on vascular endothelial growth factor. *Circ Res* 85:192, 1999.

HISTORY

A 70-year-old man with a long history of angina pectoris had been treated successfully with nitroglycerin. He entered the hospital because of short episodes of lightheadedness and occasional loss of consciousness. Physical examination was not remarkable, except for a pulse rate of 35. Blood pressure was 130/50. Electrocardiogram showed an atrial rate of 72 and a ventricular rate of 35, with complete disassociation of the P and R waves. Chest x-ray showed a moderately enlarged heart. The diagnosis was coronary artery disease with complete (third-degree) heart block. A pacemaker was inserted and he was discharged from the hospital.

QUESTIONS

1. The severe bradycardia produced
   a. Myogenic constriction of the coronary vessels
   b. Metabolic dilation of the coronary vessels
   c. Reflex dilation of the coronary vessels
   d. A decrease and an increase in coronary resistance
   e. Reversal of the endocardial to epicardial blood flow ratio

   Within 2 to 3 months after leaving the hospital the patient experienced more frequent and more severe bouts of angina pectoris, and he was admitted to the hospital for study. An angiogram showed advanced coronary disease with almost complete occlusion of the three main coronary arteries. He was then scheduled for coronary bypass surgery.

2. During the operation the surgeon electrically stimulated the right and left stellate ganglia. This stimulation resulted in
   a. No change in coronary blood flow
   b. An increase in ventricular rate and a decrease in atrial rate
   c. A decrease in ventricular rate and an increase in atrial rate
   d. A sustained coronary dilation in one of the partially occluded vessels
   e. A sustained coronary constriction in one of the partially occluded vessels

3. Shortly after bypass surgery the reactivity of his coronary vessels was tested by intracoronary administration (via a catheter) of several vasoactive agents. Which of the following substances elicited an increase in coronary resistance?
   a. Nitroglycerin
   b. Endothelin
   c. Prostacyclin
   d. Adenosine
   e. Acetylcholine

4. Despite the coronary bypass surgery the patient's cardiac function progressively deteriorated. He became severely short of breath (dyspneic) and developed intractable cardiac failure. A suitable donor was found and he had a heart transplant. After cardiac transplant which of the following is true?
   a. Coronary blood flow increased with vagus nerve stimulation
   b. Coronary blood flow decreased with sympathetic nerve stimulation
   c. Heart rate increased with inspiration
   d. Heart rate decreased with inspiration
   e. Stroke volume increased with exercise

CHAPTER 11

Special Circulations

Objectives

1. Describe the regulation of cutaneous blood flow and the role of the skin in maintaining a constant body temperature.

2. Indicate the relative importance of the local and neural factors in adjustments of skeletal muscle blood flow at rest and during exercise.

3. Describe the regulation of cerebral blood flow.

4. Explain the regulation of the pulmonary circulation.

5. Describe the characteristics of the renal circulation.

6. Relate the intestinal and hepatic components of the splanchnic circulation.

7. Explain the changes in the fetal circulation that occur at birth.

PREVIOUS CHAPTERS ON THE CIRCU-latory system describe how the heart and vessels function to provide the tissues of the body with oxygen and nutrients and to remove carbon dioxide and waste products. Because the circulations of the various organs of the body differ to some degree with respect to their function and regulation, this chapter on special circulations is included.

■ CUTANEOUS CIRCULATION

The oxygen and nutrient requirements of the skin are relatively small and, in contrast to most other body tissues, the supply of these essential materials is not the chief governing factor in the regulation of cutaneous blood flow. The pri-

mary function of the cutaneous circulation is maintenance of a constant body temperature. Consequently, the skin shows wide fluctuations in blood flow, depending on the need for loss or conservation of body heat. Mechanisms responsible for alterations in skin blood flow are primarily activated by changes in ambient and internal body temperatures.

Skin Blood Flow Is Regulated Mainly by the Sympathetic Nervous System

There are essentially two types of resistance vessels in skin: arterioles and **arteriovenous (AV) anastomoses.** The arterioles are similar to those found elsewhere in the body. AV anastomoses shunt blood from the arterioles to venules and venous plexuses; hence they bypass the capillary bed. They are found primarily in the fingertips, palms of the hands, toes, soles of the feet, ears, nose, and lips. AV anastomoses differ morphologically from the arterioles in that they are either short, straight vessels or long, coiled vessels about 20 to 40 μm in lumen diameter, with thick muscular walls richly supplied with nerve fibers (Figure 11-1). These vessels are almost exclusively under sympathetic neural control and become maximally dilated when their nerve supply is interrupted. Conversely, reflex stimulation of the sympathetic fibers to these vessels may produce constriction to the point of complete obliteration of the vascular lumen. Although AV anastomoses do not exhibit **basal tone** (tonic activity of the vascular smooth muscle independent of innervation), they are highly sensitive to vasoconstrictor agents such as epinephrine and norepinephrine. Furthermore, AV anastomoses do not appear to be under metabolic control, and they fail to show reactive hyperemia or autoregulation of blood flow. Thus *the regulation of blood flow through anastomotic channels is governed principally by the nervous system in response to reflex activation by temperature receptors or from higher centers of the central nervous system.*

In contrast to the AV anastomoses the skin resistance vessels exhibit some basal tone and are under dual control of the sympathetic nervous system and local regulatory factors, in much the same manner as are resistance vessels in other vascular beds. However, in the case of skin, neural control plays a more important role than local factors. Stimulation of sympathetic nerve fibers to skin blood vessels (arteries and veins, as well as arterioles) induces vasoconstriction, and severance of the sympathetic nerves induces vasodilation. With chronic denervation of the cutaneous blood vessels, the degree of tone that existed before denervation is gradually regained over a period of several weeks. This is accomplished by an enhancement of basal tone

that compensates for the degree of tone previously contributed by sympathetic nerve fiber activity. Epinephrine and norepinephrine elicit only vasoconstriction in cutaneous vessels. Denervation of the skin vessels results in enhanced sensitivity to circulating catecholamines **(denervation hypersensitivity).**

Parasympathetic vasodilator nerve fibers do not supply the cutaneous blood vessels. However, stimulation of the sweat glands, which are innervated by cholinergic fibers of the sympathetic nervous system, results in dilation of the skin resistance vessels. Sweat contains an enzyme that acts on a protein moiety in the tissue fluid to produce **bradykinin,** a polypeptide with potent vasodilator properties. Bradykinin formed in the tissue can act locally to dilate the arterioles and increase blood flow to the skin.

The skin vessels of certain regions, particularly the head, neck, shoulders, and upper chest, are under the influence of the higher centers of the central nervous system. Blushing, as with embarrassment or anger, and blanching, as with fear or anxiety, are examples of cerebral inhibition and stimulation, respectively, of the sympathetic nerve fibers to the affected regions.

In contrast to AV anastomoses in the skin, the cutaneous resistance vessels show autoregulation of blood flow and reactive hyperemia. If the arterial inflow to a limb is stopped with an inflated blood pressure cuff for a brief period, the skin shows a marked reddening below the point of vascular occlusion when the cuff is deflated. This increased cutaneous blood flow (reactive hyperemia) is also manifested by distension of the superficial veins in the erythematous extremity. Autoregulation of blood flow in the skin is best explained by a myogenic mechanism (see p 180).

Ambient and Body Temperature Play an Important Role in the Regulation of Skin Blood Flow *Because the primary function of the skin is to preserve the internal milieu and protect it from adverse changes in the environ-*

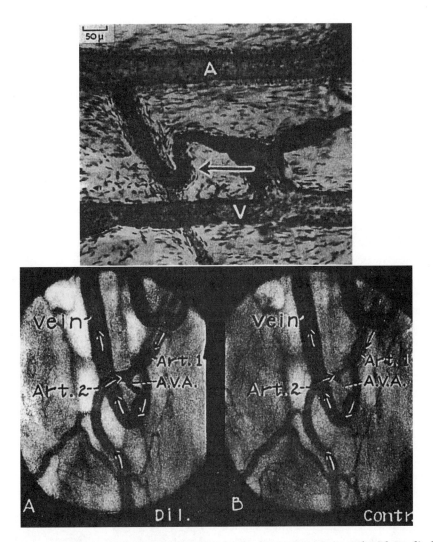

Figure 11-1 ■ *Top,* Arteriovenous *(AV)* anastomosis in the human ear injected with Berlin blue. *A,* Artery; *V,* vein; arrow points to AV anastomosis. The walls of the AV anastomosis in the fingertips are thicker and more cellular. (From Pritchard MML, Daniel PM: *J Anat* 90:309, 1956.) *Bottom,* Two frames from a motion picture record of the same relatively large arteriovenous anastomosis *(A.V.A.)* in a stable rabbit ear chamber installed 3½ months previously. *Frame A,* A.V.A. dilated; *Frame B,* A.V.A. contracted. On this day the lumen of the A.V.A. measured 51 μm dilated and 5 μm contracted at its narrowest point. (From Clark ER, Clark EL: *Am J Anat* 54:229, 1934.)

ment, and because ambient temperature is one of the most important external variables the body must contend with, it is not surprising that the vasculature of the skin is chiefly influenced by environmental temperature. Exposure to cold elicits a generalized cutaneous vasoconstriction that is most pronounced in the hands and feet. This response is chiefly mediated by the nervous system because arrest of the circulation to a hand with a pressure cuff and immersion of that hand in cold water result in vasoconstriction in the skin of the other extremities that are exposed to room temperature. With the circulation to the chilled hand unoccluded, the reflex vasoconstriction is caused in part by the cooled blood returning to the general circulation and stimulating the temperature-regulating center in the anterior hypothalamus. Direct application of cold to this region of the brain produces cutaneous vasoconstriction.

The skin vessels of the cooled hand also show a direct response to cold. Moderate cooling or exposure for brief periods to severe cold (0° to 15° C) results in constriction of the resistance and capacitance vessels, including AV anastomoses. However, prolonged exposure of the hand to severe cold has a secondary vasodilator effect. Prompt vasoconstriction and severe pain are elicited by immersion of the hand in water near 0° C but are soon followed by dilation of the skin vessels with reddening of the immersed part and alleviation of the pain. With continued immersion of the hand, alternating periods of constriction and dilation occur, but the skin temperature rarely drops to as low a degree as it did with the initial vasoconstriction. Prolonged severe cold results in tissue damage. The rosy faces of people working or playing in a cold environment are examples of cold vasodilation. However, the blood flow through the skin of the face may be greatly reduced despite the flushed appearance. The red color of the slowly flowing blood is in large measure the re-

sult of reduced oxygen uptake by the cold skin and the cold-induced shift to the left of the oxyhemoglobin dissociation curve.

Direct application of heat to the skin produces not only local vasodilation of resistance and capacitance vessels and AV anastomoses but also reflex dilation in other parts of the body. The local effect is independent of the vascular nerve supply, whereas the reflex vasodilation is a combination of anterior hypothalamic stimulation by the returning warmed blood and of stimulation of receptors in the heated part. However, evidence for a reflex from peripheral temperature receptors is not as definitive for warm stimulation as it is for cold stimulation.

*The close proximity of the major arteries and veins to each other permits considerable heat exchange (**countercurrent**) between artery and vein.* Cold blood that flows in veins from a cooled hand toward the heart takes up heat from adjacent arteries, resulting in warming of the venous blood and cooling of the arterial blood. Heat exchange is of course in the opposite direction with exposure of the extremity to heat. Thus heat conservation is enhanced and heat gain is minimized during exposure of extremities to cold and warm environments, respectively.

BOX 11-1

The fingers (and sometimes the toes) of some individuals are very sensitive to cold. When exposed to cold the arteries and arterioles to the hands constrict, producing ischemia of the fingers characterized by blanching of the skin, which is associated with tingling, numbness, and pain. The blanching is followed by cyanosis and later by redness as the arterial spasm subsides. This condition, called **Raynaud's disease,** is of unknown cause and occurs most frequently in young women.

Skin Color Depends on the Volume and Flow of Blood in the Skin and the Amount of O_2 Bound to Hemoglobin

The color of the skin is caused in large part by pigment, but in all but very dark skin, the degree of pallor or ruddiness is mainly a function of the amount of blood in the skin. With little blood in the venous plexus the skin appears pale, whereas with moderate to large quantities of blood in the venous plexus the skin shows color. Whether this color is bright red, blue, or some shade between is determined by the degree of oxygenation of the blood in the subcutaneous vessels. For example, a combination of vasoconstriction and reduced hemoglobin can produce an ashen gray color of the skin, whereas a combination of venous engorgement and reduced hemoglobin can result in a dark purple hue. Skin color provides little information about the rate of cutaneous blood flow. There may coexist rapid blood flow and pale skin when the AV anastomoses are open, and slow blood flow and red skin when the extremity is exposed to cold.

■ SKELETAL MUSCLE CIRCULATION

The rate of blood flow in skeletal muscle varies directly with the contractile activity of the tissue and the type of muscle. Blood flow and capillary density in red (slow-twitch, high-oxidative) muscle are greater than in white (fast-twitch, low-oxidative) muscle. In resting muscle the precapillary arterioles exhibit asynchronous intermittent contractions and relaxations, so that at any given moment a very large percentage of the capillary bed is not perfused. Consequently, total blood flow through quiescent skeletal muscle is low (1.4 to 4.5 ml/min/100 g). With exercise the resistance vessels relax and the muscle blood flow may increase manyfold (up to 15 to 20 times the resting level); the magnitude of the increase depends largely on the severity of the exercise.

Regulation of Skeletal Muscle Circulation Is Achieved by Neural and Local Factors

As with all tissues, physical factors such as arterial pressure, tissue pressure, and blood viscosity influence muscle blood flow. However, another physical factor comes into play during exercise—the squeezing effect of the active muscle on the vessels. With intermittent contractions, inflow is restricted and venous outflow is enhanced during each brief contraction (Figure 11-2). The presence of the venous valves prevents backflow of blood in the veins between contractions, thereby aiding in the forward propulsion of the blood (see also p 221). With strong sustained contractions the vascular bed can be compressed to the point where blood flow actually ceases temporarily.

Neural Factors Although the resistance vessels of muscle possess a high degree of basal tone, they also display tone attributable to continuous low-frequency activity in the sympathetic vasoconstrictor nerve fibers. The basal frequency of firing in the sympathetic vasoconstrictor fibers is quite low (about 1 to 2 per second), and maximal vasoconstriction is observed at frequencies as low as 8 to 10 per second. Stimulation of the sympathetic nerve fibers to skeletal muscle elicits vasoconstriction caused by the release of norepinephrine at the fiber endings. Intraarterial injection of norepinephrine elicits only vasoconstriction, whereas low doses of epinephrine produce vasodilation in muscle and large doses cause vasoconstriction.

The tonic activity of the sympathetic nerves is greatly influenced by reflexes from the baroreceptors. An increase in carotid sinus pressure results in dilation of the vascular bed of the muscle, and a decrease in carotid sinus pressure elicits vasoconstriction (Figure 11-3). When the existing sympathetic constrictor tone is high, as in the experiment illustrated in Figure 11-3, the decrease in blood flow associated with common carotid artery occlusion is small, but the in-

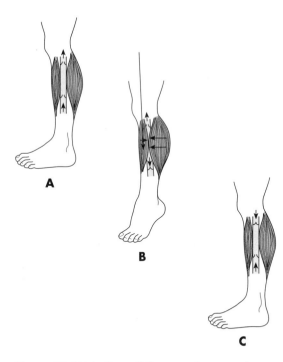

Figure 11-2 ■ Action of the muscle pump in venous return from the legs. A, Standing at rest the venous valves are open and blood flows upward toward the heart by virtue of the pressure generated by the heart and transmitted through the capillaries to the veins from the arterial side of the vascular system (vis a tergo). B, Contraction of the muscle compresses the vein so that the increased pressure in the vein drives blood toward the thorax through the upper valve and closes the lower valve in the uncompressed segment of the vein just below the point of muscular compression. C, Immediately after muscle relaxation, the pressure in the previously compressed venous segment falls, and the reversed pressure gradient causes the upper valve to close. The valve below the previously compressed segment opens because pressure below it exceeds that above it and the segment fills with blood from the foot. As blood flow continues from the foot, the pressure in the previously compressed segment rises. When it exceeds the pressure above the upper valve, this valve opens and continuous flow occurs as in A.

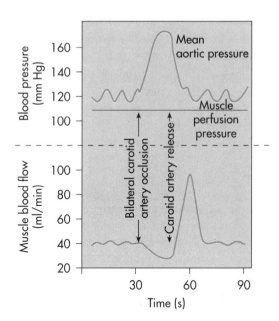

Figure 11-3 ■ Evidence for participation of the muscle vascular bed in vasoconstriction and vasodilation mediated by the carotid sinus baroreceptors after common carotid artery occlusion and release. In this preparation the sciatic and femoral nerves constituted the only direct connection between the hind leg muscle mass and the rest of the dog. The muscle was perfused by blood at a constant pressure that was completely independent of the animal's arterial pressure. (Redrawn from Jones RD, Berne RM: *Am J Physiol* 204:461, 1963.)

crease after the release of occlusion is large. The vasodilation produced by baroreceptor stimulation is caused by inhibition of sympathetic vasoconstrictor activity. Because muscle is the major body component on the basis of mass and thereby represents the largest vascular bed, the participation of its resistance vessels in vascular reflexes plays an important role in maintaining a constant arterial blood pressure.

A comparison of the vasoconstrictor and vasodilator effects of the sympathetic nerves to blood vessels of muscle and skin is summarized in Figure 11-4. Note the lower basal tone of the skin

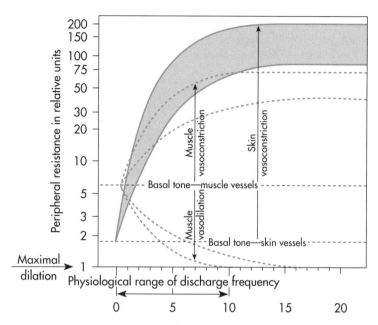

Figure 11-4 ■ **Basal tone and the range of response of the resistance vessels in muscle** *(dashed lines)* **and skin** *(shaded area)* **to stimulation and section of the sympathetic nerves. Peripheral resistance plotted on a logarithmic scale.** (Redrawn from Celander O, Folkow B: *Acta Physiol Scand* 29:241, 1953.)

vessels, their greater constrictor response, and the absence of active cutaneous vasodilation.

Local Factors Whether neural or local factors predominate in the regulation of skeletal muscle blood flow depends on the activity of the muscle. In resting muscle the neural factors predominate and superimpose neurogenic tone on the nonneural basal tone (see Figure 11-4). Section of the sympathetic nerves to muscle abolishes the neural component of vascular tone and unmasks the intrinsic basal tone of the blood vessels. *Neural and local blood flow regulating mechanisms oppose each other, and during muscle contraction the local vasodilator mechanism supervenes.* However, during exercise, strong sympathetic nerve stimulation slightly reduces the vasodilation induced by locally released metabolites.

BOX 11-2

When the valves of the superficial leg veins are incompetent, as may occur with pregnancy, thrombophlebitis, or obesity, the veins become dilated and tortuous. Such **varicose veins** can be treated by surgical removal, by injection of sclerosing solutions, or merely by the use of elastic stockings.

■ **CEREBRAL CIRCULATION**

Blood reaches the brain through the internal carotid and vertebral arteries. The latter join to form the basilar artery, which, in conjunction with branches of the internal carotid arteries, forms the **circle of Willis.** A unique feature of the cerebral circulation is that it all lies within a rigid structure, the cranium. Because intracranial contents are incompressible, any increase in arterial inflow, as with arteriolar dilation, must be associated with a comparable increase in venous outflow. The volume of blood and extravascular fluid can vary considerably in most tissues. In the brain the volume of blood and extravascular fluid is relatively constant; changes in either of these fluid volumes must be accompanied by a reciprocal change in the other. In contrast to most other organs, the rate of total cerebral blood flow is held within a relatively narrow range; in humans it averages 55 ml/min/100 g of brain.

Local Factors Predominate Over Neural Factors in the Regulation of Cerebral Blood Flow

Of the various body tissues, the brain is the least tolerant of ischemia. Interruption of cerebral blood flow for as little as 5 seconds results in loss of consciousness, and ischemia lasting just a few minutes results in irreversible tissue damage. Fortunately, regulation of the cerebral circulation is primarily under direction of the brain itself. Local regulatory mechanisms and reflexes originating in the brain tend to maintain cerebral circulation relatively constant in the presence of possible adverse extrinsic effects such as sympathetic vasomotor nerve activity, circulating humoral vasoactive agents, and changes in arterial blood pressure. Under certain conditions the brain also regulates its blood flow by initiating changes in systemic blood pressure.

Neural Factors The cerebral vessels receive innervation from the cervical sympathetic nerve fibers that accompany the internal carotid and vertebral arteries into the cranial cavity. The importance of neural regulation of the cerebral circulation is controversial, but the prevalent belief is that, relative to other vascular beds, sympathetic control of the cerebral vessels is weak and the contractile state of the cerebrovascular smooth muscle depends primarily on local metabolic factors. There are no known sympathetic vasodilator nerves to the cerebral vessels, but the vessels do receive parasympathetic fibers from the facial nerve that produce a slight vasodilation on stimulation.

Local Factors Generally, *total cerebral blood flow is constant. However, regional cortical blood flow is associated with regional neural activity.* For example, movement of one hand results in increased blood flow only in the hand area of the contralateral sensorimotor and premotor cortex. Also, talking, reading, and other stimuli to the cerebral cortex are associated with increased blood flow in the appropriate regions of the contralateral cortex (Figure 11-5). Stimulation of the retina with flashes of light increases blood flow only in the visual cortex. Glucose uptake also corresponds with regional cortical neuronal activity. For example, when the retina is stimulated by light, uptake of ^{14}C-2-deoxyglucose is enhanced in the visual cortex.

It is well known that the cerebral vessels are very sensitive to carbon dioxide tension. Increases in arterial blood CO_2 tension (Pa_{CO_2}) elicit marked cerebral vasodilation; inhalation of 7% CO_2 results in a twofold increment in cerebral blood flow. By the same token, decreases in Pa_{CO_2}, such as those elicited by hyperventilation, produce a decrease in cerebral blood flow. CO_2 evokes changes in arteriolar resistance by altering perivascular (and probably intracellular vascular smooth muscle) pH. By independently changing Pa_{CO_2} and bicarbonate concentration, it has been demonstrated that pial vessel diameter (and presumably blood flow) and pH are inversely related, regardless of the level of the Pa_{CO_2}.

Carbon dioxide can diffuse to the vascular smooth muscle from the brain tissue or from the lumen of the vessels, whereas hydrogen ions in the blood are prevented from reaching the arteriolar smooth muscle by the **blood-brain barrier.** Hence the cerebral vessels dilate when the hydrogen ion concentration of the cerebrospi-

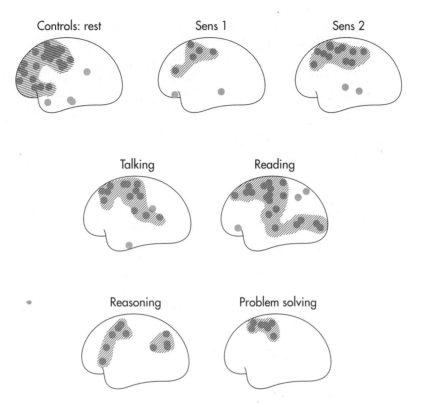

Figure 11-5 ■ **Effects of different stimuli on regional blood flow in the contralateral human cerebral cortex.** *Sens 1,* **Low-intensity electrical stimulation of the hand;** *Sens 2,* **high-intensity electrical stimulation of the hand (pain).** (Redrawn from Ingvar DH: *Brain Res* 107:181, 1976.)

nal fluid is increased but show only minimal dilation in response to an increase in the hydrogen ion concentration of the arterial blood.

With respect to K^+, such stimuli as hypoxia, electrical stimulation of the brain, and seizures elicit rapid increases in cerebral blood flow and are associated with increases in perivascular K^+. The increments in K^+ are similar to those that produce pial arteriolar dilation when K^+ is applied topically to these vessels. However, the increase in K^+ is not sustained throughout the period of stimulation. Hence only the initial increment in cerebral blood flow can be attributed to the release of K^+.

Adenosine levels of the brain increase with ischemia, hypoxemia, hypotension, hypocap-

nia, electrical stimulation of the brain, and induced seizures. When applied topically, adenosine is a potent dilator of the pial arterioles. In short, any intervention that either reduces the O_2 supply to the brain or increases the O_2 need of the brain results in rapid (within 5 seconds) formation of adenosine in the cerebral tissue. Unlike pH or K^+, the adenosine concentration of the brain increases with initiation of the stimulus and remains elevated throughout the period of O_2 imbalance. The adenosine released into the cerebrospinal fluid during conditions associated with inadequate brain O_2 supply is available to the brain tissue for reincorporation into cerebral tissue adenine nucleotides.

All three factors—pH, K$^+$, and adenosine—may act in concert to adjust the cerebral blood flow to the metabolic activity of the brain.

The cerebral circulation shows reactive hyperemia and excellent autoregulation between pressures of about 60 and 160 mm Hg. Mean arterial pressures below 60 mm Hg result in reduced cerebral blood flow and syncope, whereas mean pressures above 160 may lead to increased permeability of the blood-brain barrier and cerebral edema. Autoregulation of cerebral blood flow is abolished by hypercapnia or any other potent vasodilator, and none of the candidates for metabolic regulation of cerebral blood flow has been shown to be responsible for this phenomenon. Hence autoregulation of cerebral blood flow is probably attributable to a myogenic mechanism, although experimental proof is still lacking.

BOX 11-3

Elevation of intracranial pressure results in an increase in systemic blood pressure. This response, called **Cushing's phenomenon,** is apparently caused by ischemic stimulation of vasomotor regions in the medulla. It helps maintain cerebral blood flow in such conditions as expanding intracranial tumors.

■ THE PULMONARY AND SYSTEMIC CIRCULATIONS ARE IN SERIES WITH EACH OTHER

Under steady-state conditions, the total pulmonary and systemic blood flows are virtually identical (see Chapter 9). Despite this similarity in the rate of blood flow, the anatomic, hemodynamic, and physiological characteristics of these two sections of the cardiovascular system differ substantially.

Functional Anatomy

Pulmonary Vasculature The pulmonary vascular system is a low-resistance network of highly distensible vessels. The main pulmonary artery is much shorter than the aorta. The walls of the pulmonary artery and its branches are much thinner than the walls of the aorta, and they contain less smooth muscle and elastin. Contrary to systemic arterioles, which have very thick walls composed mainly of circularly arranged smooth muscle, the pulmonary arterioles are thin and contain little smooth muscle. The pulmonary arterioles do not have the same capacity for vasoconstriction as do their counterparts in the systemic circulation. The pulmonary venules and veins are also very thin and possess little smooth muscle.

The pulmonary capillaries differ markedly from the systemic capillaries. Whereas the systemic capillaries constitute an interconnecting network of tubular vessels, the pulmonary capillaries are aligned so that the blood flows in thin sheets between adjacent alveoli (Figure 11-6). Hence the capillary blood is exposed optimally to the alveolar gases. The total surface area for exchange between alveoli and blood is about 50 to 70 m^2. Only thin layers of vascular and alveolar endothelium separate the blood and alveolar gas. The thickness of the sheets of blood between adjacent alveoli depends on the intravascular pressure and intraalveolar pressure. Ordinarily, the width of an interalveolar sheet of blood is about equal to the diameter of a red blood cell (Figure 11-6). During pulmonary vascular congestion, as when left atrial pressure is elevated, the width of the sheet may increase several-fold. Conversely, when local alveolar pressure exceeds the adjacent capillary pressure, the capillaries may collapse and blood will not flow to those alveoli. Hydrostatic factors participate in this phenomenon, particularly with respect to the regional distribution of blood flow to the lungs, as described in the next section.

Bronchial Vasculature The bronchial arteries are branches of the thoracic aorta. These arteries and their branches, down to the arte-

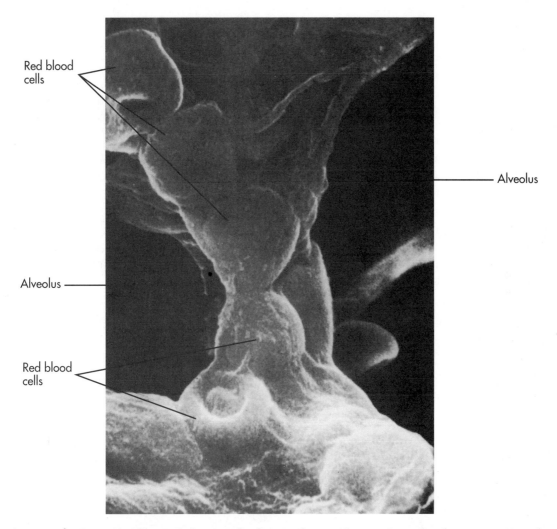

Red blood cells

Red blood cells

Alveolus

Alveolus

Figure 11-6 ■ **Scanning electron micrograph of mouse lung to show an interalveolar septum. Note that the membranes that separate an alveolus from a capillary are so thin that the shapes of the erythrocytes in the capillary can easily be discerned.** (From Greenwood MF, Holland P: *Lab Invest* 27:296, 1972.)

rioles, have the structural characteristics of most systemic arteries; that is, they have much thicker walls and more smooth muscles than do the pulmonary arterial vessels of equivalent caliber. The bronchial vessels supply blood to the tracheobronchial tree down to the terminal bronchioles.

The bronchial veins drain partly into the pulmonary venous system and partly into the azy-gos veins, which are a part of the systemic venous system. The bronchial circulation normally constitutes about 1% of the cardiac output. Therefore the fraction of the bronchial blood flow that returns to the left atrium (via the pulmonary veins) rather than to the right atrium (via the azygos veins) constitutes at most 1% of the venous return to the heart. This small quantity of bronchial venous blood, plus a small amount of coronary venous blood that drains directly into the left atrium or left ventricle, "contaminates" the pulmonary venous blood, which is ordinarily fully saturated with O_2. Hence the aortic blood is very slightly desaturated. This small quantity of venous drainage directly into the left side of the heart also accounts for the fact that, even under true equilibrium conditions, the output of the left ventricle slightly exceeds that of the right ventricle.

BOX 11-4

Sustained abridgment of the pulmonary arterial blood supply to a lung, after **pulmonary embolism,** for example, usually increases the precapillary (arterial) communications between vessels of the systemic and pulmonary circuits. Certain inflammatory and degenerative pulmonary diseases, such as **emphysema,** are often associated with increased bronchial blood flow, and significant admixtures of blood take place between the two systems.

Pulmonary Hemodynamics

Pressures in the Pulmonary Circulation
In normal individuals the average systolic and diastolic pressures in the pulmonary artery are about 25 and 10 mm Hg, respectively, and the mean pressure is about 15 mm Hg (Figure 11-7). These pressures are much lower than those in systemic arteries (Figure 11-7) because the pulmonary vascular resistance is only about one tenth the resistance of the systemic vascular bed. The mean pressure in the left atrium is normally about 5 mm Hg, and so the total pulmonary arteriovenous pressure gradient is only about 10 mm Hg. The mean hydrostatic pressure in the pulmonary capillaries lies between the pulmonary arterial and pulmonary venous values but somewhat closer to the latter.

BOX 11-5

The mean left atrial pressure is an index of the left ventricular filling pressure. To determine whether a patient suffers from **left heart failure,** it is desirable but difficult to measure the left atrial pressure directly. However, a flexible, balloon-tipped catheter can easily be guided into the pulmonary artery. If the catheter is advanced until the tip is wedged into a small branch of the pulmonary artery, the **pulmonary artery wedge pressure** serves as a useful estimate of the pressure in the left atrium. The wedged catheter halts flow in the small vessels distal to the catheter. These vessels then serve as an extension of the catheter and thereby allow the catheter to communicate with the pulmonary veins and left atrium.

Pulmonary Blood Flow At equilibrium the pulmonary and systemic blood flows are equal, except for the small disparity contributed by the bronchial circulation. Because of the low pressures in the pulmonary blood vessels and their

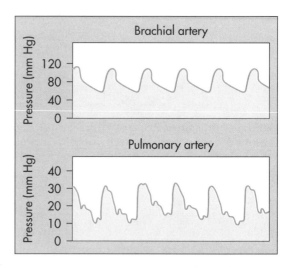

Figure 11-7 ■ **Pressures recorded in the brachial and pulmonary arteries of a normal human subject.** (Modified from Harris P, Heath D: *Human pulmonary circulation,* Edinburgh, 1962, E and S Livingstone.)

great distensibility, gravity affects the regional distribution of blood flow in the lungs.

Three distinct flow patterns may be found at different hydrostatic levels in the lung, as illustrated in Figure 11-8. Consider that the pulmonary artery delivers blood at a steady pressure of 15 mm Hg and that pulmonary venous pressure remains constant at 5 mm Hg.

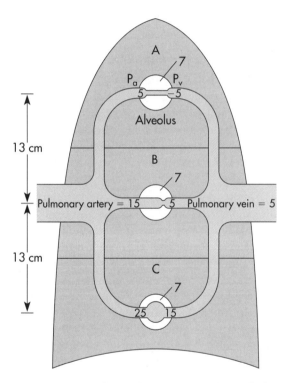

Figure 11-8 ■ **Schematic representation of the three types of flow regimens that might exist in the pulmonary circulation. In zone A, alveolar pressure exceeds intravascular pressures. Pulmonary capillaries in this zone will not be perfused. In zone B, alveolar pressure is intermediate between pulmonary arterial and venous pressures. Pulmonary capillaries will flutter between the open and closed states. In zone C, intravascular pressures exceed alveolar pressure. The pulmonary capillaries are always open, but the flow resistances in individual vessels vary with the hydrostatic pressure in the vessel.**

In those pulmonary arterial and venous branches that are 13 cm below (zone *C*) the hydrostatic level of the main pulmonary vessels, the respective pressures will be 10 mm Hg (equivalent of 13 cm of blood) greater than those in the main vessels, by virtue of gravitational effects. Conversely, in pulmonary arterial and venous branches that are 13 cm above (zone *A*) the main vessels, the respective pressures will be 10 mm Hg less than those in the main vessels. At the same hydrostatic level (zone *B*) as the main vessels, the respective pressures in the branches will be approximately equal to those in the main vessels.

Consider that the alveolar pressure equals 7 mm Hg in all alveoli. Such an alveolar pressure might exist in an individual receiving positive-pressure ventilation. In zone *A* the alveolar pressure would exceed the local arterial and venous pressures (see Figure 11-8). The pulmonary capillary pressures lie between those of the arteries and veins, and therefore alveolar pressure would also exceed capillary pressure. Capillaries lying between adjacent alveoli would collapse. Those alveoli would not be perfused, and gas would not be exchanged.

BOX 11-6

Ordinarily, the mean pressure in the alveoli is atmospheric. Therefore the conditions depicted in zone *A* do not ordinarily prevail in any region of the lungs. In **hypovolemic shock,** however, the mean pulmonary artery pressure is often very low. Therefore vascular pressures in the lung apices might be subatmospheric. The atmospheric pressure in the alveoli would then compress the apical capillaries, so that virtually no blood would flow to that zone from the pulmonary circulation. However, the bronchial circulation, which operates at much higher pressures, would be unaffected.

In zone *B* the alveolar pressure lies between the local arterial and venous pressures (see Figure 11-8). Again, if alveolar pressure equals 7 mm Hg, a capillary in that region will flutter between the open and closed states. When the capillary is open, blood will flow through it, and the capillary pressure will decrease progressively from the arterial to the venous end. The pressure at the venous end will be less than the alveolar pressure, and therefore the capillary will collapse at that end. With the cessation of flow, the arterial and capillary pressures at a given hydrostatic level will equalize. Thus the capillary pressure will quickly rise to that in the local small arteries, which exceeds the prevailing alveolar pressure. The capillary will then be forced open. With the restitution of flow, however, the pressure will drop along the length of the capillary. As the pressure at the venous end drops below the ambient alveolar pressure, the capillary will again close. Hence the capillary will flutter between the open and closed states.

The critical pressure gradient for flow in zone *B* is the arterioalveolar pressure difference, not the arteriovenous pressure difference, as it is for most vessels in the body. As long as venous pressure is less than alveolar pressure, venous pressure does not influence the flow. Such a flow condition is called a **waterfall effect** because the height of a waterfall has no influence on the flow.

In zone *C* the arterial and venous pressures both exceed the alveolar pressure. Hence the pressure everywhere along the capillary exceeds the alveolar pressure, and the capillary remains permanently open. In this zone the flow is determined by the arteriovenous pressure gradient, and the resistance may be calculated by the hydraulic analog of Ohm's law.

The large and small pulmonary vessels, including the capillaries, are very distensible, as previously noted. The pressure difference that determines the caliber of a distensible tube is the **transmural pressure,** that is, the difference between the internal and external pressures. In an erect individual the intravascular pressures in the lungs increase from apex to base. The transmural pressures increase accordingly, and the diameter of the pulmonary vessels increases from apex to base. Because resistance to flow varies inversely with vessel caliber, resistance decreases and flow increases in zone *C* in the apex-to-base direction. Such predicted changes in flow have been verified in humans.

Regulation of the Pulmonary Circulation

The total volume of blood pumped by the heart passes through the pulmonary circulation. Therefore the various cardiac and vascular factors that determine cardiac output in general also determine total pulmonary blood flow. These factors have been discussed in Chapter 9.

The autonomic nervous system innervates the pulmonary blood vessels. Although the small pulmonary vessels contain little smooth muscle, small changes in smooth muscle tone may alter vascular resistance substantially because the pressures in the pulmonary circulation are so low. Baroreceptor stimulation can dilate the pulmonary resistance vessels reflexly. Conversely, peripheral chemoreceptor stimulation constricts the pulmonary vessels; however, the importance of such neural regulation remains to be established.

Hypoxia has the most important influence on pulmonary vasomotor tone. Acute and chronic hypoxia both increase pulmonary vascular resistance (Figure 11-9). Regional reductions in alveolar O_2 tension constrict the nearby arterioles. This response helps maintain an optimal **ventilation-perfusion ratio.** The O_2 tension in poorly ventilated alveoli will approach the PO_2 in the pulmonary arterial blood. Blood flowing by such alveoli will not

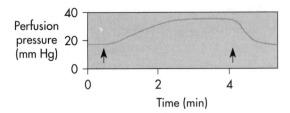

<figure>**Figure 11-9** ■ **Effect of hypoxia on vascular resistance of an isolated rat lung. The lung was perfused with blood at a constant flow. When the O$_2$ tension of the inspired air was reduced** *(between the arrows),* **the pulmonary resistance vessels constricted, as indicated by the substantial rise in perfusion pressure.** (Modified from Grover RF, Wagner WW Jr, McMurtry IF, et al: Pulmonary circulation. In *Handbook of physiology,* Section 2: *The cardiovascular system—peripheral circulation and organ blood flow,* vol III, Bethesda, MD, 1983, American Physiological Society.)</figure>

be well oxygenated, and therefore the O$_2$ tension of the blood returning to the left atrium will decrease. *Arteriolar vasoconstriction reduces the blood flow to poorly ventilated alveoli and thereby reduces the contamination of the pulmonary venous blood with poorly oxygenated blood.* Thus this mechanism shunts pulmonary blood flow from the poorly ventilated regions to the better ventilated regions of the lungs and thereby improves the O$_2$ saturation of the systemic arterial blood. The mechanism by which hypoxia raises pulmonary vascular resistance has not yet been established. Electrophysiological studies on pulmonary vascular smooth muscle cells indicate that hypoxia inhibits an outward potassium current. The resulting depolarization of the cell membrane augments the influx of calcium into the smooth muscle cells and thereby induces contraction. These results therefore suggest that in an intact pulmonary blood vessel, hypoxia would lead to vasoconstriction.

■ THE RENAL CIRCULATION ACCOUNTS FOR ABOUT 20% OF THE CARDIAC OUTPUT

Anatomy

The primary branches of the **renal artery** divide into a number of **interlobar arteries.** These interlobar branches (Figure 11-10) proceed radially from the hilus toward the corticomedullary junction between adjacent medullary pyramids. As an interlobar artery approaches the corticomedullary junction, it branches into a number of arcuate arteries, which travel in various directions over the bases of the adjacent medullary pyramids, in the zone between the cortex and the medulla. The arcuate branches that arise from adjacent interlobar arteries do not interconnect. Hence occlusion of an interlobar artery destroys a pyramid-shaped region of the kidney.

From the arcuate arteries, a number of **interlobular branches** travel toward the capsular surface of the kidney (see Figure 11-10). The **afferent arterioles** to the **glomeruli** are branches of these interlobular arteries. Each human kidney has approximately 1 million glomeruli. The afferent arteriole to each glomerulus divides into several vessels that form discrete capillary loops (Figure 11-11). The proximal and distal limbs of each loop are interconnected by many smaller capillaries. The distal limbs of each capillary loop within a glomerulus rejoin to form the **efferent arteriole,** the diameter of which is usually less than that of the afferent arteriole. The entire glomerular capillary tuft is enveloped by **Bowman's capsule,** which collects the glomerular filtrate.

The efferent arterioles divide into another capillary network, the **peritubular capillaries** (Figure 11-12). The architecture of the peritubular capillary network varies, depending on whether the efferent arteriole arises from glomeruli close to the medullary border (the **juxtamedullary glomeruli**) or from glomeruli in the more peripheral regions of the renal cortex (see Figure 11-10).

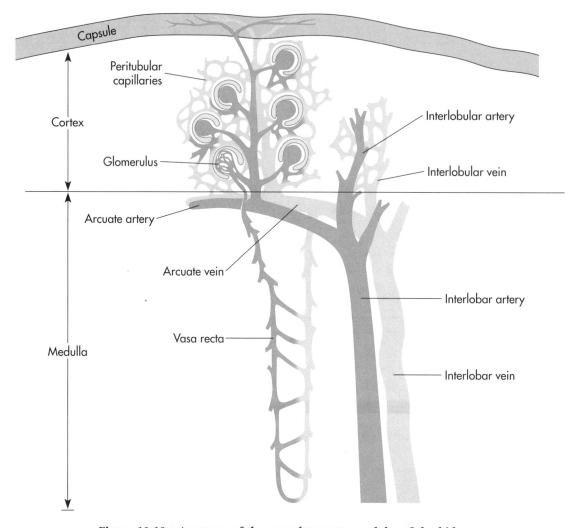

Figure 11-10 ■ **Anatomy of the vasculature to one lobe of the kidney.**

Capillaries that originate from the regular cortical glomeruli surround relatively short renal tubules, which are located almost entirely in the renal cortex itself. The capillary networks of neighboring cortical nephrons freely communicate with one another. Most of the capillaries arising from the efferent arterioles of juxtamedullary glomeruli form long hairpin loops **(vasa recta)** that accompany the loops of Henle deep into the renal medulla, sometimes to the tips of the renal papillae (see Figure 11-10). The vasa recta participate in the countercurrent exchange system responsible for concentrating the urine. In general, the renal venous system parallels the arterial distribution to the renal tissues.

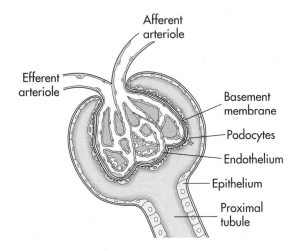

Figure 11-11 ■ **Anatomy of the mammalian glomerulus.**

Afferent arteriole

Efferent arteriole

Basement membrane

Podocytes

Endothelium

Epithelium

Proximal tubule

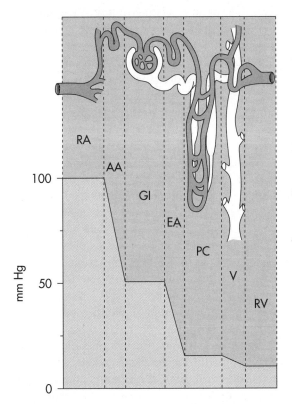

Figure 11-12 ■ **Intravascular pressures in the renal artery *(RA)*, afferent arterioles *(AA)*, glomerular capillaries *(GI)*, efferent arterioles *(EA)*, peritubular capillaries *(PC)*, venules *(V)*, and renal vein *(RV)*.** (From Frohnert PP: Renal blood flow. In Knox FG, editor: *Textbook of renal pathophysiology,* Hagerstown, MD, 1978, Harper & Row. Based on data from Brenner BM: *J Clin Invest* 50:1776, 1971.)

Renal Hemodynamics

Segmental Resistance The pressure drops only slightly in the interlobar, arcuate, and interlobular arteries: the main preglomerular resistance resides in the afferent arterioles (see Figure 11-12). The pressure in the glomerular capillaries is normally about 50 to 60 mm Hg. Thus the net balance of forces across the capillary wall favors the outward filtration of plasma water along the entire length of the capillary loop. The filtration coefficient of the glomerular capillaries exceeds that of most other capillaries in the body. Hence *about 20% of the plasma water that enters the glomerular capillaries is filtered into Bowman's capsule.* The greatest hydraulic resistance in the renal circulation is in the efferent arterioles. Consequently, the pressure in the peritubular capillaries is normally about 10 to 20 mm Hg. Such pressures favor net reabsorption of the large quantities of fluid that pass from the renal tubules to the interstitial spaces of the kidney. The peritubular capillaries are also considerably more permeable than most of the other capillaries in the body.

Renal Blood Flow *The weight of the kidneys constitutes only about 0.5% of total body weight, yet the kidneys receive about 20% of cardiac output.* Most of this rich blood supply perfuses the renal cortex; blood flow per unit weight to the inner medulla and papillae is only about one tenth of that to the cortex. Nevertheless, even these medullary tissues receive as much blood per unit weight as does the brain.

The kidney has one of the highest metabolic rates in the body. However, the large renal blood flow is not essential to subserve the great metabolic rate. The kidney extracts less than 10% of the O_2 present in the renal arterial blood. Therefore the renal blood flow is at least ten times greater than that needed to deliver the required O_2 and nutrients. The excessively high renal blood flow is so important because it delivers large volumes of blood to the glomeruli for the process of ultrafiltration.

The Renal Circulation Is Regulated Mainly by Intrinsic Mechanisms

Autoregulation Renal blood flow tends to remain constant, despite fluctuations in arterial perfusion pressure. In the experiment represented in Figure 11-13, for example, arterial pressure was suddenly raised from 140 to 190 mm Hg. This stepwise change in pressure rapidly increased the renal blood flow, from 135 to 165 ml/min. The rise in renal blood flow was transitory, however, and flow returned close to the control level in less than 1 minute. Over a pressure range of about 75 to 170 mm Hg, the steady-state level of renal blood flow is relatively insensitive to changes in arterial pressure (Figure 11-14). Beyond this range, however, renal blood flow varies directly with perfusion pressure.

This ability of the renal blood flow to remain constant, despite fluctuations in perfusion pressure, is a process intrinsic to the kidney itself; it has been demonstrated even in isolated kidney preparations (see Figure 11-13). Concomitant measurement of glomerular filtration rate (GFR) reveals that the tendency for GFR to be autoregulated is equally pronounced (see Figure 11-14). Therefore the resistance change induced by an alteration in perfusion pressure must occur mainly in the afferent arteriole. As the perfusion pressure is raised, for example, afferent arteriolar constriction not only limits the increase in renal blood flow but also restricts the rise in glomerular capillary pressure and the concomitant increment in GFR.

Renal autoregulation has been studied extensively, but the mechanism remains controversial. The two principal mediators appear to be the **myogenic mechanism** and **tubuloglomerular feedback.** The myogenic mechanism is the intrinsic property of vascular smooth muscle to contract in response to a stretching

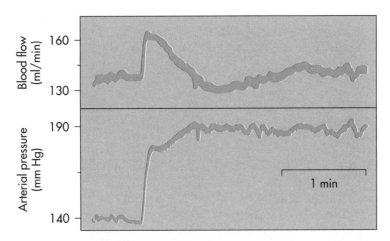

Figure 11-13 ■ **Changes in renal blood flow evoked by a sudden increase in arterial perfusion pressure from 140 to 190 mm Hg in an isolated dog kidney. The kidney was perfused from a peripheral artery of another dog.** (Modified from Semple SJG, deWardener HE: *Circ Res* 7:643, 1959.)

force, such as an increase in transmural pressure (see Chapter 8). Tubuloglomerular feedback involves a feedback loop in which a change in the flow of renal tubular fluid is detected by the **macula densa** of the **juxtaglomerular apparatus,** and the juxtaglomerular apparatus then sends a signal to the afferent arterioles to restore basal levels of renal blood flow and GFR. The precise nature of the signal that regulates the caliber of the afferent arterioles is controversial. Many vasoactive substances, such as prostaglandins, catecholamines, adenosine, nitric oxide, and the components of the renin-angiotensin system, may participate in the process of tubuloglomerular feedback.

The juxtaglomerular apparatus is the source of one of the principal humoral mechanisms, the **renin-angiotensin system,** involved in the regulation of blood volume and blood pressure. In response to various types of signals, such as a reduction in GFR, the juxtaglomerular apparatus releases the enzyme **renin.** This enzyme acts on a substrate, **angiotensinogen,** which circulates in the blood, to release the dec-

apeptide **angiotensin I.** This peptide is then split by a **converting enzyme,** mainly in the lungs, to form an octapeptide, **angiotensin II.** This peptide is not only a potent arteriolar vasoconstrictor, but it also affects many other vital functions, such as the regulation of certain renal tubular transport processes and the release of adrenocortical hormones.

Neural Regulation Stimulation of the renal sympathetic nerves decreases renal blood flow substantially but reduces GFR only slightly. The neural activity constricts the afferent and efferent arterioles and the proximal segments of the vasa recta. Presumably, the reduction of renal blood flow exceeds the reduction of GFR because the postglomerular constriction is greater than the preglomerular constriction.

In resting subjects the basal level of renal sympathetic tone is low; abolition of that tone scarcely affects renal blood flow. The arterial baroreceptor reflexes influence the renal vasculature only slightly. Activation of low-pressure vascular receptors elicits much larger reflex effects on the renal circulation. A reduction in

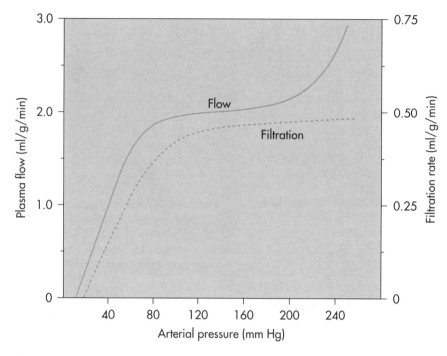

Figure 11-14 ■ Renal plasma flow and glomerular filtration rate as a function of arterial perfusion pressure in an anesthetized dog. (Adapted from Shipley RE, Study RS: *Am J Physiol* 167:676, 1951.)

left atrial pressure, for example, increases renal nerve activity and renal vascular resistance greatly. Emotional reactions, such as anxiety, fear, and rage, also curtail renal blood flow dramatically.

■ THE SPLANCHNIC CIRCULATION PROVIDES BLOOD FLOW TO THE GASTROINTESTINAL TRACT, LIVER, SPLEEN, AND PANCREAS

Several features distinguish the splanchnic circulation, the most noteworthy being that two large capillary beds are partially in series with one another. The small splanchnic arterial branches supply the capillary beds in the gastrointestinal tract, spleen, and pancreas. From these capillary beds, the venous blood ultimately flows into the portal vein, which nor-

mally provides most of the blood supply to the liver. However, the hepatic artery also supplies blood to the liver.

Intestinal Circulation

Anatomy The gastrointestinal tract is supplied by the celiac, superior mesenteric, and inferior mesenteric arteries. The superior mesenteric artery is the largest of all the aortic branches and carries over 10% of the cardiac output. Small mesenteric arteries form an extensive vascular network in the submucosa (Figure 11-15). Their branches penetrate the longitudinal and circular muscle layers and give rise to third- and fourth-order arterioles. Some third-order arterioles in the submucosa become the main arterioles to the tips of the villi.

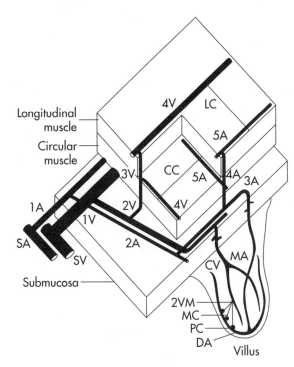

Figure 11-15 ■ **Distribution of small blood vessels to the rat intestinal wall.** *SA,* **Small artery;** *SV,* **small vein:** *1A* **to** *5A,* **first- to fifth-order arterioles;** *1V* **to** *4V,* **first- to fourth-order venules;** *CC* **and** *LC,* **capillaries in circular and longitudinal muscle layers;** *MA* **and** *CV,* **main arteriole and collecting venule of a villus;** *DA,* **distribution arteriole;** *2VM,* **second-order mucosal venule;** *PC,* **precapillary sphincter;** *MC,* **mucosal capillary.** (From Gore RW, Bohlen HG: *Am J Physiol* 233:H685, 1977.)

The direction of the blood flow in the capillaries and venules in a villus is opposite to that in the main arteriole (Figure 11-16). This arrangement constitutes a **countercurrent exchange system.** An effective countercurrent multiplier in the villus facilitates the absorption of sodium and water. The countercurrent exchange also permits diffusion of O_2 from arterioles to venules. At low flow rates, a substantial fraction of the O_2 may be shunted from arterioles to venules near the base of the villus. Thus the supply of O_2 to the mucosal cells at the tip of the villus may be curtailed. When intestinal blood flow is reduced, the shunting of O_2 is exaggerated, which may cause extensive necrosis of the intestinal villi.

Neural Regulation The neural control of the mesenteric circulation is almost exclusively sympathetic. Increased sympathetic activity constricts the mesenteric arterioles, precapillary sphincters, and capacitance vessels. These responses are mediated by α-adrenergic receptors, which are prepotent in the mesenteric circulation; however, β-adrenergic receptors are also present. Infusion of a β-receptor agonist, such as isoproterenol, causes vasodilation.

During fighting or in response to artificial stimulation of the hypothalamic "defense" area, pronounced vasoconstriction occurs in the mesenteric vascular bed. This shifts blood flow from the temporarily less important intestinal circulation to the more crucial skeletal muscles, heart, and brain.

Autoregulation Autoregulation in the intestinal circulation is not as well developed as in certain other vascular beds, such as those in the brain and kidney. The principal mechanism responsible for autoregulation is metabolic, although a myogenic mechanism probably also participates (see Chapter 8). The adenosine concentration in the mesenteric venous blood rises fourfold after brief arterial occlusion. Adenosine is a potent vasodilator in the mesenteric vascular bed and may be the principal metabolic mediator of autoregulation. However, potassium and altered osmolality may also contribute to the overall response.

The O_2 consumption of the small intestine is more rigorously controlled than is the blood flow. In one series of experiments, the O_2 uptake of the small intestine remained constant when arterial perfusion pressure was varied between 30 and 125 mm Hg.

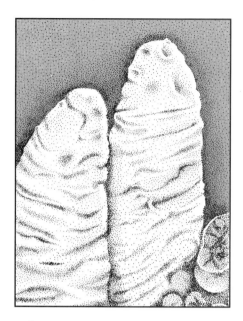 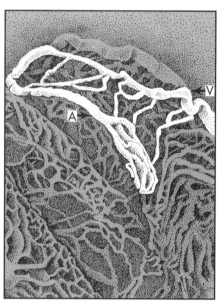

Figure 11-16 ■ **Scanning electron micrographs of rabbit intestinal villi** *(left panel)* **and corrosion cast of the microcirculation in the villus** *(right panel).* **A,** Arteriole; **V,** venule. (From Gannon BJ, Gore RW, Rogers PAW: *Biomed Res* 2(suppl):235, 1981.)

Functional Hyperemia Food ingestion increases intestinal blood flow. The secretion of certain gastrointestinal hormones contributes to this hyperemia. Gastrin and cholecystokinin augment intestinal blood flow, and they are secreted when food is ingested. The absorption of food affects intestinal blood flow. Undigested food has no vasoactive influence, whereas several products of digestion are potent vasodilators. Among the various constituents of chyme, the principal mediators of mesenteric hyperemia are glucose and fatty acids.

Hepatic Circulation

Anatomy The blood flow to the liver is normally about 25% of cardiac output. The flow is derived from two sources, the portal vein and the hepatic artery. Ordinarily, the portal vein provides about three fourths of the blood flow.

The portal venous blood has already passed through the gastrointestinal capillary bed, and therefore much of the O_2 has already been extracted. The hepatic artery delivers the remaining one fourth of the blood, which is fully saturated with O_2. Hence about three fourths of the O_2 used by the liver is derived from the hepatic arterial blood.

The small branches of the portal vein and hepatic artery give rise to terminal portal venules and hepatic arterioles (Figure 11-17). These terminal vessels enter the hepatic acinus (the functional unit of the liver) at its center. Blood flows from these terminal vessels into the sinusoids, which constitute the capillary network of the liver. The sinusoids radiate toward the periphery of the acinus, where they connect with the terminal hepatic venules. Blood from these terminal venules drains into progressively larger

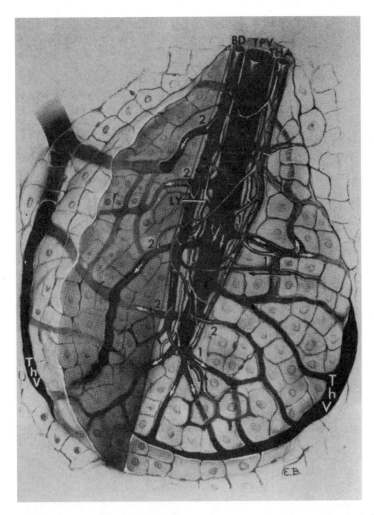

Figure 11-17 ■ **Microcirculation to a hepatic acinus.** *THA,* Terminal hepatic arteriole; *TPV,* terminal portal venule; *BD,* bile ductule; *THV,* terminal hepatic venule; *LY,* lymphatic. The hepatic arterioles empty either directly *(1)* or through the peribiliary plexus *(2)* into the sinusoids that run from the terminal portal venule to the terminal hepatic venules. (From Rappaport AM: *Microvasc Res* 6:212, 1973.)

branches of the hepatic veins, which are tributaries of the inferior vena cava.

Hemodynamics The mean blood pressure in the portal vein is about 10 mm Hg and that in the hepatic artery about 90 mm Hg. The resistance of the vessels upstream to the hepatic sinusoids is considerably greater than that of the downstream vessels. Consequently, the pressure in the sinusoids is only 2 or 3 mm Hg greater than that in the hepatic veins and inferior vena cava. The ratio of presinusoidal to postsinusoidal resistance in the liver is much greater than is the ratio of precapillary to postcapillary resistance for almost any other vascular bed. Hence drugs and other interventions that alter the presinusoidal resistance usually affect the pressure in the sinusoids only slightly. Such changes in presinusoidal resistance have little effect on the fluid exchange across the sinusoidal wall. Conversely, changes in hepatic venous (and in central venous) pressure are transmitted almost quantitatively to the hepatic sinusoids and profoundly affect the transsinusoidal exchange of fluids.

Regulation of Flow Blood flows in the portal venous and hepatic arterial systems vary reciprocally. When blood flow is curtailed in one system, the flow increases in the other system. However, the ensuing increase in flow in one system usually does not fully compensate for the initiating reduction in flow in the other system.

The portal venous system does not autoregulate. As portal venous pressure and flow are raised, resistance either remains constant or decreases. However, the hepatic arterial system does autoregulate.

The liver tends to maintain a constant O_2 consumption because the extraction of O_2 from the hepatic blood is very efficient. As the rate of O_2 delivery to the liver is varied, the liver compensates by an appropriate change in the fraction of O_2 extracted from the blood. This extraction is facilitated by the distinct separation of the presinusoidal vessels at the acinar center from the postsinusoidal vessels at the periphery of the acinus (Figure 11-17). The substantial distance between these types of vessels prevents a countercurrent exchange of O_2, contrary to the condition that exists in an intestinal villus (see Figure 11-16).

The sympathetic nerves constrict the presinusoidal resistance vessels in the portal venous and hepatic arterial systems. Neural effects on the capacitance vessels are more important, however. The liver contains about 15% of the total blood volume of the body. Under appropriate conditions, such as in response to hemor-

rhage, about half of the hepatic blood volume can be rapidly expelled by virtue of a constriction of the capacitance vessels. Hence the liver constitutes an important blood reservoir in humans. In certain other species, such as the dog, the spleen is a more important blood reservoir.

BOX 11-7

When central venous pressure is elevated, as in **congestive heart failure,** large quantities of plasma water transude from the liver into the peritoneal cavity; such a fluid accumulation in the abdomen is known as **ascites.** Extensive fibrosis of the liver, as in the various types of **hepatic cirrhosis,** leads to a pronounced increase in hepatic vascular resistance, which raises the pressure substantially in the portal venous system. The consequent increase in capillary hydrostatic pressure throughout the splanchnic circulation also leads to extensive fluid transudation into the abdominal cavity (i.e., ascites). Furthermore, the pressure may rise substantially in other veins that anastomose with the portal vein. A noteworthy example is that of the esophageal veins. These veins may enlarge considerably to form **esophageal varices,** which may rupture and thereby lead to severe, and frequently fatal, internal bleeding. To obviate these grave problems associated with elevated portal venous pressure, an anastomosis **(portacaval shunt)** is often created surgically between the portal vein and the inferior vena cava to lower portal venous pressure.

■ **FETAL CIRCULATION**

The circulation of the fetus shows a number of differences from that of the postnatal infant. The fetal lungs are functionally inactive, and the fetus depends completely on the placenta for O_2 and nutrient supply. Oxygenated fetal blood from the placenta passes through the umbilical vein to the liver. Approximately half passes through the liver, and the remainder bypasses the liver and reaches the inferior vena cava through the **ductus venosus** (Figure 11-18). In the inferior vena cava, blood from the ductus venosus joins blood returning from the lower trunk and extremities, and this combined stream is in turn joined by blood from the liver through the hepatic veins.

The streams of blood tend to maintain their identity in the inferior vena cava and are divided into two streams of unequal size by the edge of the interatrial septum **(crista dividens).** The larger stream, which is mainly blood from the umbilical vein, is shunted to the left atrium through the **foramen ovale,** which lies between the inferior vena cava and the left atrium (inset, Figure 11-18). The other stream passes into the right atrium, where it is joined by superior vena caval blood returning from the upper parts of the body and by blood from the myocardium.

In contrast to the adult, in whom the right and left ventricles pump in series, the ventricles in the fetus operate essentially in parallel. Because of the large pulmonary resistance, only one tenth of right ventricular output goes through the lungs. The remainder passes through the **ductus arteriosus** from the pulmonary artery to the aorta at a point distal to the origins of the arteries to the head and upper extremities. Blood flows from pulmonary artery to aorta because the pulmonary resistance is high and the diameter of the ductus arteriosus is as large as that of the descending aorta.

The large volume of blood coming through the foramen ovale into the left atrium is joined by blood returning from the lungs, and it is pumped out by the left ventricle into the aorta. Most of the blood in the ascending aorta goes to the head, upper thorax, and arms; the remainder joins blood from the ductus arteriosus and supplies the rest of the body and the placenta. The amount of blood pumped by the left ventricle is about half of that pumped by the right ventricle. The major fraction of the blood that passes down the descending aorta comes from the ductus arteriosus and right ventricle and flows by way of the two umbilical arteries to the placenta.

Figure 11-18 indicates the O_2 saturations of the blood at various points of the fetal circulation. Fetal blood leaving the placenta is 80% saturated, but the saturation of the blood passing through the foramen ovale is reduced to 67% by mixing with desaturated blood returning from the lower part of the body and the liver. Addition of the desaturated blood from the lungs reduces the O_2 saturation of left ventricular blood to 62%, which is the level of saturation of the blood reaching the head and upper extremities.

The blood in the right ventricle, a mixture of desaturated superior vena caval blood, coronary venous blood, and inferior vena caval blood, is only 52% saturated with O_2. When the major portion of this blood traverses the ductus arteriosus and joins that pumped out by the left ventricle, the resulting O_2 saturation of blood traveling to the lower part of the body and back to the placenta is 58%. Thus it is apparent that the tissues receiving blood of the highest O_2 saturation are the liver, heart, and upper parts of the body, including the head.

At the placenta the chorionic villi dip into the maternal sinuses, and O_2, CO_2, nutrients, and metabolic waste products exchange across the membranes. The barrier to exchange is quite large, and the equilibrium of P_{O_2} between the two circulations is not reached at normal rates of blood flow. Therefore the O_2 tension of the fetal blood leaving the placenta is very low. Were it not for the fact that fetal hemoglobin has a greater affinity for O_2 than does adult hemoglobin, the fetus would not receive an adequate O_2 supply. The fetal oxyhemoglobin dissociation curve is shifted to the left so that at

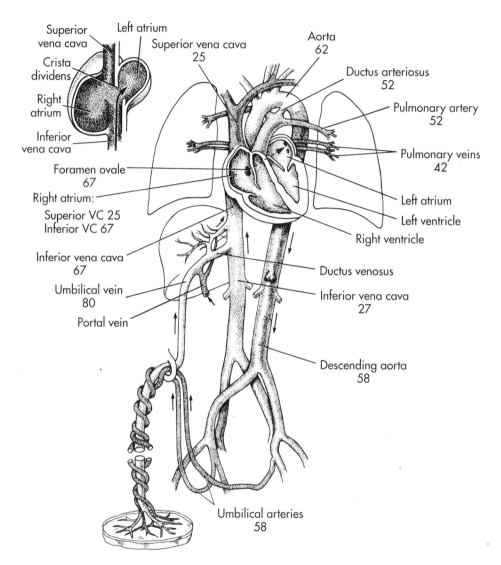

Superior vena cava
Crista dividens
Right atrium
Inferior vena cava

Left atrium
Superior vena cava
25

Aorta
62

Ductus arteriosus
52

Pulmonary artery
52

Pulmonary veins
42

Foramen ovale
67

Right atrium:
Superior VC 25
Inferior VC 67

Left atrium

Left ventricle

Right ventricle

Inferior vena cava
67

Umbilical vein
80

Portal vein

Ductus venosus

Inferior vena cava
27

Descending aorta
58

Umbilical arteries
58

Figure 11-18 ■ Schematic diagram of the fetal circulation. The numbers represent the percentage of O$_2$ saturation of the blood flowing in the indicated blood vessel. The inset at upper left illustrates the direction of flow of a major portion of the inferior vena cava blood through the foramen ovale to the left atrium. (Values for O$_2$ saturations are from Dawes GS, Mott JC, Widdicombe JG: *J Physiol* 126:563, 1954.)

equal pressures of O_2, fetal blood carries significantly more O_2 than does maternal blood.

In early fetal life the high cardiac glycogen levels that prevail may protect the heart from acute periods of hypoxia. The glycogen levels decrease in late fetal life and reach adult levels by term.

BOX 11-8

If the mother is subjected to hypoxia, the reduced blood O_2 tension is reflected in the fetus by tachycardia and an increase in blood flow through the umbilical vessels. If the hypoxia persists or if flow through the umbilical vessels is impaired, fetal distress occurs and is first manifested as bradycardia.

Several Changes Occur in the Circulatory System at Birth

The umbilical vessels have thick muscular walls that are very reactive to trauma, tension, sympathomimetic amines, bradykinin, angiotensin, and changes in Po_2. In animals in which the umbilical cord is not tied, hemorrhage of the newborn is prevented by constriction of these large vessels in response to one or more of these stimuli. Closure of the umbilical vessels produces an increase in total peripheral resistance and of blood pressure. When blood flow through the umbilical vein ceases, the ductus venosus, a thick-walled vessel with a muscular sphincter, closes. The event that initiates closure of the ductus venosus is still unknown.

The asphyxia that starts with constriction or clamping of the umbilical vessels, together with the cooling of the body, activates the respiratory center of the newborn infant. As the lungs fill with air, pulmonary vascular resistance decreases to about one tenth of the value existing before lung expansion. This resistance change is not caused by the presence of O_2 in the lungs because the change is just as great if the lungs are filled with nitrogen. However, filling the lungs with liquid does not reduce pulmonary vascular resistance.

The left atrial pressure is raised above the pressure in the inferior vena cava and right atrium by (1) the decrease in pulmonary resistance, with the resulting large flow of blood through the lungs to the left atrium, (2) the reduction of flow to the right atrium caused by occlusion of the umbilical vein, and (3) the increased resistance to left ventricular output produced by occlusion of the umbilical arteries. This reversal of the pressure gradient across the atria abruptly closes the valve over the foramen ovale, and the septal leaflets fuse over several days.

With the decrease in pulmonary vascular resistance, the pressure in the pulmonary artery falls to about one half its previous level (to about 35 mm Hg). This change in pressure, coupled with a slight increase in aortic pressure, reverses the flow of blood through the ductus arteriosus. However, within several minutes the large ductus arteriosus begins to constrict, producing turbulent flow, which is manifested as a murmur in the newborn. Constriction of the ductus arteriosus is progressive and is usually complete within 1 to 2 days after birth. Closure of the ductus arteriosus appears to be initiated by the high O_2 tension of the arterial blood passing through it; pulmonary ventilation with O_2 closes the ductus, whereas ventilation with air low in O_2 opens this shunt vessel. Whether O_2 acts directly on the ductus or through the release of a vasoconstrictor substance is not known.

BOX 11-9

The ductus arteriosus occasionally fails to close after birth. This constitutes a congenital cardiovascular abnormality that is amenable to surgical correction.

At birth the walls of the two ventricles are approximately of the same thickness, with a possibly slight preponderance of the right ventricle. Also in the newborn, the muscle layer of the pulmonary arterioles is thick, which is partly responsible for the high pulmonary vascular resistance of the fetus. After birth the thickness of the walls of the right ventricle diminishes, as does the muscle layer of the pulmonary arterioles; the left ventricular walls become thicker. These changes are progressive over a period of weeks after birth.

Summary

Skin Circulation

- Most of the resistance vessels in the skin are under dual control of the sympathetic nervous system and local vasodilator metabolites, but the arteriovenous anastomoses found in the hands, feet, and face are solely under neural control.
- The main function of skin blood vessels is to aid in the regulation of body temperature by constricting to conserve heat and dilating to lose heat.
- Skin blood vessels dilate directly and reflexly in response to heat, and constrict directly and reflexly in response to cold.

Skeletal Muscle Circulation

- Skeletal muscle blood flow is regulated centrally by the sympathetic nerves and regulated locally by the release of vasodilator metabolites.
- At rest, neural regulation of blood flow is paramount, but it yields to metabolic regulation during muscle contractions.

Cerebral Circulation

- Cerebral blood flow is predominantly regulated by metabolic factors, especially CO_2, K^+, and adenosine.
- Increased regional cerebral activity produced by stimuli such as touch, pain, hand motion, talking, reading, reasoning, and problem solving is associated with enhanced blood flow in the activated areas of the contralateral cerebral cortex.

Pulmonary Circulation

- The pulmonary circulation consists of the pulmonary vasculature, whose function is to promote the exchange of O_2 and CO_2 across the pulmonary capillaries, and the bronchial vasculature, whose function is to deliver O_2 and nutrients to the airways.
- The resistance of the pulmonary vasculature is low. Because of the low pulmonary vascular pressures, the distribution of blood flow to different regions of the lungs is affected by the body's position in space.
- The smooth muscles in the pulmonary arterioles constrict in response to hypoxia. This response tends to shift blood flow to the well-ventilated alveoli and away from the poorly ventilated alveoli.

Renal Circulation

- Renal blood flow is very high (about 20% of cardiac output), and the chief resistance to blood flow in the kidneys resides in the afferent and efferent arterioles.
- Glomerular capillary pressure is high (about 50 to 60 mm Hg), and the glomerular capillaries are very permeable to water; these two factors favor the filtration of large quantities of water from the blood to Bowman's capsule.

Intestinal Circulation

- The microcirculation in the intestinal villi constitutes a countercurrent exchange system for O_2. This places the villi in jeopardy in states of low blood flow.
- The splanchnic resistance and capacitance vessels are very responsive to changes in sympathetic neural activity.

Hepatic Circulation

- The liver receives about 25% of cardiac output; about three fourths of this comes via the portal vein and about one fourth via the hepatic artery. When flow is diminished in either the portal or hepatic system, flow in the other system usually increases, but not proportionately.
- The liver tends to maintain a constant O_2 consumption, in part because its mechanism for extracting O_2 from the blood is so efficient.

- The liver normally contains about 15% of total blood volume. It serves as an important blood reservoir for the body.

Fetal Circulation

- In the fetus a large percentage of right atrial blood passes through the foramen ovale to the left atrium, and a large percentage of pulmonary artery blood passes through the ductus arteriosus to the aorta.
- At birth the umbilical vessels, ductus venosus, and ductus arteriosus close by contraction of their muscle layers. The reduction in pulmonary vascular resistance caused by lung inflation is the main factor that reverses the pressure gradient between the atria, thereby closing the foramen ovale.

■ BIBLIOGRAPHY

1. Escourrou P, Raffestin B, Papelier Y, et al: Cardiopulmonary and carotid baroreflex control of splanchnic and forearm circulations, *Am J Physiol* 264:H777, 1993.
2. Faraci FM, Heistad DD: Regulation of the cerebral circulation: role of endothelium and potassium channels. *Physiol Rev* 78:53-97, 1998.
3. Granger DN, Kvietys PR, Korthuis RJ, et al: Microcirculation of the intestinal mucosa. In *Handbook of physiology*, Section 6: *The gastrointestinal system—motility and circulation*, vol I, Bethesda, MD, 1989, American Physiological Society.
4. Greenway CV, Lautt WW: Hepatic circulation. In *Handbook of physiology*, Section 6: *The gastrointestinal system—motility and circulation*, vol I, Bethesda, MD, 1989, American Physiological Society.
5. Griendling KK, Murphy TJ, Alexander RW: Molecular biology of the renin-angiotensin system. *Circulation* 87:1816, 1993.
6. Guissani DA, Unno N, Jenkins SL, et al: Dynamics of cardiovascular responses to repeated partial umbilical cord compression in late-gestation sheep fetus. *Am J Physiol* 273:H2351-H2360, 1997.
7. Ito S: Role of nitric oxide in glomerular arterioles and macula densa. *News Physiol Sci* 9:115, 1994.
8. Leeman M, de Beyl VZ, Delcroix M, et al: Effects of endogenous nitric oxide on pulmonary vascular tone in intact dogs. *Am J Physiol* 266:H2343, 1994.
9. Maass-Moreno R, Rothe CF: Contribution of large hepatic veins to postsinusoidal vascular resistance. *Am J Physiol* 262:G14, 1992.
10. Phillis JW, editor: *The regulation of cerebral blood flow*, Boca Raton, FL, 1993, CRC Press.
11. Schwartz LM, McKenzie JE: Adenosine and active hyperemia in soleus and gracilis muscle of cats. *Am J Physiol* 259:H1295, 1990.
12. Stamler JS, Loh E, Roddy M-A, et al: Nitric oxide regulates basal systemic and pulmonary vascular resistance in healthy humans. *Circulation* 89:2035, 1994.
13. van Tilborg KA, Rabelink TJ, van Rijn HJM, et al: Arterial baroreflex control of renal hemodynamics in humans. *Circulation* 90:1883, 1994.
14. Wagner WW Jr, Weir EK, editors: *Pulmonary circulation and gas exchange*, Armonk, NY, 1994, Futura Publishing.
15. Weir EK, Archer SL: Mechanism of acute hypoxic pulmonary vasoconstriction: the tale of two channels. *FASEB J* 9:183, 1995.

■ CASE 11-1

HISTORY

A 35-year-old woman went to see her family physician because of repeated episodes of severe pain in the fingers of both hands when she went on a skiing vacation. These "attacks" were usually followed by dark blue color and then bright red color. Physical examination was negative, as was visualization of the arteries of the hands by angiography. She was diagnosed as having Raynaud's disease.

QUESTION

1. Which of the following treatments would <u>not</u> be recommended?
   a. Stop smoking
   b. Sympathetic nerve inhibitors
   c. Sympathectomy
   d. Epinephrine
   e. Nifedipine, a calcium uptake blocker

■ CASE 11-2

HISTORY

A 53-year-old man has consumed substantial amounts of alcohol over the past 3 decades. For the past 2 or 3 years, he has noticed that his belt size has progressively increased, and that his abdomen has distended. His physician was able to evoke a fluid wave across the abdomen when he tapped the patient's abdomen. His doctor made the diagnosis of hepatic cirrhosis, which is associated with extensive fibrosis of the liver.

QUESTION

1. The reason for the large accumulation of fluid in the patient's abdomen is that
   a. The hydrostatic pressure in the splanchnic capillaries was abnormally high.
   b. The hydrostatic pressure in the hepatic artery was abnormally high.
   c. The hydrostatic pressure in the hepatic veins exceeded that in the portal vein.
   d. The hydrostatic pressure in the hepatic veins exceeded that in the splenic vein.
   e. The hepatic resistance was subnormal.

■ CASE 11-3

HISTORY

A 6-year-old boy was referred by his family physician to a pediatric cardiologist because of chronic fatigue, effort intolerance, and a heart murmur. On physical examination, the boy appeared slightly small for his age, had normal skin color, no clubbing of the fingers, and a harsh murmur throughout systole that was heard best in the fourth intercostal space to the left of the sternum but extending over the entire precordium. X-ray revealed an enlarged heart, especially the right ventricle. An ear oximeter showed normal oxygenation of arterial blood. Hematocrit was normal. Cardiac catheterization data were:

Mean right atrial pressure: 5 mm Hg
Right ventricular systolic pressure: 30 mm Hg
Right ventricular diastolic pressure: 3 mm Hg
Right atrial blood P_{O_2}: 40 mm Hg
Right ventricular blood P_{O_2}: 60 mm Hg

QUESTION

1. The patient was admitted to the cardiac surgery unit for repair of
   a. Coarctation of the aorta
   b. Interventricular septal defect
   c. Pulmonic stenosis
   d. Tetralogy of Fallot
   e. Patent ductus arteriosus

CHAPTER 12

Interplay of Central and Peripheral Factors in the Control of the Circulation

Objectives

1. Describe the sequence of cardiovascular events during exercise.

2. Describe how most cardiovascular functions are integrated in exercise.

3. Describe the effects of blood loss on the cardiovascular system.

4. Explain the various compensatory mechanisms that protect against hemorrhagic shock.

5. Explain the various decompensatory mechanisms that intensify the effects of blood loss.

THE PRIMARY FUNCTION OF THE CIRculatory system is to deliver the supplies needed for tissue metabolism and growth and to remove the products of metabolism. To explain how the heart and blood vessels serve this function, it has been necessary to analyze the system morphologically and functionally and to discuss the mechanisms of action of the component parts in their contribution to maintaining adequate tissue perfusion under different physiological conditions.

Once the functions of the various components are understood, it is essential that their interrelationships in the overall role of the circulatory system be considered. Tissue perfusion depends on arterial pressure and local vascular resistance, and arterial pressure in

turn depends on cardiac output and total peripheral resistance (TPR). Arterial pressure is maintained within a relatively narrow range in the normal individual, a feat accomplished by reciprocal changes in cardiac output and TPR. However, cardiac output and peripheral resistance are each influenced by a number of factors, and it is the interplay among these factors that determines the level of these two variables. The autonomic nervous system and the baroreceptors play the key role in regulating blood pressure. However, from the long-range point of view, the control of fluid balance by the kidney, adrenal cortex, and central nervous system, with maintenance of a constant blood volume, is of the greatest importance.

In a well-regulated system, one way to study the extent and sensitivity of the regulatory mechanism is to disturb the system and observe its response in restoring the preexisting steady state. Disturbances in the form of physical exercise and hemorrhage will be used to illustrate the effects of the various factors that go into regulation of the circulatory system.

■ EXERCISE

The cardiovascular adjustments in exercise consist of a combination and integration of neural and local (chemical) factors. The neural factors consist of (1) central command, (2) reflexes originating in the contracting muscle, and (3) the baroreceptor reflex. **Central command** is the cerebrocortical activation of the sympathetic nervous system that produces cardiac acceleration, increased myocardial contractile force, and peripheral vasoconstriction. Reflexes can be activated intramuscularly by stimulation of mechanoreceptors (by stretch, tension) and chemoreceptors (by products of metabolism) in response to muscle contraction. Impulses from these receptors travel centrally via small myelinated (group III) and unmyelinated (group IV) afferent nerve fibers. The group IV unmyelinated fibers may represent the muscle chemoreceptors; no morphological chemoreceptor has been identified. The central connections of this reflex are unknown, but the efferent limb is the sympathetic nerve fibers to the heart and peripheral blood vessels. The baroreceptor reflex and the local factors that influence skeletal muscle blood flow (metabolic vasodilators) are described in Chapter 8. Vascular chemoreceptors do not play a significant role in regulation of the cardiovascular system in exercise. The pH, P_{CO_2}, and P_{O_2} of arterial blood are normal during exercise, and the vascular chemoreceptors are located on the arterial side of the circulatory system.

Mild-to-Moderate Exercise

In humans or in trained animals, anticipation of physical activity inhibits the vagal nerve impulses to the heart and increases sympathetic discharge. The concerted inhibition of parasympathetic areas and activation of sympathetic areas of the medulla on the heart result in an increase in heart rate and myocardial contractility. The tachycardia and the enhanced contractility increase cardiac output, which in turn increases arterial pressure.

Peripheral Resistance Declines During Exercise At the same time that cardiac stimulation occurs, the sympathetic nervous system also elicits vascular resistance changes in the periphery. In skin, kidneys, splanchnic regions, and inactive muscle, sympathetic-mediated vasoconstriction increases vascular resistance, which diverts blood away from these areas. This increased resistance in vascular beds of inactive tissues persists throughout the period of exercise.

The increase in blood flow in the active muscles at the onset of exercise cannot be attributed to a neural mechanism because chemical block of the autonomic nervous system does not alter this blood flow response. This increase in muscle blood flow may be caused by the modest elevation of blood pressure or by some unknown mechanism.

As cardiac output and blood flow to active muscles increase with progressive increments in the intensity of exercise, visceral blood flow (to the splanchnic and renal vasculatures) decreases. Blood flow to the myocardium increases, whereas that to the brain is unchanged. Skin blood flow initially decreases during exercise and then increases as body temperature rises with increments in duration and intensity of exercise. Skin blood flow finally decreases when the skin vessels constrict as the total body O_2 consumption nears maximum.

The major circulatory adjustment to prolonged exercise involves the vasculature of the active muscles. Local formation of vasoactive metabolites induces marked dilation of the resistance vessels, which progresses with increases in the intensity level of exercise. Potassium is one of the vasodilator substances released by contracting muscle, and it may be in part responsible for the initial decrease in vascular resistance in the active muscles. Other contributing factors may be the release of adenosine and a decrease in pH during sustained exercise. The local accumulation of metabolites relaxes the terminal arterioles. Blood flow through the muscle may increase 15 to 20 times above the resting level. This metabolic vasodilation of the precapillary vessels in active muscles occurs very soon after the onset of exercise, and the decrease in TPR enables the heart to pump more blood at a lesser load and more efficiently (less pressure work, p 234) than if TPR were unchanged. Only a small percentage of the capillaries is perfused at rest, whereas in actively contracting muscle all or nearly all of the capillaries contain flowing blood (**capillary recruitment**). The surface available for exchange of gases, water, and solutes is increased manyfold. Furthermore, the hydrostatic pressure in the capillaries is increased because of the relaxation of the resistance vessels. Hence there is a net movement of water and solutes into the muscle tissue. Tissue pressure rises and remains elevated during exercise as fluid continues to move out of the capillaries and is carried away by the lymphatics. Lymph flow is increased as a result of the increase in capillary hydrostatic pressure and the massaging effect of the contracting muscles on the valve-containing lymphatic vessels (see p 171).

The contracting muscle avidly extracts O_2 from the perfusing blood (increased AV-O_2 difference, Figure 12-1), and the release of O_2 from

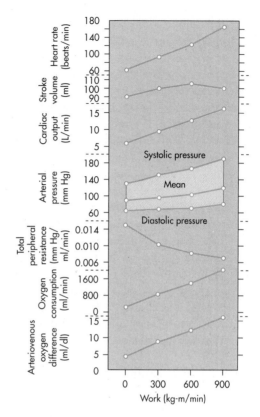

Figure 12-1 ■ **Effect of different levels of exercise on several cardiovascular variables.** (From Carlsten A, Grimby G: *The circulatory response to muscular exercise in man,* Springfield, IL, 1966, Charles C Thomas.)

the blood is facilitated by the nature of oxyhemoglobin dissociation. The reduction in pH caused by the high concentration of CO_2 and the formation of lactic acid and the increase in temperature in the contracting muscle contribute to shifting the oxyhemoglobin dissociation curve to the right. At any given partial pressure of O_2, less O_2 is held by the hemoglobin in the red cells, and consequently there is more effective O_2 removal from the blood. Oxygen consumption may increase as much as sixtyfold with only a fifteenfold increase in muscle blood flow. Muscle myoglobin serves as a limited O_2 store in exercise and can release attached O_2 at very low partial pressures. Hence it facilitates O_2 transport from capillaries to mitochondria by serving as an O_2 carrier.

Cardiac Output Can Increase Substantially in Exercise The enhanced sympathetic drive and the reduced parasympathetic inhibition of the sinoatrial node continue during exercise, and consequently tachycardia persists. If the workload is moderate and constant, the heart rate will reach a certain level and remain there throughout the period of exercise. However, if the workload increases, a concomitant increase in heart rate occurs until a plateau is reached in severe exercise at about 180 beats per minute (see Figure 12-1). In contrast to the large increment in heart rate, the increase in stroke volume is only about 10% to 35% (see Figure 12-1), the larger values occurring in trained individuals. (In very well-trained distance runners, whose cardiac outputs can reach six to seven times the resting level, stroke volume reaches about twice the resting value.)

Thus it is apparent that the increase in cardiac output observed with exercise is correlated principally with an increase in heart rate. If the baroreceptors are denervated, the cardiac output and heart rate responses to exercise are sluggish compared with the changes in animals with normally innervated baroreceptors. However, in the absence of autonomic innervation of the heart, as produced experimentally in dogs by total cardiac denervation, exercise still elicits an increment in cardiac output comparable with that observed in normal animals, but chiefly by means of an elevated stroke volume. However, if a β-adrenergic receptor blocking agent is given to dogs with denervated hearts, exercise performance is impaired. The β-adrenergic receptor blocker apparently prevents the cardiac acceleration and enhanced contractility caused by increased amounts of circulating catecholamines

and hence limits the increase in cardiac output necessary for maximal exercise performance.

Venous Return Is Enhanced in Exercise In addition to the contribution made by sympathetically mediated constriction of the capacitance vessels in both exercising and nonexercising parts of the body, venous return is aided by the working skeletal muscles and the muscles of respiration. The intermittently contracting muscles compress the vessels that course through them and, in the case of veins with their valves oriented toward the heart, pump blood back toward the right atrium. The flow of venous blood to the heart is also aided by the increase in the pressure gradient developed by the more negative intrathoracic pressure produced by deeper and more frequent respirations. In humans, there is little evidence that blood reservoirs, such as skin, lungs, and liver, contribute much to circulating blood volume. In fact, blood volume is usually reduced slightly during exercise, as evidenced by a rise in the hematocrit ratio, because of water loss externally by sweating and enhanced ventilation, and fluid movement into the contracting muscle. The fluid loss from the vascular compartment into contracting muscle reaches a plateau as interstitial fluid pressure rises and opposes the increased hydrostatic pressure in the capillaries of the active muscle. The fluid loss is partially offset by movement of fluid from the splanchnic regions and inactive muscle into the bloodstream. This influx of fluid occurs as a result of a decrease of hydrostatic pressure in the capillaries of these tissues and of an increase in plasma osmolarity because of movement of osmotically active particles into the blood from the contracting muscle. In addition, reduced urine formation by the kidneys helps to conserve body water.

The large volume of blood returning to the heart is so rapidly pumped through the lungs and out into the aorta that central venous pressure remains essentially constant. Thus the Frank-Starling mechanism of a greater initial fiber length does not account for the greater stroke volume in moderate exercise. Chest x-ray films of individuals at rest and during exercise reveal a decrease in heart size in exercise, which is in harmony with the observations of a constant ventricular filling pressure. However, in maximal or near-maximal exercise, right atrial pressure and end-diastolic ventricular volume do increase. Thus the Frank-Starling mechanism contributes to the enhanced stroke volume in very vigorous exercise.

Arterial Pressure Increases Slightly During Exercise If the exercise involves a large proportion of the body musculature, such as in running or swimming, the reduction in total vascular resistance can be considerable (see Figure 12-1). Nevertheless, arterial pressure starts to rise with the onset of exercise, and the increase in blood pressure roughly parallels the severity of the exercise performed (see Figure 12-1). Therefore the increase in cardiac output is proportionally greater than the decrease in TPR. The vasoconstriction produced in the inactive tissues by the sympathetic nervous system (and to some extent by the release of catecholamines from the adrenal medulla) is important for maintaining normal or increased blood pressure because sympathectomy or drug-induced block of the adrenergic sympathetic nerve fibers results in a decrease in arterial pressure **(hypotension)** during exercise.

Some sympathetic-mediated vasoconstriction occurs in active muscle and increases in strenuous exercise when more than half of the total body musculature is contracting. In experiments in which one leg is working at maximal levels and then the other leg starts to work, blood flow decreases in the first working leg. Furthermore, blood levels of norepinephrine rise significantly in exercise, and most of it comes from sympathetic nerves in the active muscles.

As body temperature rises during exercise, the skin vessels dilate in response to thermal stimulation of the heat-regulating center in the hypothalamus, and TPR decreases further. This would result in a decline in blood pressure were it not for the increasing cardiac output and constriction of arterioles in the renal, splanchnic, and other tissues.

In general, mean arterial pressure rises during exercise as a result of the increase in cardiac output. However, the effect of enhanced cardiac output is offset by the overall decrease in TPR, so that the mean blood pressure increase is relatively small. Vasoconstriction in the inactive vascular beds contributes to the maintenance of a normal arterial blood pressure for adequate perfusion of the active tissues. The actual pressure attained represents a balance between cardiac output and TPR (p 141). Systolic pressure usually increases more than diastolic pressure, which results in an increase in pulse pressure (see Figure 12-1). The larger pulse pressure is primarily attributable to a greater stroke volume, and to a lesser degree to a more rapid ejection of blood by the left ventricle with less peripheral runoff during the brief ventricular ejection period.

Severe Exercise

In severe exercise taken to the point of exhaustion, the compensatory mechanisms begin to fail. Heart rate attains a maximal level of about 180 beats per minute, and stroke volume reaches a plateau and often decreases, resulting in a fall in blood pressure. Dehydration occurs. Sympathetic vasoconstrictor activity supersedes the vasodilator influence on the cutaneous vessels and has the hemodynamic effect of a slight increase in effective blood volume. However, cutaneous vasoconstriction also decreases the rate of heat loss. Body temperature is normally elevated in exercise, and reduction in heat loss through cutaneous vasoconstriction can, under these conditions, lead to very high body temperatures with associated feelings of acute distress. The tissue and blood pH decrease as a result of increased lactic acid and CO_2 production. The reduced pH is probably the key factor that determines the maximal amount of exercise a given individual can tolerate because of muscle pain, subjective feeling of exhaustion, and inability or loss of will to continue. A summary of the neural and local effects of exercise on the cardiovascular system is schematized in Figure 12-2.

Postexercise Recovery

When exercise stops, sympathetic activity to the heart ceases and the heart rate and cardiac output decrease. Peripheral sympathetic activity also decreases, and coupled with resistance vessel dilation (caused by the accumulated vasodi-

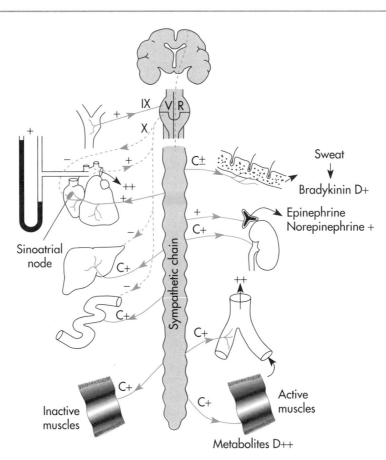

Figure 12-2 ■ **Cardiovascular adjustments in exercise.** *VR,* Vasomotor region; *C,* vasoconstrictor activity; *D,* vasodilator activity; *IX,* glossopharyngeal nerve; *X,* vagus nerve; +, increased activity; −, decreased activity.

lator metabolites), arterial pressure falls, often below the preexercise level. This hypotension is brief, and the baroreceptor reflexes restore the blood pressure to normal levels.

Limits of Exercise Performance

The two main forces that could limit skeletal muscle performance in the human body are the rate of O_2 utilization by the muscles and the O_2 supply to the muscles. Muscle O_2 usage is probably not critical because during exercise maximum O_2 consumption ($\dot{V}O_{2max}$) by a large percentage of the body muscle mass is unchanged or increases slightly when additional muscles are activated. In fact, during exercise of a large muscle mass, as in vigorous bicycling, commencement of bilateral arm exercise without change in the cycling efforts produces only a small increment in cardiac output and $\dot{V}O_{2max}$. However, it causes a decrease in blood flow to the legs. This centrally mediated (baroreceptor reflex) vasoconstriction during maximal cardiac output prevents a fall in blood pressure that would otherwise be caused by metabolically induced vasodilation in the active muscles. If muscle O_2 utilization were limiting, recruitment of more contracting muscle would use much more O_2 to meet the enhanced O_2 requirements (about the amount equal to the sum of oxygen consumption of the arms and legs exercised alone).

Limitation of O_2 supply could be caused by inadequate oxygenation of blood in the lungs or by limitation of the supply of O_2-laden blood to the muscles. Failure to fully oxygenate blood by the lungs can be excluded because even with the most strenuous exercise at sea level, arterial blood is fully saturated with O_2. Therefore O_2 delivery (or blood flow because arterial blood O_2 content is normal) to the active muscles appears to be the limiting factor in muscle performance. This limitation could be caused by the inability to increase cardiac output beyond a certain level as a result of a limitation of stroke volume because heart rate reaches maximal levels before $\dot{V}O_{2max}$ is reached. Hence *the major factor is the pumping capacity of the heart.*

With exercise of a small group of muscles, such as those found in the hand, when the cardiovascular system is not severely taxed, the limiting factor is unknown but lies within the muscle.

Physical Training and Conditioning

The response of the cardiovascular system to regular exercise is to increase its capacity to deliver O_2 to the active muscles and to improve the ability of the muscle to utilize O_2. The $\dot{V}O_{2max}$ is quite reproducible in a given individual and varies with the level of physical conditioning. Training progressively increases the $\dot{V}O_{2max}$, which reaches a plateau at the highest level of conditioning. Highly trained athletes have a lower resting heart rate, greater stroke volume, and lower peripheral resistance than they had before training or after deconditioning (becoming sedentary). The low resting heart rate is caused by a higher vagal tone and a lower sympathetic tone. With exercise, the maximal heart rate of the trained individual is the same as that in the untrained person but is attained at a higher level of exercise.

The trained person also exhibits a low vascular resistance that is inherent in the muscle. For example, if an individual exercises one leg regularly over an extended period and does not exercise the other leg, the vascular resistance is lower and the $\dot{V}O_{2max}$ is higher in the "trained" leg than in the "untrained" leg. Physical conditioning is associated with greater extraction of O_2 from the blood (greater AV-O_2 difference) by the muscles. With long-term training, capillary density and the numbers of mitochondria increase, as does the activity of the oxidative enzymes in the mitochondria. Also, it appears that ATPase activity, myoglobin, and enzymes involved in lipid metabolism increase with physical conditioning.

■ HEMORRHAGE

In an individual who has lost a large quantity of blood, the principal system affected is the cardiovascular system. The arterial systolic, diastolic, and pulse pressures diminish and the arterial pulse is rapid and feeble. The cutaneous veins collapse and fill slowly when compressed centrally. The skin is pale, moist, and slightly cyanotic. Respiration is rapid, but the depth of respiration may be shallow or deep.

Hemorrhage Evokes Compensatory and Decompensatory Effects on the Arterial Blood Pressure

Cardiac output decreases as a result of blood loss (see Chapter 9). The changes in mean arterial pressure evoked by an acute hemorrhage in experimental animals are illustrated in Figure 12-3. If sufficient blood is withdrawn rapidly to bring mean arterial pressure to about 50 mm Hg, the pressure tends to rise spontaneously toward control over the subsequent 20 or 30 minutes. In some animals (curve *A*, Figure 12-3), this

trend continues, and normal pressures are regained within a few hours. In other animals (curve *B*), after an initial pressure rise, the pressure begins to decline and it continues to fall at an accelerating rate until death ensues. This progressive deterioration of cardiovascular function is termed **hemorrhagic shock.** At some point the deterioration becomes irreversible; a lethal outcome can be retarded only temporarily by any known therapy, including massive transfusions of donor blood.

The Compensatory Mechanisms Are Neural and Humoral

The changes in arterial pressure immediately after an acute blood loss (see Figure 12-3) indicate that certain compensatory mechanisms must be operating. Any mechanism that senses the level of blood pressure and raises the pressure to-

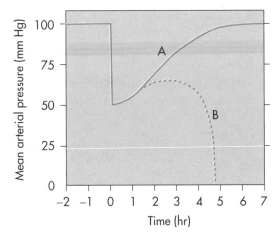

Figure 12-3 ■ Changes in mean arterial pressure after a rapid hemorrhage. At time zero, the animal is bled rapidly to a mean arterial pressure of 50 mm Hg. After a period in which the pressure returns toward the control level, some animals continue to improve until the control pressure is attained (curve *A*). However, in other animals the pressure will begin to decline until death ensues (curve *B*).

ward normal in response to the reduction in pressure may be designated a **negative feedback mechanism.** It is termed "negative" because the direction of the secondary change in pressure is opposite to that of the initiating change. The following negative feedback responses are evoked: (1) baroreceptor reflexes, (2) chemoreceptor reflexes, (3) cerebral ischemic responses, (4) reabsorption of tissue fluids, (5) release of endogenous vasoconstrictor substances, and (6) renal conservation of salt and water.

Baroreceptor Reflexes The reduction in mean arterial pressure and in pulse pressure during hemorrhage decreases the stimulation of the baroreceptors in the carotid sinuses and aortic arch (see Chapter 8). Several cardiovascular responses are thus evoked, all of which tend to restore the normal level of arterial pressure. Reduction of vagal tone and enhancement of sympathetic tone increase heart rate and enhance myocardial contractility.

The increased sympathetic discharge also produces generalized venoconstriction, which has the same hemodynamic consequences as a transfusion of blood (see Chapter 9). Sympathetic activation constricts the vasculature in certain blood reservoirs. This vasoconstriction provides an autotransfusion of blood into the circulating bloodstream. In the dog, considerable quantities of blood are mobilized by contraction of the spleen. In humans, the cutaneous, pulmonary, and hepatic vasculatures probably constitute the principal blood reservoirs.

Generalized arteriolar vasoconstriction is a prominent response to the diminished baroreceptor stimulation during hemorrhage. The reflex increase in peripheral resistance minimizes the fall in arterial pressure that results from reduction of cardiac output. Figure 12-4 shows the effect of an 8% blood loss on mean aortic pressure in a group of dogs. If both vagi are cut to eliminate the influence of the aortic arch baroreceptors, and only the carotid sinus

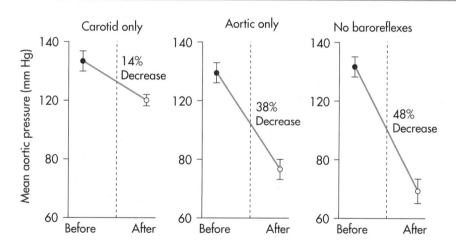

Figure 12-4 ■ Changes in mean aortic pressure in response to an 8% blood loss in a group of eight dogs. *Left panel,* **The carotid sinus baroreceptor reflexes were intact and the aortic reflexes were interrupted.** *Middle panel,* **The aortic reflexes were intact and the carotid sinus reflexes were interrupted.** *Right panel,* **All sinoaortic reflexes were abrogated.** (From Shepherd JT: *Circulation* 50:418, 1974; derived from the data of Edis AJ: *Am J Physiol* 221:1352, 1971.)

baroreceptors are operative (left panel), this hemorrhage decreases mean aortic pressure by 14%. This pressure change did not differ significantly from the pressure decline (12%) evoked by the same hemorrhage before vagotomy (not shown). When the carotid sinuses are denervated and the aortic baroreceptor reflexes are intact, the 8% blood loss decreases mean aortic pressure by 38% (middle panel). Hence the carotid sinus baroreceptors are more effective than the aortic baroreceptors in attenuating the fall in pressure. The aortic baroreceptors must also be operative, however, because when both sets of afferent baroreceptor pathways are interrupted, an 8% blood loss reduces arterial pressure by 48%.

Although the arteriolar vasoconstriction is widespread during hemorrhage, it is by no means uniform. Vasoconstriction is most severe in the cutaneous, skeletal muscle, and splanchnic vascular beds, and it is slight or absent in the cerebral and coronary circulations. In many instances the cerebral and coronary vascular resistances are diminished. Thus *the reduced cardiac output is redistributed to favor flow through the brain and the heart.*

In the early stages of mild-to-moderate hemorrhage, the changes in renal resistance are usually slight. The tendency for increased sympathetic activity to constrict the renal vessels is counteracted by autoregulatory mechanisms (see Chapter 11). With more prolonged and severe hemorrhages, however, renal vasoconstriction becomes intense. The reductions in renal circulation are most severe in the outer layers of the renal cortex. The inner zones of the cortex and outer zones of the medulla are spared.

The severe renal and splanchnic vasoconstriction during hemorrhage favors the heart and brain. However, if such constriction persists too long, it may be detrimental. Frequently, patients survive the acute hypotensive period only

to die several days later from the kidney failure that results from renal ischemia. Intestinal ischemia may also have dire effects. In the dog, for example, intestinal bleeding and extensive sloughing of the mucosa occur after only a few hours of hemorrhagic hypotension. Furthermore, the diminished splanchnic flow swells the centrilobular cells in the liver. The resulting obstruction of the hepatic sinusoids raises the portal venous pressure, which intensifies the intestinal blood loss. Fortunately, the pathological changes in the liver and in the intestine are usually much less severe in humans than in dogs.

Chemoreceptor Reflexes Reductions in arterial pressure below about 60 mm Hg do not evoke any additional responses through the baroreceptor reflexes because this pressure level constitutes the threshold for stimulation (see Chapter 8). However, low arterial pressure may stimulate peripheral chemoreceptors because of hypoxia in the chemoreceptor tissue consequent to inadequate local blood flow. Chemoreceptor excitation enhances the already existent peripheral vasoconstriction evoked by the baroreceptor reflexes. Also, respiratory stimulation assists venous return by the auxiliary pumping mechanism described in Chapter 9.

Cerebral Ischemia When the arterial pressure is below about 40 mm Hg, the resulting cerebral ischemia activates the sympathoadrenal system. The sympathetic nervous discharge is several times greater than the maximal neural activity that occurs when the baroreceptors cease to be stimulated. Therefore the vasoconstriction and facilitation of myocardial contractility may be pronounced. With more severe degrees of cerebral ischemia, however, the vagal centers also become activated. The resulting bradycardia may aggravate the hypotension that initiated the cerebral ischemia.

Reabsorption of Tissue Fluids The arterial hypotension, arteriolar constriction, and re-

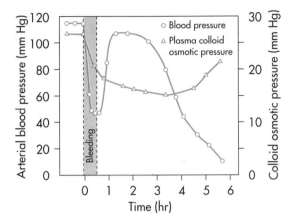

Figure 12-5 ■ Changes in arterial blood pressure and plasma colloid osmotic pressure in response to withdrawal of 45% of the estimated blood volume over a 30-minute period, beginning at time zero. The data are the average values for 23 cats. (Redrawn from Zweifach BW: *Anesthesiology* 41:157, 1974.)

duced venous pressure during hemorrhagic hypotension lower the hydrostatic pressure in the capillaries. The balance of transmural forces promotes the net reabsorption of interstitial fluid into the vascular compartment (see Chapter 7). The rapidity of this response is displayed in Figure 12-5. In a group of cats, 45% of the estimated blood volume was removed over a 30-minute period. The mean arterial blood pressure declined rapidly to about 45 mm Hg. The pressure then returned quickly, but only temporarily, to near the control level. The plasma colloid osmotic pressure declined markedly during the bleeding and continued to decrease more gradually for several hours. The reduction in colloid osmotic pressure reflects the dilution of the blood by tissue fluids that contain little protein.

Considerable quantities of fluid may thus be drawn into the circulation during hemorrhage. About 0.25 ml of fluid per minute per kilogram of body weight may be reabsorbed. Approximately 1 L of fluid per hour might be autoinfused into the circulatory system of an average individual from the interstitial spaces after an acute blood loss.

Considerable quantities of fluid may also be slowly shifted from intracellular to extracellular spaces. This fluid exchange is probably mediated by secretion of cortisol from the adrenal cortex in response to hemorrhage. Cortisol appears to be essential for a full restoration of plasma volume after hemorrhage.

Endogenous Vasoconstrictors The **catecholamines** epinephrine and norepinephrine are released from the adrenal medulla in response to the same stimuli that evoke widespread sympathetic nervous discharge. Blood levels of catecholamines are high during and after hemorrhage. When animals are bled to an arterial pressure level of 40 mm Hg, the catecholamines increase as much as 50 times.

Epinephrine comes almost exclusively from the adrenal medulla, whereas norepinephrine is derived from both the adrenal medulla and the peripheral sympathetic nerve endings. These humoral substances reinforce the effects of sympathetic nervous activity listed previously.

Vasopressin, a potent vasoconstrictor, is actively secreted by the posterior pituitary gland in response to hemorrhage. The plasma concentration of vasopressin rises progressively as the arterial blood pressure diminishes (Figure 12-6). The receptors responsible for the augmented release are the sinoaortic baroreceptors and stretch receptors in the left atrium.

The diminished renal perfusion during hemorrhagic hypotension leads to the secretion of **renin** from the juxtaglomerular apparatus (see Chapter 11). This enzyme acts on a plasma protein, **angiotensinogen,** to form **angiotensin,** a very powerful vasoconstrictor.

Renal Conservation of Salt and Water
Fluid and electrolytes are conserved by the kid-

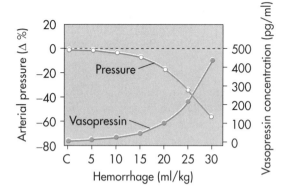

Figure 12-6 ■ **Mean percentage changes in arterial blood pressure and in plasma vasopressin concentration in response to blood loss (0.5 ml/kg/min) in a group of 12 dogs; the maximal volume of blood withdrawn was 30 ml/kg.** (Redrawn from Shen Y-T, Cowley AW Jr, Vatner SF: *Circ Res* 68:1422, 1991.)

neys during hemorrhage in response to various stimuli, including the increased secretion of vasopressin (antidiuretic hormone) noted previously (see Figure 12-6). The lower arterial pressure decreases the glomerular filtration rate and thus curtails the excretion of water and electrolytes. Also, the diminished renal blood flow raises the blood levels of angiotensin, as previously described. This polypeptide accelerates the release of **aldosterone** from the adrenal cortex. Aldosterone in turn stimulates sodium reabsorption by the renal tubules, and water accompanies the sodium that is actively reabsorbed.

The Decompensatory Mechanisms Are Mainly Humoral, Cardiac, and Hematological

In contrast to the negative feedback mechanisms just described, latent **positive feedback mechanisms** are also evoked by hemorrhage. Such mechanisms exaggerate any primary change initiated by the blood loss. Specifically,

positive feedback mechanisms aggravate the hypotension induced by blood loss and tend to initiate vicious cycles, which may lead to death. The operation of positive feedback mechanisms is illustrated in curve *B* of Figure 12-3.

Whether a positive feedback mechanism will lead to a vicious cycle depends on the **gain** of that mechanism. Gain is defined as the ratio of the secondary change evoked by a given mechanism to the initiating change itself. A gain greater than 1 induces a vicious cycle; a gain less than 1 does not. For example, consider a positive feedback mechanism with a gain of 2. If, for any reason, mean arterial pressure were to decrease by 10 mm Hg, the positive feedback mechanism with a gain of 2 would then evoke a secondary pressure reduction of 20 mm Hg, which in turn would cause a further decrement of 40 mm Hg; that is, each change would induce a subsequent change that was twice as great. Hence mean arterial pressure would decline at an ever-increasing rate until death supervened, much as is depicted by curve *B* in Figure 12-3.

Conversely, a positive feedback mechanism with a gain of 0.5 would indeed exaggerate any change in mean arterial pressure but would not necessarily lead to death. For example, if arterial pressure suddenly decreased by 10 mm Hg, the positive feedback mechanism would initiate a secondary, additional fall of 5 mm Hg. This in turn would provoke a further decrease of 2.5 mm Hg. The process would continue in ever-diminishing steps, with the arterial pressure approaching an equilibrium value asymptotically.

Some of the more important positive feedback mechanisms include (1) cardiac failure, (2) acidosis, (3) central nervous system depression, (4) aberrations of blood clotting, and (5) depression of the reticuloendothelial system.

Cardiac Failure The role of cardiac failure in the progression of shock during hemorrhage is controversial. All investigators agree that the heart fails terminally, but opinions differ con-

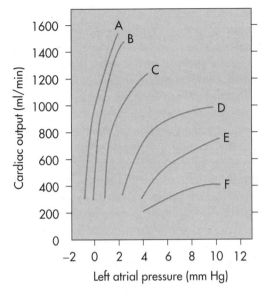

Figure 12-7 ■ Ventricular function curves for the left ventricles during the course of hemorrhagic shock. Curve *A* represents the control function curve; curve *B*, 117 min; curve *C*, 247 min; curve *D*, 280 min; curve *E*, 295 min; and curve *F*, 310 min after the initial hemorrhage. (Redrawn from Crowell JW, Guyton AC: *Am J Physiol* 203:248, 1962.)

Figure 12-8 ■ Reduction in arterial blood pH (mean ± SD) in a group of 11 dogs whose blood pressure had been held at a level of 35 mm Hg by bleeding into a reservoir, beginning at time zero. (Modified from Markov AK, Oglethorpe N, Young DB, et al: *Circ Shock* 8:9, 1981.)

cerning the importance of cardiac failure during earlier stages of hemorrhagic hypotension. Shifts to the right in ventricular function curves (Figure 12-7) constitute experimental evidence of a progressive depression of myocardial contractility during hemorrhage.

The hypotension induced by hemorrhage reduces the coronary blood flow and therefore depresses ventricular function. The consequent reduction in cardiac output leads to a further decline in arterial pressure, a classic example of a positive feedback mechanism. Furthermore, the reduced blood flow to the peripheral tissues leads to an accumulation of vasodilator metabolites. These substances decrease peripheral re-

sistance and therefore aggravate the fall in arterial pressure.

Acidosis The inadequate blood flow during hemorrhage affects the metabolism of all cells in the body. The resulting stagnant anoxia accelerates the production of lactic acid and other acid metabolites by the tissues. Furthermore, impaired kidney function prevents adequate excretion of the excess H^+, and generalized metabolic acidosis ensues (Figure 12-8). The resulting depressant effect of acidosis on the heart (see Chapter 4) further reduces tissue perfusion and thus aggravates the metabolic acidosis. Acidosis also diminishes the reactivity of the heart and resistance vessels to neurally released and circulating catecholamines, and thereby intensifies the hypotension.

Central Nervous System Depression The hypotension in shock reduces cerebral blood flow. Moderate degrees of cerebral ischemia induce a pronounced sympathetic nervous stimulation of the heart, arterioles, and veins, as stated previously. With severe degrees of hypotension, however, the cardiovascular centers in the brainstem eventually become depressed because of inadequate blood flow to the brain. The resulting loss of sympathetic tone then reduces cardiac output and peripheral resistance. The consequent reduction in mean arterial pressure intensifies the inadequate cerebral perfusion.

Various endogenous **opioids,** such as **enkephalins** and β-**endorphin,** may be released into the brain substance or into the circulation in response to hemorrhage. Opioids exist along with catecholamines in secretory granules in the adrenal medulla and sympathetic nerve terminals, and they are released together in response to stress. Similar stimuli release β-endorphin and adrenocorticotropic hormone (ACTH) from the anterior pituitary gland. The opioids depress the centers in the brainstem that mediate some of the compensatory autonomic adaptations to blood loss, endotoxemia, and other shock-provoking stresses. Conversely, the opioid antagonist **naloxone** improves cardiovascular function and survival in various forms of shock.

Aberrations of Blood Clotting *The alterations of blood clotting after hemorrhage are typically biphasic—an initial phase of hypercoagulability followed by a secondary phase of hypocoagulability and fibrinolysis.* In the initial phase, platelets and leukocytes adhere to the vascular endothelium, and intravascular clots, or **thrombi,** develop within a few minutes of the onset of severe hemorrhage. Coagulation may be extensive throughout the minute blood vessels.

Thromboxane A_2 may be released from various ischemic tissues. It aggregates platelets, and

more thromboxane A_2 is released from the trapped platelets, which serve to trap additional platelets. This form of positive feedback intensifies and prolongs the clotting tendency. The mortality from certain standard shock-provoking procedures has been reduced considerably by anticoagulants such as heparin.

In the later stages of hemorrhagic hypotension, the clotting time is prolonged and fibrinolysis is prominent. As stated previously, hemorrhage into the intestinal lumen is common after several hours of hemorrhagic hypotension in dogs. Blood loss into the intestinal lumen would aggravate the hemodynamic effects of the original hemorrhage.

Reticuloendothelial System During the course of hemorrhagic hypotension, reticuloendothelial system (RES) function becomes depressed. The phagocytic activity of the RES is modulated by an opsonic protein. The opsonic activity in plasma diminishes during shock; this process may account in part for the depression of RES function. As a consequence, the antibacterial and antitoxic defense mechanisms are impaired. Endotoxins from the normal bacterial flora of the intestine constantly enter the circulation. Ordinarily they are inactivated by the RES, principally in the liver. When the RES is depressed, these endotoxins invade the general circulation. *Endotoxins produce profound, generalized vasodilation, mainly by inducing the abundant synthesis of an isoform of nitric oxide synthase in the smooth muscle of blood vessels throughout the body.* The profound vasodilation aggravates the hemodynamic changes caused by blood loss.

In addition to their role in inactivating endotoxin, the macrophages release many of the mediators that are associated with shock. These mediators include acid hydrolases, neutral proteases, oxygen free radicals, certain coagulation factors, and arachidonic acid derivatives: prostaglandins, thromboxanes, and leukotrienes. Macrophages also release certain **monokines** that modulate temperature regulation, intermediary metabolism, hormone secretion, and the immune system.

The Positive and Negative Feedback Mechanisms Interact

Hemorrhage provokes a multitude of circulatory and metabolic derangements. Some of these changes are compensatory; others are decompensatory. Certain feedback mechanisms possess a high gain, others a low gain. Furthermore, the gain of any specific mechanism varies with the severity of the hemorrhage. For example, with only a slight loss of blood, mean arterial pressure is within the range of normal and the gain of the baroreceptor reflexes is high. With greater losses of blood, when mean arterial pressure is below about 60 mm Hg (i.e., below the threshold for the baroreceptors), further reductions of pressure have no additional influence through the baroreceptor reflexes. Hence below this critical pressure, the baroreceptor reflex gain is zero or near zero.

As a general rule, with minor degrees of blood loss, the gains of the negative feedback mechanisms are high, whereas those of the positive feedback mechanisms are low. The converse is true with more severe hemorrhages. The gains of the various mechanisms are additive algebraically. Therefore, whether a vicious cycle develops depends on whether the sum of the various gains exceeds 1. Total gains in excess of 1 are more likely with severe losses of blood. To avert a vicious cycle, serious hemorrhages must be treated quickly and intensively, preferably by whole blood transfusions, before the process becomes irreversible.

Summary

Exercise

- In anticipation of exercise, the vagus nerve impulses to the heart are inhibited and the sympathetic nervous system is activated by central command. The result is an increase in heart rate, myocardial contractile force, cardiac output, and arterial pressure.
- With exercise, vascular resistance increases in skin, kidneys, splanchnic regions, and inactive muscles, and decreases in active muscles.
- The increase in cardiac output is mainly accomplished by the increase in heart rate. Stroke volume increases only slightly.
- Total peripheral resistance decreases, oxygen consumption and blood oxygen extraction increase, and systolic and mean blood pressure increase slightly.
- As body temperature rises during exercise, the skin blood vessels dilate. However, when heart rate becomes maximal during severe exercise, the skin vessels constrict. This increases the effective blood volume but causes greater increases in body temperature and a feeling of exhaustion.
- The limiting factor in exercise performance is the delivery of blood to the active muscles.

Hemorrhage

- Acute blood loss induces tachycardia, hypotension, generalized arteriolar vasoconstriction, and generalized venoconstriction.
- Acute blood loss invokes a number of negative feedback (compensatory) mechanisms, such as baroreceptor and chemoreceptor reflexes, responses to moderate cerebral ischemia, reabsorption of tissue fluids, release of endogenous vasoconstrictors, and renal conservation of water and electrolytes.

• Acute blood loss also induces a number of positive feedback (decompensatory) mechanisms, such as cardiac failure, acidosis, central nervous system depression, aberrations of blood coagulation, and depression of the reticuloendothelial system.

• The outcome of acute blood loss depends on the gains of the various feedback mechanisms and on the interactions between the positive and negative feedback mechanisms.

■ BIBLIOGRAPHY

1. Astiz ME, Rackow EC, Weil MH: Pathophysiology and treatment of circulatory shock. *Crit Care Clin* 9:183, 1993.
2. Buckwalter JB, Clifford PS: α-Adrenergic vasoconstriction in active skeletal muscles during dynamic exercise. *Am J Physiol* 277:H33, 1999.
3. Buckwalter JB, Clifford PS: Autonomic control of skeletal muscle blood flow at the onset of exercise. *Am J Physiol* 277:H1872, 1999.
4. Cameron JD, Dart AM: Exercise training increases total systemic arterial compliance in humans. *Am J Physiol* 266:H693, 1994.
5. Geerdes BP, Frederick KL, Brunner MJ: Carotid baroreflex control during hemorrhage in conscious and anesthetized dogs. *Am J Physiol* 265:R195, 1993.
6. Herbertson MJ, Werner HA, Walley KR: Nitric oxide synthesis inhibition partially prevents decreased LV contractility during endotoxemia. *Am J Physiol* 270:H1979, 1996.
7. Iellamo F, Legramante JM, Raimandi G, et al: Baroflex control of sinus node during dynamic exercise in humans: effects of central command and muscle reflexes. *Am J Physiol* 272:H1157, 1997.
8. Kulecs JM, Collins HL, Dicarlo SE: Postexercise hypertension is mediated by reductions in sympathetic nerve activity. *Am J Physiol* 276:H27, 1999.
9. Laughlin MH, Korthuis RJ, Duncker DJ, et al: Control of blood flow to cardiac and skeletal muscles during exercise. In *Handbook of physiology*, Section 12: *Exercise: regulation and integration of multiple systems*, Bethesda, MD, 1996, Oxford University Press, p 705.
10. Lefer AM, Lefer DJ: Pharmacology of the endothelium in ischemia-reperfusion and circulatory shock. *Annu Rev Pharmacol Toxicol* 33:71, 1993.
11. Mitaka C, Hitata Y, Ichikawa K, et al: Effects of nitric oxide synthase inhibitor on hemodynamic change and O_2 delivery in septic dogs. *Am J Physiol* 268:H2017, 1995.
12. O'Leary DS, Robinson ED, Butler JL, et al: Is active skeletal muscle functionally vasoconstricted during dynamic exercise in conscious dogs? *Am J Physiol* 272:R386, 1997.
13. Szabo C: Alterations in nitric oxide production in various forms of circulatory shock. *New Horizons* 3:2, 1995.
14. Tschakorsky ME, Hughson RL: Ischemic muscle chemoreflex response elevates blood flow in nonischemic exercising human forearm muscle. *Am J Physiol* 277:H635, 1999.
15. Yao Y-M, Bahrami S, Leichtfried G, et al: Significance of NO in hemorrhage-induced hemodynamic alterations, organ injury, and mortality in rats. *Am J Physiol* 270:H1616, 1996.

■ CASE 12-1

HISTORY

A 23-year-old male track star decided to enter the Boston Marathon. He had only run in short distance events, up to 10 K (6.21 miles), before entry in the marathon. At the 15-mile mark, he was leading the race, but he was soon passed by one of his competitors. This inspired him to make a strong effort to retake the lead, but he was unable to increase his speed. At the 20-mile mark he began to feel faint and within the next mile he became sick to his stomach, somewhat disoriented, and he finally staggered and fell to the ground, exhausted.

QUESTIONS

1. When the runner was at the 17-mile mark, what limited him from achieving his goal of retaking the lead?
   a. His leg muscles were unable to use more oxygen.
   b. His respiratory system was unable to saturate the arterial blood with oxygen.

c. He had inadequate vasoconstriction in the splanchnic regions and in the inactive muscles.

d. His cardiac output became inadequate.

e. His arteriovenous oxygen difference was decreased.

2. At the time of his collapse, which of the following did <u>not</u> occur?

a. Body temperature fell

b. Heart rate reached a maximal level

c. Skin blood vessels constricted

d. Blood pH decreased

e. Blood pressure decreased

■ CASE 12-2

HISTORY

A 47-year-old woman had an acute episode of severe abdominal pain, and she suddenly vomited a large amount of bloody material. Her husband called for an ambulance to take her to the hospital. The emergency room physician learned that the patient had frequent, severe episodes of upper abdominal pain over the past 6 weeks. Physical examination revealed that the patient's skin was very pale and cold, her heart rate was 110 beats/min, and her blood pressure was 85/65 mm Hg. Examination of the patient's blood revealed that the hematocrit ratio (i.e., the ratio of red cell volume to whole blood volume) was 40%. The physician made the tentative diagnosis of a bleeding peptic ulcer.

QUESTIONS

1. The patient's skin was pale and cold because

a. The arterial baroreceptors reflexively induced the parasympathetic nerves to the skin to release acetylcholine.

b. The arterial chemoreceptors reflexively induced the parasympathetic nerves to the skin to release vasoactive intestinal peptide.

c. The arterial chemoreceptors reflexively induced the parasympathetic nerves to the skin to release neuropeptide Y.

d. The arterial baroreceptors reflexively induced the sympathetic nerves to the skin to release nitric oxide.

e. The arterial baroreceptors reflexively induced the sympathetic nerves to the skin to release norepinephrine.

2. The patient's arterial blood pressure of 85/65 mm Hg indicates that

a. The patient's left ventricle was pumping an abnormally low cardiac output and low stroke volume.

b. The patient's left ventricle was pumping more blood than was her right ventricle.

c. The patient's left ventricle was pumping an abnormally low cardiac output but a normal stroke volume.

d. The patient's left ventricle was pumping a normal cardiac output and an abnormally low stroke volume.

e. The patient's left ventricle was pumping less blood than was her right ventricle.

3. If the patient's bleeding had stopped before she arrived at the hospital, which of the following changes would be expected in the patient's blood 1 hour after she had arrived at the hospital?

a. The individual red blood cells would be larger than normal.

b. The hematocrit ratio would be reduced.

c. The lymphocyte count would be abnormally high.

d. The plasma albumin concentration would be increased.

e. The plasma globulin concentration would be increased.

Case Study Answers

■ **CASE 1**

b is correct. The circulation time will be shortened because some blood passes through the shunt (short circuit).

■ **CASE 2**

1. **c** is correct. When the extracellular K^+ concentration increases, the Nernst equation indicates that the transmembrane potential will become less negative.

2. **b** is correct. When the slope of the slow diastolic depolarization is increased, the firing threshold of the automatic cells is reached more quickly.

3. **d** is correct. The Purkinje fibers are automatic fibers, and they generate action potentials at a low frequency whenever they are not depolarized by action potentials that originate in higher frequency pacemaker sites.

4. **a** is correct. When ventricular pacing at 75 beats/min was discontinued, spontaneous pacemaker activity in the ventricles was suppressed for several seconds because the preceeding period of artificial pacing had hyperpolarized the ventricular pacemaker cells (Purkinje fibers).

■ **CASE 3**

1. **d** is correct. The murmur is characteristic of mitral stenosis.

2. **c** is correct. The pulse is totally irregular.

3. **b** is correct. A phlebotomy would relieve the excessive preload and allow the cardiac output to improve and the edema and ascites to subside.

4. **b** is correct. The elevated left atrial pressure would be transmitted back to the wedged catheter (wedge pressure).

5. **e** is correct. Nitroglycerin is prescribed for angina pectoris due to myocardial ischemia and not prescribed for congestive heart failure.

6. **c** is correct. $\dfrac{300}{0.18 - 0.08} = \dfrac{300}{0.10} =$ 3000 ml/min = 3 L/min

■ CASE 4

1. **a** is correct. A decrease in arterial pressure would reflexly increase sympathetic activity and thereby increase the neuronal release of norepinephrine.

2. **d** is correct. The Ach released from vagal fibers acts on muscarinic receptors on SA node automatic cells, and these receptors interact very quickly with specific K^+ channels because no second messenger intervenes.

3. **a** is correct. The cardiac responses to vagal stimulation develop and decay rapidly, but the responses to sympathetic stimulation develop and decay very slowly. Hence respiratory dysrhythmia is mediated almost entirely by the vagus nerves, and this dysrhythmia would be abolished by a potent muscarinic antagonist.

4. **a** is correct. Heart rate increases during inspiration in this dysrhythmia, and this increase is mediated mainly by a reduction in vagal activity.

5. **e** is correct. Acetylcholinesterase is abundant in atrial tissues, and especially in the SA and AV nodes.

■ CASE 5

1. **b** is correct. $(P_a - P_v)/Q$ (i.e., [100 − 10]/ 300) equals 0.30 mm Hg/ml/min.

2. **d** is correct. The left ([100 − 10]/500) and right ([100 − 10]/300) vascular resistances were 0.18 and 0.30 mm Hg/ml/min, respectively, and the reciprocals of those resistances were 5.56 and 3.33 ml/min/mm Hg, respectively. Hence the reciprocal of the sum (8.89 ml/min/mm Hg) of these reciprocals equals 0.11 mm Hg/ml/min.

3. **a** is correct. The pressure difference across the plaque (100 − 80 mm Hg), divided by

the flow past the plaque (300 ml/min), equals 0.066 mm Hg/ml/min.

■ CASE 6

1. **a** is correct. The mean arterial pressure in the systemic and pulmonary vascular beds depends on the outputs of the left and right ventricles and the systemic vascular resistances. Over any substantial time interval, the outputs of the two ventricles are equal, but the systemic vascular resistance far exceeds the pulmonary vascular resistance.

2. **c** is correct. When the arterial pressure rises, the arteries become less compliant (as does a balloon), and also the arterial compliance decreases with age.

■ CASE 7-1

1. **d** is correct. (44 + 2) − (23 + 8) = 15.

2. **c** is correct. Portal-caval shunt (portal vein to inferior vena cava) could reduce the high venous pressure in the mesentery by allowing mesenteric blood to bypass the high vascular resistance in the liver. This would aid in eliminating the ascites.

3. **b** is correct. Albumin is small enough (low molecular weight) to exert the main osmotic force of plasma and large enough to remain within the vascular compartment.

■ CASE 7-2

1. **e** is correct. The albumin concentration in the patient's blood is low because of the loss of albumin from the burned tissues. This results in a decreased plasma oncotic pressure, and that plus the loss of fluid from the damaged microvessels leads to a decreased blood volume and an increased red cell concentration. Therefore a plasma transfusion, which supplies albumin plus saline without red cells, is the most effective treatment.

2. **d** is correct. The small diameter (or radius) of the capillaries is responsible for the low wall

tension, according to the law of Laplace, where T (wall tension) = P (pressure) × r (radius of capillary). The low wall tension protects against capillary rupture.

■ CASE 8-1

1. *b* is correct. The arterioles are maximally dilated secondary to the inadequate blood flow that causes the local release of vasodilator metabolites.
2. *a* is correct. Use of tobacco is believed to be a contributing factor to the cause and exacerbation of thromboangiitis obliterans.

■ CASE 8-2

1. *e* is correct. Diabetic coma is not characterized by repeating brief bouts of unconsciousness.
2. *c* is correct. Digitalis is not prescribed for SVT unless there is also impaired myocardial function.

■ CASE 9

1. *c* is correct. The blood loss would decrease the central venous pressure, and this reduction in cardiac preload would decrease the cardiac output.
2. *a* is correct. A drug that improves cardiac contractility would increase cardiac output, which would tend to increase the arterial blood volume. Hence if total blood volume remains constant, the venous blood volume would decrease. Consequently, the central venous pressure would decline.
3. *e* is correct. Gravity acts to pool blood in the compliant, dependent veins, and hence the pressure in the foot veins will increase. The redistribution of the venous blood volume will cause the central venous volume and pressure to diminish. The consequent reduction in preload decreases the cardiac output.
4. *b* is correct. When the heart rate is abnormally high, cardiac filling is inadequate, and

therefore stroke volume and cardiac output are decreased.

■ CASE 10

1. *d* is correct. Two factors operate in bradycardia. At the slower rate, more time is spent in diastole, which decreases coronary resistance (less extravascular compression). However, at the slower rate the heart uses less oxygen and fewer vasodilator metabolites are present, which permits greater expression of basal tone (coronary constriction). The end result is the algebraic sum of these two opposing factors.
2. *a* is correct. The coronary vessels are maximally dilated as a result of the accumulation of vasodilator metabolites consequent to an inadequate oxygen supply to the myocardial cells. If any vasoconstriction occurred, it would be transient.
3. *b* is correct. Endothelin is a powerful vasoconstrictor.
4. *e* is correct. With exercise a denervated heart increases stroke volume more than heart rate to meet the required cardiac output. Any increase in heart rate must come from release of epinephrine and norepinephrine from the adrenal medulla.

■ CASE 11-1

d is correct. Epinephrine would enhance the vasoconstriction and make the symptoms worse, whereas the alternative choices would help to alleviate the attacks.

■ CASE 11-2

a is correct. The hepatic fibrosis increases the hepatic vascular resistance, and therefore the pressure in the vessels downstream to the liver is elevated. Consequently, the balance of Starling forces in the splanchnic capillaries favors the movement of fluid out of the capillaries and into the abdominal cavity.

■ CASE 11-3

b is correct. The murmur, the high right ventricular systolic pressure with a normal right atrial pressure, the elevated PO_2 of the right ventricular blood, and the absence of cyanosis indicated a left-to-right shunt through an interventricular septal defect.

■ CASE 12-1

1. *d* is correct. His heart became unable to pump enough blood per unit time due to a decrease in stroke volume, and hence in cardiac output.

2. *a* is correct. His body temperature reached an alarmingly high level due to inadequate heat loss via the skin (vasoconstriction secondary to decrease in blood pressure) in the face of the great heat production in the active muscles.

■ CASE 12-2

1. *e* is correct. The hypotension would act via the arterial baroreceptors to activate the sympathetic nerves to the skin. The consequent release of norepinephrine would constrict the cutaneous arterioles, and the skin temperature would drop.

2. *a* is correct. The abnormally low mean arterial pressure (about 72 mm Hg) would signify an abnormally small cardiac output. The low mean arterial pressure could not have been caused by arterial vasodilation because the baroreceptor reflex response to a low mean arterial pressure would be vasoconstriction, not dilation. The low pulse pressure (20 mm Hg) would signify an abnormally small stroke volume.

3. *b* is correct. The decrease in capillary hydrostatic pressure draws interstitial fluid into the plasma compartment and thereby dilutes the red cell component of whole blood.

Index

Artery; *see* Arterial *entries*
Artificial respiration
    discontinuation, effects on heart rate, 95, 97
    effect on cardiac output, 224
Ascending aorta, 117
Asphyxia, 191
Asthma, 67
Atherosclerosis, 140, 141, 235
Athlete
    cardiovascular system of, 277-278
    pulse pressure in, 146
Atrial fibrillation, 49-51
Atrial flutter, 50
Atrial natriuretic peptide, 92
Atrial pacemaker complex, 28
Atrial pressure during exercise, 273, 275
Atrial septal defect, 101
Atrial systole, 76-77
Atrioventricular block, 35, 36, 37, 38, 218
Atrioventricular node, 8-9
    automaticity, 31-32
    conduction, 33-36, 38, 39
    parasympathetic influences, 86-87, 88
    transmission block, 47
Atrioventricular pathway, accessory, 35
Atrioventricular stenosis, 77
Atrioventricular valve, 70-72
Atrium, 68
    action potentials during final repolarization, 23
    baroreceptors of, 191
    conduction in, 33, 34
    fetal, 265, 266
    heart sounds, 74, 75
    paroxysmal tachycardias of, 48
    premature depolarization, 47, 48
    receptors in heart rate regulation, 91-92
Atropine, 86
Auscultatory blood pressure measurement, 150-151
Automaticity, 28, 30-32
Autonomic nervous system
    in blood flow regulation
        coronary, 232-233
        cutaneous, 241-244
        peripheral, 185-193
        pulmonary, 254
    in heart rate regulation, 85-97
        Bainbridge reflex and atrial receptors in, 91-92
        baroreceptor reflex in, 90-91
        chemoreceptor reflex in, 95, 96, 97
        higher cerebral centers in, 90
        parasympathetic pathways, 86-87, 88
        sympathetic pathways, 88-89
        ventricular receptor reflexes in, 95-97
    in myocardial performance regulation, 105-109
Autoregulation
    cerebral, 250
    cutaneous, 242

Autoregulation—cont'd
    intestinal, 261
    peripheral, 180-181
    renal, 258-259
Auxiliary pump, 223
Auxiliary pumping mechanism, 223
AV; *see* Atrioventricular *entries*
Azygos vein, 251

B

B receptor, 191
Bachmann's bundle, 33
Bainbridge reflex
    in heart rate regulation, 91-92
    in respiratory cardiac dysrhythmia, 93, 94
Balloon angioplasty, 236, 237, 238
Baroreceptor reflex
    in heart rate regulation, 90-91
    in hemorrhage, 279-280
    in myocardial performance, 108-109
    in pulmonary circulation, 254
    in rapid adjustments of blood pressure, 187-190
    in respiratory cardiac dysrhythmia, 94
    in skeletal muscle circulation, 245-246
Baroreceptors
    arterial, 187-190
    cardiopulmonary, 191
Basal tone, 184, 186-187, 242, 246-247, 259
Beta-adrenergic receptor, 88-89
    coronary blood flow and, 232
    effects on calcium currents, 20
    gastrointestinal blood flow and, 261
    vascular resistance and, 187
Beta-adrenergic receptor blocking agents, 232
Beta-endorphin, 284
Bile duct, 263
Birth, circulatory changes, 267-268
Blanching, 242
Block
    atrioventricular, 35, 36, 37, 38, 47
    bundle branch, 37
    unidirectional, 39-40
Blood
    loss; *see* Hemorrhage
    rheologic properties of, 126-131, 132
Blood clotting in hemorrhage, 284
Blood flow, 115-133, 155-174
    arterial
        elasticity and, 139-141
        pulsatile, 3
    arterioles in, 155-156
    autoregulation, 180-181
    capillary, 156-157
    cerebral, 247-250
    coronary, 227-240
        cardiac efficiency and, 235
        cardiac oxygen consumption and, 234

Glycogen level, fetal, 267
Graves disease, 3
Gravitational forces in cardiac output, 218
Growth factors, vascular endothelial, 170-171, 237

H

h gate, 14-16
Heart; *see also* Cardiac *entries*
   anatomy and structures, 55-78
      cardiac output, 78-81
      cycle, 74-78
      excitation-contraction coupling mediation, 61-65
      heart sounds, 73-74
      myocardial cell, 55-61
      pericardium, 73
      preload and afterload, 65-68, 69
      valves, 68-72, 73-74
   circuitry, 1-6
   coupling with blood vessels, 208-212
   electrical activity of, 7-53
      afterdepolarization leading to triggered activity, 41-43
      cardiac action potentials, 7-27, 28
      cardiac excitability, 26-27, 28
      conduction, 24-26
      dysrhythmias and, 43-46
      electrocardiographic examination, 43-46
      pacemaking, 28-39
      reentry, 39-41
Heart attack; *see* Cardiac arrest
Heart block
   atrioventricular, 35, 36, 38, 47, 218
   bundle branch, 37
   unidirectional, 39-40
Heart failure, 93
   cardiac and vascular function curves in, 213-216
   congestive, 93
      calcium channel antagonists for, 21
      cervical venous distension in, 222
      pulse pressure in, 146
   in hemorrhage, 282-283
   pericardial pressure-volume relations in, 100
   preload in, 66
   pulmonary artery wedge pressure in, 252
   residual volume *versus* stroke volume in, 76
   right, 215, 216
   ventricular function curve shift and, 100-101
Heart murmur, 74, 75
Heart rate
   afterdepolarizations and, 41, 42
   in cardiac output, 85, 141, 199, 200, 216-218
   during exercise, 273, 274, 275
   intrinsic, 86
   normal, 85
   regulation of, 85-114
      Bainbridge reflex and atrial receptors in, 91-92
      baroreceptor reflex in, 90-91
      chemoreceptor reflex in, 95, 96, 97

Heart rate—cont'd
   regulation of—cont'd
      higher cerebral centers in, 90
      myocardial performance and, 97-112; *see also*
         Myocardium
      parasympathetic pathways in, 86-87, 88
      sympathetic pathways, 88-89
      ventricular receptor reflexes in, 95-97
      rhythmic variations in; *see* Dysrhythmia
   in well-trained athlete, 277
Heart sounds, 73-74
Heart valves, 68-72
   closure of in production of heart sounds, 73-74
Heartbeat; *see* Heart rate
Heat exposure, cutaneous response to, 244
Hematocrit ratio, 127-129, 130
Hemiblock, left, 37
Hemodynamics, 115-133
   bloodstream velocity and vascular area, 115-116
   hepatic, 263-264
   laminar *versus* turbulent, 125-126
   pressure and flow relationship dependent on conduit,
      118-122
   pressure gradient in, 116-118, 119
   pulmonary, 252-254
   renal, 258
   resistance to flow, 122-125
   rheologic properties of blood, 126-131, 132
   sheer stress on vessel wall, 126
Hemoglobin
   fetal, 265
   skin color and, 245
Hemorrhage, 278-285
   capillary hydrostatic pressure in, 170
   effects on cardiac output, heart rate, and stroke volume,
      91, 92
   pulse pressure in, 146
   vascular function curve and, 206, 211, 212
Hemorrhagic shock, 187, 278, 284
Hepatic artery, 262
   mean blood pressure of, 263
   regulation of flow, 264
Hepatic circulation, 262-264
   blood reservoirs in, 207
   in hemorrhage, 280
His bundle, 33
   electrogram, 47
Hormones
   gastrointestinal, 262
   in myocardial performance regulation, 109-112
   vascular resistance and, 187
HR; *see* Heart rate
H-V interval, 47
Hydraulic conductance, 125
Hydraulic filtering, 135-139
Hydraulic resistance, 122-124, 125
Hydraulic resistance equation, 123-124

Hydrogen ion concentration
central chemoreceptors and, 193
in cerebral blood flow regulation, 248-249, 250
in hemorrhage, 283-284
in myocardial ischemia, 235
in myocardial performance, 111-112
Hydrogen ions in coronary blood flow, 233
Hydrostatic regulation of capillary filtration, 166-169
Hypercapnia, 191
cerebral circulation and, 250
Hyperemia
active, 183
functional in intestinal circulation, 262
reactive, 182, 183, 184
vasoactive metabolites in, 233
Hyperpolarization current in automaticity, 30-31
Hypersensitivity, denervation, 242
Hypertension
afterload in, 66
arterial pressure in, 148
blood viscosity in, 128
drugs for, interfering with reflex adaptation to standing, 221
Hyperthyroidism, 3, 110
Hypertrophy, ventricular, 46
Hyperventilation, 95
cerebral blood flow and, 248
Hypervolemia, 206
Hypotension
arterial, 187
endocardial *versus* epicardial blood flow, 230
during exercise, 275
hemorrhagic, 280, 283
orthostatic, 221
Hypothalamus
in heart rate control, 90
in vascular reflexes, 193
Hypothyroidism, 110
Hypovolemia, 206
Hypovolemic shock, 253
Hypoxia, 191, 192
cerebral blood flow and, 249
maternal, 267
pulmonary vasomotor tone and, 254-255

I

I band, 56, 58, 59
Idioventricular pacemaker, 28-29
Impulse propagation or initiation disturbances, 46
Inactivation gate, 14-16
Inactivation of fast sodium current, 13
Incisura, 76, 148
Independent stimulus, 200, 209
Independent variable, 200, 209
Indicator dilution technique for measuring cardiac output, 79-80
Infarction, myocardial, 205

Inferior vena cava, fetal, 265, 266
Inspiration
cardiac output and, 222, 223
in respiratory cardiac dysrhythmia, 93
Insulin in cardiac performance regulation, 111
Interatrial myocardial band, anterior, 33
Intercalated disk, 56, 58, 59, 60, 61
Interlobar artery, 255, 256
Interlobar branches, 255, 256
Intermittent claudication, 185
Internodal pathway, 33
Intestinal circulation, 260-262
Intrathoracic pressure, 222-223
Intravascular pressure, renal, 257
Intrinsic heart rate, 86
Intubation, tracheal, 95, 97
Inward current
calcium, 19
potassium, 11
sodium, 16
transient, 43
Inwardly rectified potassium channel, 21, 23
Inwardly rectifying potassium current, 10, 11
Ion; *see also* Calcium; Potassium; Sodium
automaticity and, 30-32
concentration restoration during fast response action potential, 23
conductance of, 12
resting potential and, 9-13
Ion channel, 10
Ischemia
cerebral, 193, 248, 280
hemorrhage and, 280
myocardial, 235-236
Ischemic cell, 9
Isoelectric line, 43
Isometric contraction, 75
Isoproterenol, 20, 89, 105, 107
Isovolumic contraction, 74-75
Isovolumic relaxation, 76

J

Junctional processor, 62
Juxtaglomerular apparatus, 259
Juxtamedullary glomeruli, 255

K

K^+; *see* Potassium
Kidney
circulation, 255-260
in hemorrhage, 280
salt and water conservation during hemorrhage, 281-282

L

Lactic acid, 233
Laminar flow, 118-122, 125-126
Laplace's law, 62, 158-159

Myocardium
  cells of, 55-57, 58, 59, 60, 61
  contractility of
    in cardiac output, 199, 200
    during exercise, 272
    in hemorrhage, 283
  death of tissue, 205
  oxygen consumption, 139, 234
    cardiac efficiency and, 235
    coronary blood flow and, 232, 233
  performance regulation, 97-112
    Frank-Starling mechanism in, 98-101, 102
    heart rate and, 101-104, 105
    hormones in, 109-112
    nervous system in, 105-109
  resting fiber length in force of cardiac contraction, 57-61
  vascular and cardiac function curves in contractility of, 210-211
Myoendothelial junction, 176, 177
Myofibrils, 58, 59
Myogenic mechanism, 180-181
  in renal circulation, 258-259
Myosin, 55, 177-178

N

Na⁺; *see* Sodium
Natural pacemaker, 28
Negative feedback mechanism, 279, 285
Nephrosis, 171
Nernst equation, 11, 12
Nervous system
  in arteriovenous anastomoses regulation, 242
  in atrioventricular conduction, 36
  in blood flow regulation
    cerebral, 248
    coronary, 232-233
    cutaneous, 241-244
    in hemorrhage, 279
    hepatic, 264
    mesenteric, 261
    peripheral, 185-193
    pulmonary, 254
    renal, 259-260
    skeletal muscle, 245-247
  cardiovascular regulation in exercise, 272
  in heart rate regulation, 85-97
    Bainbridge reflex and atrial receptors in, 91-92
    baroreceptor reflex in, 90-91
    chemoreceptor reflex in, 95, 96, 97
    higher cerebral centers in, 90
    parasympathetic pathways, 86-87, 88
    sympathetic pathways, 88-89
    ventricular receptor reflexes in, 95-97
  in myocardial performance regulation, 105-109
Neuropeptide Y, 108

Newborn, circulatory changes, 267-268
Newtonian fluid, 118, 122
Nexi, 56, 58, 59
Nifedipine, 19
  effects on sinoatrial node, 32
Nitrates, 237
Nitric oxide, 159-160, 184
  coronary blood flow and, 233-234
Nitrites, 237
Nitroprusside, 90
NO; *see* Nitric oxide
Nonnutritional flow, 157
Norepinephrine
  calcium conductance and, 20
  in cardiac performance regulation, 109, 110
  in cutaneous vasoconstriction, 242
  effect on arterioles, 156, 157
  in heartbeat regulation, 89
  in hemorrhage, 281
  overflow in sympathetic and vagal stimulation, 108
  peripheral circulation and, 185
  in respiratory cardiac dysrhythmia, 93
  role in atrioventricular conduction, 36
  vascular resistance and, 187
  ventricular function curve and, 100, 101
Normal sinus rhythm, 46
Normovolemia, 206
NPY; *see* Neuropeptide Y
NTS; *see* Tractus solitarius
Nucleus ambiguus, 86
Nutritional flow, 156-157

O

Occlusion, coronary artery
  endocardial *versus* epicardial blood flow, 230
  myocardial hibernation in, 236
  myocardial stunning in, 236
Oncotic pressure, 166-167
Opioids, 284
Ordered reentry, 39
Orthostatic hypotension, 221
Osmolarity in vasodilation, 182-184
Osmotic regulation of capillary filtration, 166-169
Outward potassium current, 11
  in automaticity, 31
  transient, 18
Overdrive suppression, 32-33
Overshoot of action potential, 16
Oxygen
  movement, 165-166
  in myocardial performance, 111
  skin color and, 245
Oxygen consumption
  cardiac, 234
  cardiac output and, 78-79
  during exercise, 273-274, 277
    in well-trained athlete, 277

Oxygen consumption—cont'd
  gastrointestinal, 261
  hepatic, 262, 264
  intestinal, 261
  myocardial, 139, 234
    cardiac efficiency and, 235
    coronary blood flow and, 232, 233
Oxygen partial pressure
  in cardiac performance, 111
  central chemoreceptors and, 193
  metabolic regulation of blood flow and, 182
  peripheral chemoreceptors and, 191-192
Oxygen saturation
  fetal, 265, 266
  in systemic arterial blood, 255
Oxygen tension
  fetal, 265, 267
  mixed venous, 139
  peripheral chemoreceptor stimulation with decrease of,
    191-192
  pulmonary, 254-255
Oxyhemoglobin dissociation curve
  during exercise, 273
  fetal, 265-267

P

P wave, 34, 43
  of premature atrial depolarization, 47, 48
  in third-degree heart block, 38
Pacemaker, 28-39
  atrioventricular conduction, 33-36, 38, 39
  automaticity, 30-32
  ectopic, 28-29
  idioventricular, 28-29
  overdrive suppression, 32-33
  of sinoatrial node, 29-30
  ventricular conduction, 37-39, 40
Pacemaker potential, 29
Pacemaker shift, 30
$Paco_2$; see Arterial carbon dioxide tension
Palpatory blood pressure measurement, 150
Pancreas, blood flow to, 260-264
Pao_2; see Oxygen partial pressure
Papillary muscle, 102
Parallel, resistance in, 124-125
Parasympathetic nervous system
  in heart rate regulation, 86-87, 88
  in myocardial performance regulation, 107-108
  in peripheral circulation control, 187
Parasystole, 47
Paroxysmal supraventricular tachycardia, 48-49
Paroxysmal tachycardia, 48-49
  ectopic pacemakers in development of, 28
Paroxysmal ventricular tachycardia, 48-49
Patch-clamping technique, 17
Peptide, atrial natriuretic, 92

Perfusion pressure
  coronary blood flow and, 229, 231
  intestinal, 261
  renal blood flow and, 258, 259, 260
Pericardium, 73, 100
Peripheral chemoreceptor stimulation, 95, 96
Peripheral circulation, 175-197
  autonomic nervous system in control of, 185-193
  autoregulation and myogenic mechanism in,
    180-181
  contraction and relaxation of arteriolar vascular smooth
    muscle in, 177-178, 179
  endothelium and, 182, 183
  tissue metabolic activity in, 182-185
Peripheral resistance
  arterial pressure and, 141, 142, 143, 144-145
    diastolic, 147-148, 149
  cardiac function curve and, 212
  during exercise, 272-274, 275
  vascular function curve and, 200-205, 207-208, 212
Peripheral runoff, 142, 143, 201, 202
Peritubular capillaries, 255, 257
Permeability of cell, 8-9
pH
  central chemoreceptors and, 193
  in cerebral blood flow regulation, 248-249, 250
  during exercise, 273
  in hemorrhage, 283-284
  in myocardial performance, 111-112
Pharmacomechanical coupling, 178, 179
Phenocardiogram, 73, 74
Phenylephrine, 90
Phosphate in vasodilation, 182-184
Phospholamban, 64, 105
Phospholipase C, 178, 179
Physical training, 277-278
Physiological shunting of blood flow, 157
Pinocytosis, 171
Pitot tubes, 116
Placenta, 264, 265
Plasma fibrinogen, 132
Plateau phase of action potential, 8, 19-22
  early afterdepolarization appearing at end of, 41-42
Platelets in hemorrhage, 284
Poiseuille's law, 118
Pores, transcapillary diffusion across, 161-166
Portal vein, 262
  mean blood pressure of, 263
  regulation of flow, 264
Positive feedback mechanism, 282, 285
Positive inotropic effect, 67
Posterior division of left bundle branch, 37
Posterior hemiblock, left, 37
Posterior internodal pathway, 33
Postextrasystolic potentiation, 103-104
Postrepolarization refractoriness, 27

Venous valve, muscular activity and, 221-222, 245, 246
Ventilation-perfusion ratio, 254
Ventricle, 68
  action potentials during final repolarization, 23
  conduction, 37-39, 40
  diastole, 76-78
  ejection phase, 75-76
  fetal, 265, 266
  fiber angles of, 68, 70
  hypertrophic, mean electrical axis in, 46
  premature depolarization, 48, 103-104
  pulmonary blood flow and central venous pressure
      regulation by, 212-216
  sympathetic nerve stimulation and, 89
    cardiac and vascular function curves and, 210-211
  systole, 74-76
    coronary blood flow and, 230-232
Ventricular fibrillation, 50, 223
  coronary blood flow and, 230-232
Ventricular function curve, 100, 101
  carotid sinus pressure and, 109
  in hemorrhage, 283
Ventricular pressure curve, 67, 68, 76
Ventricular receptor reflex, 95-97
Ventricular tachycardia
  heart rate and cardiac output in, 218
  paroxysmal, 48-49
Venules
  flow resistance, 2
  gastrointestinal, 260
  hepatic, 262, 263
  hydraulic resistance equation, 123
  pulmonary, 250
  renal, 257
Verapamil, 19
Vessel wall tension, 158-159
Villi, gastrointestinal, 261, 262
Viscera in vascular reflexes, 193
Viscosity, 121-122
  of blood, 127-131, 132
Viscous drag, 126, 127
V_m; see Transmembrane potential
Voltage clamping, 11
Voltage-dependent phenomenon, 16

Voltage-dependent sodium channel, fast response action
    potentials depending on, 13-23
  ionic concentration restoration, 23
  plateau phase, 19-22
  repolarization
    early, 18-19
    final, 22-23
  statistical characteristics of gate concept, 17-18
  upstroke in, 13-17
Volume
  blood, 5
    arterial blood pressure and, 141, 142
    cerebral, 248
    effect on vascular function curve, 205-206, 211-212
    during exercise, 274
    in hemorrhage, 281
    hepatic, 264
    in right ventricular failure, 215
    skin color and, 245
  residual, 76
  stroke, 68
    arterial function and, 135-137, 139
    atrial pacing and, 217
    in cardiac output, 85
    during exercise, 273, 274
    in heart failure, 76
    pulse pressure and, 145-146
  urine, 92
Volume flow, 115
Vulnerable point in fibrillation, 50

W

Walking, venous pressure during, 222
Wall tension, 158-159
Water
  renal conservation during hemorrhage, 281-282
  transcapillary exchange, 161-165
Waterfall effect, 254
Windkessels, 135
Wolff-Parkinson-White syndrome, 35

Z

Z line, 55, 56, 57, 58, 59